Case Studies in Nursing Management

PRACTICE, THEORY, AND RESEARCH

Nursing Management

[CASE STUDIES IN

PRACTICE, THEORY, AND RESEARCH

Ann Marriner-Tomey, RN, PhD, FAAN

Professor, Indiana University School of Nursing;
Nursing Management Consultant,
Indianapolis, Indiana

73

The C. V. Mosby Company

St. Louis • Baltimore • Philadelphia • Toronto   1990

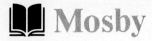 Mosby

Editor: Darlene Como
Developmental Editor: Laurie Sparks
Designer: Susan Lane
Production and Editing: Editing, Design & Production, Inc.

Printed in the United States of America

The C.V. Mosby Company
11830 Westline Industrial Drive, St. Louis, Missouri 63146

Library of Congress Cataloging in Publication Data

Case studies in nursing management: practice, theory, and research /
    [edited by] Ann Marriner-Tomey.
        p.   cm.
    Includes bibliographical references.
    ISBN 0-8016-5848-9
    1. Nursing services — Administration — Case studies.   I.   Marriner
-Tomey, Ann
    RT89.C33   1990
    362.1′73′068 — dc20   89-28666
                                                                 CIP

GW/D/D   9   8   7   6   5   4   3   2   1

Contributors

Mary C. Alderson
Patient Care Coordinator,
Indiana University Hospital,
Indianapolis, Indiana

Lorraine B. Anderson
Assistant Professor,
Indiana University School of Nursing,
Indianapolis, Indiana

Jan Austin
Nurse Recruiter,
Clark County Hospital,
Jeffersonville, Indiana

Debra Barker
Staff Nurse,
Indiana University Hospital,
Indianapolis, Indiana

Regina K. Bennett
Major, Army Nurse Corps

Joycelyn K. Blackmon
Graduate Student,
Georgia College School of Nursing,
Milledgeville, Georgia

Sylvia L. Bond
Vice-President, Inpatient Services,
Medical Center of Central Georgia,
Macon, Georgia

Diana Boyer
Director of Materials and Environmental
  Services,
Bartholomew County Hospital,
Columbus, Indiana

Constance F. Buran
Assistant Professor of Nursing,
University of Indianapolis,
Indianapolis, Indiana

Patricia Lynn Burgamy
Inservice Coordinator, Med-Surgical Division,
Central State Hospital,
Milledgeville, Georgia

Phyllis Chafin
Head Nurse, Critical Care Area,
Fairview Park Hospital,
Dublin, Georgia

Genevieve E. Chandler
Assistant Professor,
University of Massachusetts,
Amherst, Massachusetts

Janet Chorpenning
Assistant Professor,
Indiana University School of Nursing,
Indianapolis, Indiana

Jo Anne Clanton
LCDR, NC, United States Navy

Kathleen Kay Clevenger
Staff Development Coordinator, Critical Care,
Indiana University Hospital,
Indianapolis, Indiana

Carol Deets
Professor,
Indiana University School of Nursing,
Indianapolis, Indiana

Marilyn Sue Doub
Long Term Care Consultant,
Bloomington, Indiana

Glenda C. Floyd
Supervisor, Carl Vinson, VAMC
Dublin, Georgia

Linda Holbrook Freeman
Associate Professor of Nursing,
University of Louisville,
Louisville, Kentucky

Christine M. Gelb
Clinical Director, Maternal Child Nursing,
Methodist Hospital,
Indianapolis, Indiana

Carol Lavonne Harn
Director, Medical Surgical Nursing,
Medical Center of Central Georgia,
Macon, Georgia

Mary C. Harrell
Unit Director, Medical Intensive Care Units,
Indiana University Hospital,
Indianapolis, Indiana

Leta M. Holder
Associate Professor,
Georgia College School of Nursing,
Milledgeville, Georgia

D. Jean Holley
Director of Inservice Education,
Fairview Park Hospital,
Dublin, Georgia

Kathleen A. Holmes
Unit Director,
Indiana University Hospital,
Indianapolis, Indiana

David Eugene Hunt
Administrative Coordinator,
Reid Memorial Hospital,
Richmond, Indiana

Debbie Reese Hutchinson
Discharge Planning Coordinator,
Medical Center of Central Georgia,
Macon, Georgia

Kay Ann Jackson-Frankl
Consultant in Nursing,
Aurora, Indiana

Tamilyn Jones
Doctoral Student,
Indiana University School of Nursing,
Indianapolis, Indiana

M. Jan Keffer
Doctoral Candidate,
University of Illinois at Chicago,
Chicago, Illinois

Pamela C. Levi
Dean and Professor,
Georgia College School of Nursing,
Milledgeville, Georgia

Cheryl Pope Long
Associate Professor and Coordinator,
Maternal-Child Health,
Georgia College School of Nursing,
Milledgeville, Georgia

Jude A. Magers
Director, Nursing Clinical Services,
St. Vincent Stress Center,
Indianapolis, Indiana

Ann Marriner-Tomey
Professor,
Indiana University School of Nursing;
Nursing Management Consultant,
Indianapolis, Indiana

Darla D. Meyers
Assistant Director of Nursing,
HCA Fairview Park Hospital,
Dublin, Georgia

Carol S. Millay
Director, Maternal/Child Nursing,
Carle Foundation Hospital,
Urbana, Illinois

Vicki H. Morgan
OB/GYN Nurse Practitioner,
Public Health, State of Georgia,
Sparta, Georgia

Glenda G. Ridley
Director of Nursing,
Central State Hospital,
Milledgeville, Georgia

Mary Lorraine Riegner
Head Nurse, ICU,
Community Hospitals, Inc.,
Indianapolis, Indiana

Katherine S. Russell
Assistant Professor,
Coordinator, Nursing Administration,
Georgia College School of Nursing,
Milledgeville, Georgia

Robert M. Saywell, Jr.
Associate Professor and Director,
Graduate Program in Health Administration,
Indiana University School of Public and
    Environmental Affairs,
Indianapolis, Indiana

Lou Ellen Sears
Nursing Consultant,
Cloverleaf Healthcare,
Indianapolis, Indiana

Sharon Holcombe Servais
Nursing Director, Emergency Services.
Medical Center of Central Georgia,
Macon, Georgia

Alice F. Smith
Staff Nurse,
Fairview Park Hospital,
Dublin, Georgia

Joanne C. Stratton
Associate Director of Nursing,
Porter Memorial Hospital,
Valparaiso, Indiana

Deborah B. Wilson
Assistant Unit Manager,
Wishard Memorial Hospital,
Indianapolis, Indiana

Andrea L. Ziegert
Assistant Professor,
Indiana University,
School of Public and Environmental Affairs,
Indianapolis, Indiana

To **Keith**
my husband and best friend

Preface

Nothing is so practical as a good theory. *Case Studies in Nursing Management: Practice, Theory, and Research* applies management theories to nursing administration situations and then reviews related research. Each chapter begins with a case study or critical incident that can be used at any level of education or administrative practice to stimulate thinking and learning. Then a theory is presented. Although the case study can be analyzed by any number of approaches, the author analyzes the situation using the theory presented, thus applying theory to practice. The last section of each chapter reports related research in general and in nursing specifically.

To identify the theories to include, a content analysis was done on 23 nursing administration books that were published during the 1980s to determine what theories were most commonly used. Many of the books focused on how to administer but were quite atheoretical. Motivation theories were the most frequently mentioned and included the following in descending order of frequency: hierarchy of needs; motivation-hygiene; management by objectives; expectancy; achievement motivation; existence, relatedness, growth; intrinsic-extrinsic; attribution; behavior modification; equity; and social learning. The leadership theories most frequently discussed in descending order of frequency were theory x and y; managerial grid, contingency theory, four systems; path-goal; life cycle; and situational. Other theories identified included planned change; French and Raven's power typology; Vroom and Yetton's decision making; and transactional analysis; and most recently nursing theories have been incorporated into nursing administration textbooks.

These theories were organized by the management process. Parts of the book are plan, organize, lead, motivate, and evaluate. An article on "The validity and usefulness of theories in an emerging organizational science" by Miner* was used to validate the theories in the classification system. "Theoretical frameworks cited in nursing research from January 1974 to June 1985"† were also used.

This book presents many of the classical organizational behavior theories, several of which have received relatively little attention in the nursing literature and consequently nursing practice. The need to test theory in nursing administration is apparent. The dearth of research support for the theories in general suggests a need to refine research methodologies and change paradigms.

Guba‡ indicates that we need to have a paradigm shift from positive to naturalist. We need to move from simple to complex because the diversity and interactivity of the real world make focusing on one element while holding others constant improbable. The whole is more

---

* Miner, J.B. (1984). *Academy of Management Review, 9*(2), 296-306.
† Beck, C.T. (1985). *Nurse Educator, 10*(6), 36-38.
‡ Guba, E.C. (1985). The context of emergent paradigm research. In Y.S. Lincoln (Ed.), *Organizational theory and inquiry: The paradigm revolution.* Beverly Hills, CA: Sage Publications.

than the sum of its parts. We need to move from hierarchical to heterarchical concepts of order because order is affected by a number of interacting and rapidly changing factors. We need to move from determinancy to indeterminancy because ambiguity is the condition of nature. We need to move from linear to mutual causality because we are affected by simultaneous influencing of factors over time. We need to move from assembly to morphogenesis, which is unpredictable change, to create higher-order forms from lower-order forms. We need to move from objective to perspectival views, as efforts to understand truth can only be partial. Even the accumulation of all perspectives does not provide the total picture.

Ann Marriner-Tomey

Contents

PART I
PLAN

1   Decision-Making Model: Victor H. Vroom and Arthur G. Jago, 1
     Jude A. Magers

2   Planned Change: Kurt Lewin, 19
     Carol S. Millay

3   Theories of Justice, 30
     M. Jan Keffer

4   Language in Organizations: Louis R. Pondy, 42
     Kay Ann Jackson-Frankl

5   Symbolic Interactionism: Herbert Blumer, 54
     Kathleen Kay Clevenger and Mary C. Alderson

6   Attribution Theory: Fritz Heider, 58
     Jan Austin and Kathleen A. Holmes

7   Group Process: Bruce W. Tuckman, 63
     Diana Boyer

8   Economic Theories, 68
     Robert M. Saywell, Jr., and Andrea L. Ziegert

PART II
ORGANIZE

9   Theory of Bureaucracy: Max Weber, 93
     Pamela C. Levi

10   Classical Management Theory: Henri Fayol, 102
     Cheryl Pope Long

11   Contingency Theory: Differentiation and Integration: Paul R. Lawrence and Jay W. Lorsch, 113
     Christine M. Gelb

12   Theory of System 4: Rensis Likert, 123
     Ann Marriner-Tomey

13   Systems Theory: Ludwig von Bertalanffy, 129
     Linda Holbrook Freeman and Debra Barker

14   Job Characteristics Theory: Edward E. Lawler III, J. Richard Hackman, and
      Greg Oldham, 136
      Phyllis Chafin

PART III
LEAD

15   Theory X and Y: Douglas McGregor, 147
      Vicki H. Morgan

16   Contingency Theory of Leadership: Fred Fiedler, 154
      Regina K. Bennett and Joanne C. Stratton

17   Path-Goal Theory of Leadership: Robert J. House, 166
      Constance F. Buran and Deborah B. Wilson

18   Situational Leadership: Paul Hersey and Kenneth Blanchard, 174
      Leta M. Holder

19   Control Theory: Arnold S. Tannenbaum, 183
      Katherine S. Russell

20   The Bases of Social Power: John R.P. French, Jr., and Bertram Raven, 192
      Carol Deets and Tamilyn Jones

21   Structural Theory: Women in Management: Roasabeth Moss Kanter, 204
      Genevieve E. Chandler

PART IV
MOTIVATE

22   Hierarchy of Needs: A.H. Maslow, 211
      Alice F. Smith

23   Existence, Relatedness, and Growth Theory: Clayton P.
      Alderfer, 222
      Darla D. Meyers

24   Motivation-Hygiene Theory: Frederick Herzberg, 229
      Glenda C. Floyd

25   Achievement-Motivation Theory: John Atkinson, David
      McClelland, and Joseph Veroff, 238
      Debbie Reese Hutchinson

26   Expectancy Theory: Victor Vroom, 245
      Sharon Holcombe Servais

27   Equity Theory: J. Stacy Adams, 256
      Joycelyn K. Blackmon

28   Intrinsic and Extrinsic Motivation: Edward L. Deci, 264
      Carol Lavonne Harn

29   Goal-Setting Theory: Edwin Locke, 270
      D. Jean Holley

30   Management by Objectives, 281
      Glenda G. Ridley

31   Goal Congruence Theory: Chris Argyris, 288
      Ann Marriner-Tomey and Janet Chorpenning

32   Behavior Modification: B.F. Skinner, 293
      Patricia Lynn Burgamy

33   Social Learning Theory: Modeling: Albert Bandura, 303
      Sylvia L. Bond

PART V
EVALUATE

34   Budget as Control, 309
      Lorraine B. Anderson

35   Analyzing Performance Problems: Robert F. Mager and Peter Pipe, 320
      Jo Anne Clanton and Marilyn Sue Doub

36   Maier's Appraisal Interviewing Model: Norman R:F. Maier, 325
      Marilyn Sue Doub and Jo Anne Clanton

37   Role Theories, 330
      Mary C. Harrell and Lou Ellen Sears

38   Conflict Mode Model: K.W. Thomas and R.H. Kilmann, 337
      David Eugene Hunt

39   Integrative Stress Theory: John M. Ivancevich and Michael T. Matteson, 344
      Mary Lorraine Riegner

Case Studies in Nursing Management

PRACTICE, THEORY, AND RESEARCH

PART I

PLAN

Chapter 1

Decision-Making Model
Victor H. Vroom and Arthur G. Jago

Jude A. Magers

▌▌ CASE STUDY

A nurse manager, responsible for five acute mental health adult units, observed a negative change in the 5-East unit operations. The manager receives weekly risk management reports monitoring quality-of-care facility-wide indicators. Over a 5-week period an increased incidence of procedural errors for the 5-East unit was noted. The error rates were approaching thresholds of unsafe practice in the areas of restraint, seclusion, and medication administration. The manager realized the need for an immediate response to the risk management findings.

During the same period of increasing risk indicators on the 5-East unit, the manager observed significant behavioral changes in the unit's patient care coordinator, most notably excessive absenteeism and tardiness. A reduction in problem-solving abilities was also recorded. In addition, her peers had noted increased irritability and a withdrawal from professional interactions. Before her promotion, the patient care coordinator was a staff nurse for 5 years. Her performance evaluations were excellent. She was well-liked and respected among the interdisciplinary team of health care professionals. The change in the patient care coordinator's performance appeared to be a recent development.

The manager suspected a correlation between the coordinator's leadership style on the unit and the trends in patient care indicators reported by the risk management department. The decision-making processes to be chosen by the manager would need to be immediate and effective at both an individual and a unit (group) level of performance. The manager decided to use the decision-making model of Vroom and Jago (1988) to analyze options in responding to the situational problem. She chose the Vroom and Jago model because it emphasizes subordinate participation and leadership styles in decision making.

|||||||||||||||||||||||||||||||||||||||||||||||||||||||||||||||||||||||||

VROOM AND JAGO DECISION-MAKING MODEL

Vroom and Jago (1988) describe a decision-making model that is a social process. The model is a revision of the Vroom and Yetton model (1973). A detailed description of the model is necessary to appreciate the transition from the Vroom and Yetton model to the Vroom and Jago model.

The Vroom and Jago model proposes an additional number of problem attributes, deletion of the decision rules, change from dichotomous variables to continuous variables, and mathematical formulas to arrive at a decision-making model of greater complexity than the Vroom and Yetton model. The new model is computer-friendly. The additions and revisions suggest that the new model has addressed some of the weaknesses of the 1973 model.

Vroom and Yetton (1973) cite Norman R.F. Maier as a significant influence on their early interest in behavior (p. xiii). Central to Vroom's interest in organizational behavior were questions regarding situational attributes of decision making and choice of leadership style (p. 4). Tannenbaum and Schmidt (1973) contributed critical insight into the discussion of leadership style and the leader's relationship to the subordinate (p. 163). These authors suggested a continuum of choices available to a manager. This was one of several concepts that countered the Taylor theory of management, which dominated the industrial world from 1911 to 1960 (Vroom & Jago, 1988, p. 10). Vroom and Jago (1988) credit behavioral scientists for the evolution of the principles of participative management, in particular, Mayo, Lewin, Argyris, and McGregor (pp. 11, 12). Vroom and Jago depart from the extremes of the social scientists in the belief that the situational approach must recognize attributes that determine a desired leadership style.

Vroom and Jago (1988) define 12 problem attributes. The model retains seven attributes of the Vroom and Yetton model: quality requirement, leader information, problem structure, commitment requirement, commitment probability, goal congruence, and subordinate conflict. The problem attributes are central to the understanding and utilization of the decision-making model. The attributes could be described as critical questions asked by the manager in each problem situation that requires a decision. To use the list of attributes, the manager must first clarify whether the situational problem affects an individual or a group. She will answer the 12 attribute questions and arrive at one of five decision processes (leadership styles or methods). The decision processes fall on a continuum that is inclusive of autocratic, consultative, delegative, and consensus. Principles of group dynamics and outcomes by Maier form the foundation of the group decision processes found in both the Vroom and Yetton model and the Vroom and Jago model (Vroom & Jago, 1988, p. 38).

A significant change from the Vroom and Yetton model was the use of continuous variables. The earlier model used dichotomous variables of "yes" and "no" in answering the attribute questions. This method led to feasible sets of decision processes, but its menu-type approach suggested more than one preferred choice. The structure of dichotomous variables was a weakness in the model, because it restricted specific measurable outcomes. Vroom and Jago believed that continuous variables were necessary to provide a stronger prescriptive role in a decision-making model. The new model places 10 of the 12 problem attributes on a 5-point Likert scale. Two of the 12 problem attributes maintain a yes or no format. A manager confronted with a situational problem analyzes the event as individual or group, scores the attribute scales using the available information, and arrives at a preferred decision process. The model specifies the most desirable method (prescription) in response to the information provided by the manager. The complexity of the model lies in the mathematical formulas developed by Vroom and Jago. The introduction of mathematical functions to the attribute structure provides support to research methodology, improves prescriptive outcomes, and allows computerization in management decision making. The weakness of the new model's mathematical functions is the lack of ease in manually scoring the attributes on the 5-point scales without the use of computers. Vroom and Jago adpated the revised model to accommodate the manager who has no access to computers. The decision to adapt the model was made realizing that the complexity inherent in the continuous variables would be lost (1988, p. 183). A decision-tree concept, used in the Vroom and Yetton model (1973), was chosen by Vroom and Jago. The adapted decision-tree format deletes the Likert scale and four attributes: time constraint, geographical dispersion of participants, time as a motivator, and subordinate development. Without the ability to computerize the model, the problem situations must be conducive to a yes or no format (Vroom & Jago, 1988, p. 183).

It is important to note that the model prescribes methods, rather than skills, within the decision processes. Methods may range from autocratic styles to delegative styles. Vroom and Jago (1988) delineate the differences between the choice of a preferred method and the ability to favorably implement the method (prescription) (p. 37).

The choice of the preferred method is evaluated by outcome criteria. Vroom and Jago (1988) have developed criteria that measure overall effectiveness of the choice: decision quality, commitment, costs, and subordinate development. The quantitative values compare outcomes across all decision-making processes (see Figures 1-15 and 1-20). The manipulation of decision processes with the evaluation of outcome before actual implementation is a strength of the model. "Manipulation is used to test the impact of proposed changes [choice] on the system without disturbing the subject of the model" (Marriner-Tomey, 1988, p. 10). The ability to generate quantitative data adds utility to the model. Its complexity in structure reflects a manager's challenge in choosing decision-making processes. The Vroom and Jago model continues to contribute to the discussion of leadership and its dynamic phenomena. The analysis of the case study in the next section demonstrates its utility.

CASE ANALYSIS

"Three major behavioral characteristics influence decision making: (1) perception of the problem, (2) a personal value system, and (3) the ability to process data" (Marriner-Tomey, 1988, p. 22). These behavioral characteristics are intrinsic in the Vroom and Jago model's functions. Application of the model to the case study demonstrates the importance of perception, values, and ability to process data.

The nurse manager observed a behavioral change in the performance of the 5-East unit patient care coordinator and a trend in declining unit operations. The perceived need for management intervention to help problem-solve directed the manager to consider the most appropriate leadership style that would support resolution of the problem with the greatest overall gains.

The manager first assessed the individual situational problem. She entered her perceived values into the problem attributes scales for individual situations. This required answering each attribute question as defined in the model (Figures 1-1 through 1-11).* Mathematical values were ranked 1 through 5 for the attributes except for time constraint. Time constraint retained a dichotomous variable of yes or no (1 or 5 value for measurement outcome). The manager wanted feedback on preferred decision processes that considered need of timely response,

Text continued on p. 9.

---

* Information regarding the availability of this software may be obtained from Leadership Software, Inc., P.O. Box 271848, Houston, TX 77277-1848.

PROBLEM ATTRIBUTE: QUALITY REQUIREMENT (LIKERT SCALE 1-5)

(c) 1986, 1987 by Leadership Software, Inc.	ENTER PROBLEM ATTRIBUTES	PROBLEM ATTRIBUTES
Aside from any need to generate commitment, this question refers to the need to find a rational, wise or technically correct solution. Some decisions lack such a requirement (e.g., what colors to paint the cafeteria). Virtually any alternative will do, providing it is successfully implemented. Most problems, however, do possess some sort of a quality requirement (i.e., you expect that some alternatives will be more likely than others to attain external objectives). Remember ..... this question is independent of any commitment requirement that exists.		- 5 - QR - Quality Requirement ‖ 1 - CP - Commitment Requirement ‖ 1 - LI - Leader Information 1 - ST - Problem Structure 1 - CP - Commitment Probability 1 - GC - Goal Congruence 1 - CO - Subordinate Conflict 1 - SI - Subordinate Information 1 - TC - Time Constraints 1 - MT - Motivation-Time 1 - MD - Motivation-Development
		DECISION PROCESSES
		AI - Autocratic Decision AII - AI with Info. Collection CI - One-on-One Consultation GI - Joint Decision-Making DI - Delegation

PRESS A NUMBER OR 'H' FOR MORE HELP OR <ESC> TO QUIT

FIGURE 1-1 The manager scored Quality Requirement as a value of 5 (Critical Import). *Reproduced from* Managing Participation in Organizations — MPO *[Computer Program]. Copyright 1986, 1987 by Leadership Software, Inc. Used with permission. Decision processes adapted from Vroom, V.H., & Yetton, P.W. (1973).* Leadership and decision-making. *Pittsburgh: University of Pittsburgh Press.*

PROBLEM ATTRIBUTE: COMMITMENT REQUIREMENT (LIKERT SCALE 1-5)

(c) 1986, 1987 by Leadership Software, Inc.	ENTER PROBLEM ATTRIBUTES	PROBLEM ATTRIBUTES
This refers to the importance of getting acceptance or commitment to the decision from the subordinate. Even high quality decisions can fail if they are resisted or opposed. Look for either of two things: Does the success of the decision hinge on how well the subordinate executes it? Is the person likely to 'feel strongly' about the issues involved such that he/she might resist some solutions? Remember, however, to judge the importance of acceptance without regard to the importance of decision quality (i.e., this is independent of Question 'QR').		5 - QR - Quality Requirement ‖ - 4 - CR - Commitment Requirement ‖ 1 - LI - Leader Information 1 - ST - Problem Structure 1 - CP - Commitment Probability 1 - GC - Goal Congruence 1 - CO - Subordinate Conflict 1 - SI - Subordinate Information 1 - TC - Time Constraints 1 - MT - Motivation-Time 1 - MD - Motivation-Development
		DECISION PROCESSES
		AI - Autocratic Decision AII - AI with Info. Collection CI - One-on-One Consultation GI - Joint Decision-Making DI - Delegation

PRESS A NUMBER OR 'H' FOR MORE HELP OR <ESC> TO QUIT

FIGURE 1-2 The manager scored Commitment Requirement as a value of 4 (High Import). *Reproduced from* Managing Participation in Organizations — MPO *[Computer Program]. Copyright 1986, 1987 by Leadership Software, Inc. Used with permission. Decision processes adapted from Vroom, V.H., & Yetton, P.W. (1973).* Leadership and decision-making. *Pittsburgh: University of Pittsburgh Press.*

PROBLEM ATTRIBUTE: LEADER INFORMATION (LIKERT SCALE 1-5)

(c) 1986, 1987 by Leadership Software, Inc.	ENTER PROBLEM ATTRIBUTES	PROBLEM ATTRIBUTES
This attribute refers to the degree to which you believe you have sufficient information and expertise to solve the problem by yourself without the aid of your subordinate. The information referred to is that which is relevant to the technical side of the problem, not information as to what solution would most please the subordinate. Note that what is called for is a judgment about your knowledge in relation to the demands of the problem, not a relative judgment of your knowledge versus that of the subordinate.		5 - QR - Quality Requirement 4 - CR - Commitment Requirement - 1 - LI - Leader Information ‖ 1 - ST - Problem Structure 1 - CP - Commitment Probability 1 - GC - Goal Congruence 1 - CO - Subordinate Conflict 1 - SI - Subordinate Information 1 - TC - Time Constraints 1 - MT - Motivation-Time 1 - MD - Motivation-Development
		DECISION PROCESSES
		AI - Autocratic Decision AII - AI with Info. Collection CI - One-on-One Consultation GI - Joint Decision-Making DI - Delegation

PRESS A NUMBER OR 'H' FOR MORE HELP OR <ESC> TO QUIT

FIGURE 1-3   The manager scored Leader Information as a value of 1 (No–Not sufficient). *Reproduced from* Managing Participation in Organizations — MPO *[Computer Program]. Copyright 1986, 1987 by Leadership Software, Inc. Used with permission. Decision processes adapted from Vroom, V.H., & Yetton, P.W. (1973).* Leadership and decision-making. *Pittsburgh: University of Pittsburgh Press.*

PROBLEM ATTRIBUTE: PROBLEM STRUCTURE (LIKERT SCALE 1-5)

(c) 1986, 1987 by Leadership Software, Inc.	ENTER PROBLEM ATTRIBUTES	PROBLEM ATTRIBUTES
A problem is structured if the present state, the desired state, and the mechanisms for transforming the former into the latter are all known. Such problems are potentially programmable: once certain specific information is obtained, an optimal solution can easily be determined. Unstructured problems are those for which the present state, the desired state, or the transformation processes are unclear or unknown. Creativity is required to identify goals or potential solutions. The less familiar a problem, the less structured it is.		5 - QR - Quality Requirement 4 - CR - Commitment Requirement 1 - LI - Leader Information - 2 - ST - Problem Structure ‖ 1 - CP - Commitment Probability 1 - GC - Goal Congruence 1 - CO - Subordinate Conflict 1 - SI - Subordinate Information 1 - TC - Time Constraints 1 - MT - Motivation-Time 1 - MD - Motivation-Development
		DECISION PROCESSES
		AI - Autocratic Decision AII - AI with Info. Collection CI - One-on-One Consultation GI - Joint Decision-Making DI - Delegation

PRESS A NUMBER OR 'H' FOR MORE HELP OR <ESC> TO QUIT

FIGURE 1-4   The manager scored Problem Structure as a value of 2 (Probably No). *Reproduced from* Managing Participation in Organizations — MPO *[Computer Program]. Copyright 1986, 1987 by Leadership Software, Inc. Used with permission. Decision processes adapted from Vroom, V.H., & Yetton, P.W. (1973).* Leadership and decision-making. *Pittsburgh: University of Pittsburgh Press.*

PROBLEM ATTRIBUTE: COMMITMENT PROBABILITY (LIKERT SCALE 1-5)

(c) 1986, 1987 by Leadership Software, Inc.	ENTER PROBLEM ATTRIBUTES	PROBLEM ATTRIBUTES
This refers to your estimate of the prior probability that an autocratic decision would be accepted. Do you have enough 'power' to 'sell' your decision to the subordinate? There are three types of power: LEGITIMATE (authority vested in the position), EXPERT (respected wisdom concerning the technical issues), ATTRACTION (charismatic qualities). Some situations require more power than others: some alternatives need more power if they are to be sold. Think of how the most rational of alternatives is likely to be received if selected by you alone.		5 - QR - Quality Requirement 4 - CR - Commitment Requirement 1 - LI - Leader Information 2 - ST - Problem Structure - 2 - CP - Commitment Probability ‖ 1 - GC - Goal Congruence 1 - CO - Subordinate Conflict 1 - SI - Subordinate Information 1 - TC - Time Constraints 1 - MT - Motivation-Time 1 - MD - Motivation-Development
		DECISION PROCESSES
		AI - Autocratic Decision AII - AI with Info. Collection CI - One-on-One Consultation GI - Joint Decision-Making DI - Delegation

PRESS A NUMBER OR 'H' FOR MORE HELP OR <ESC> TO QUIT

FIGURE 1-5 The manager scored Commitment Probability as a value of 3 (Maybe). *Reproduced from* Managing Participation in Organizations — MPO *[Computer Program]. Copyright 1986, 1987 by Leadership Software, Inc. Used with permission. Decision processes adapted from Vroom, V.H., & Yetton, P.W. (1973).* Leadership and decision-making. *Pittsburgh: University of Pittsburgh Press.*

PROBLEM ATTRIBUTE: GOAL CONGRUENCE (LIKERT SCALE 1-5)

(c) 1986, 1987 by Leadership Software, Inc.	ENTER PROBLEM ATTRIBUTES	PROBLEM ATTRIBUTES
This refers to the extent to which the subordinate will be motivated to pursue a solution to the problem which is rational from the standpoint of the goals of the organization, rather than from his or her own self-interests. Answer 'YES' if you and the subordinate share a common goal or objective; you are both 'in the same boat.' 'NO' if goals of the organization and the individual are likely to conflict. Mixed motive situations (some, but not all goals, are congruent) should be answered with a MAYBE, PROBABLY YES, or PROBABLY NO.		5 - QR - Quality Requirement 4 - CR - Commitment Requirement 1 - LI - Leader Information 2 - ST - Problem Structure 2 - CP - Commitment Probability - 5 - GC - Goal Congruence ‖ 1 - CO - Subordinate Conflict 1 - SI - Subordinate Information 1 - TC - Time Constraints 1 - MT - Motivation-Time 1 - MD - Motivation-Development
		DECISION PROCESSES
		AI - Autocratic Decision AII - AI with Info. Collection CI - One-on-One Consultation GI - Joint Decision-Making DI - Delegation

PRESS A NUMBER OR 'H' FOR MORE HELP OR <ESC> TO QUIT

FIGURE 1-6 The manager scored Goal Congruence as a value of 5 (Yes–Shared). *Reproduced from* Managing Participation in Organizations — MPO *[Computer Program]. Copyright 1986, 1987 by Leadership Software, Inc. Used with permission. Decision processes adapted from Vroom, V.H., & Yetton, P.W. (1973).* Leadership and decision-making. *Pittsburgh: University of Pittsburgh Press.*

PROBLEM ATTRIBUTE: SUBORDINATE CONFLICT (LIKERT SCALE 1-5)

(c) 1986, 1987 by Leadership Software, Inc.	ENTER PROBLEM ATTRIBUTES	PROBLEM ATTRIBUTES
This refers to the likelihood of conflict between you and your subordinate over a preferred solution to the problem. At least initially, are you likely to have differing opinions about what should be done? These differences may be due to differences in training, expertise, or to the fact that the situation is, in itself, highly controversial. Note the difference between this question and that dealing with goal congruence (Question GC). The two are distinct, one dealing with goals and the other with their agreement over means to attain these goals.		5 - QR - Quality Requirement 4 - CR - Commitment Requirement 1 - LI - Leader Information 2 - ST - Problem Structure 2 - CP - Commitment Probability 5 - GC - Goal Congruence - 3 - CO - Subordinate Conflict ‖ 1 - SI - Subordinate Information 1 - TC - Time Constraints 1 - MT - Motivation-Time 1 - MD - Motivation-Development
		DECISION PROCESSES
		AI - Autocratic Decision AII - AI with Info. Collection CI - One-on-One Consultation GI - Joint Decision-Making DI - Delegation

PRESS A NUMBER OR 'H' FOR MORE HELP OR <ESC> TO QUIT

FIGURE 1-7   The manager scored Subordinate Conflict as a value of 3 (Maybe). *Reproduced from* Managing Participation in Organizations—MPO *[Computer Program]. Copyright 1986, 1987 by Leadership Software, Inc. Used with permission. Decision processes adapted from Vroom, V.H., & Yetton, P.W. (1973).* Leadership and decision-making. *Pittsburgh: University of Pittsburgh Press.*

PROBLEM ATTRIBUTE: SUBORDINATE INFORMATION SCALE 1-5

(c) 1986, 1987 by Leadership Software, Inc.	ENTER PROBLEM ATTRIBUTES	PROBLEM ATTRIBUTES
This attribute refers to the likelihood that the subordinate has sufficient information and expertise to solve the problem alone. What is called for is a judgment of the subordinate's knowledge in relation to the demands of the problem, not a relative judgment of the person's knowledge versus yours. Note that you are making a judgment about your subordinate's information and expertise, not about his or her motivation to use that information and expertise in the pursuit of organizational goals. That is dealt with in Question GC.		5 - QR - Quality Requirement 4 - CR - Commitment Requirement 1 - LI - Leader Information 2 - ST - Problem Structure 2 - CP - Commitment Probability 5 - GC - Goal Congruence 3 - CO - Subordinate Conflict - 4 - SI - Subordinate Information ‖ 1 - TC - Time Constraints 1 - MT - Motivation-Time 1 - MD - Motivation-Development
		DECISION PROCESSES
		AI - Autocratic Decision AII - AI with Info. Collection CI - One-on-One Consultation GI - Joint Decision-Making DI - Delegation

PRESS A NUMBER OR 'H' FOR MORE HELP OR <ESC> TO QUIT

FIGURE 1-8   The manager scored Subordinate Information as a value of 4 (Probably Yes). *Reproduced from* Managing Participation in Organizations—MPO *[Computer Program]. Copyright 1986, 1987 by Leadership Software, Inc. Used with permission. Decision processes adapted from Vroom, V.H., & Yetton, P.W. (1973).* Leadership and decision-making. *Pittsburgh: University of Pittsburgh Press.*

PROBLEM ATTRIBUTE: TIME CONSTRAINTS (YES OR NO)

(c) 1986, 1987 by Leadership Software, Inc.	ENTER PROBLEM ATTRIBUTES	PROBLEM ATTRIBUTES	
A time constraint exists if BOTH of the following are true: (1) any reasonable decision would be better than a decision that comes too late (doing something is better than missing the deadline), (2) working with the subordinate, even if he/she were available, is likely to cause the decision to be too late. These conditions exist in true emergencies when time is in extremely short supply—a situation that is extremely rare. Notice that this question can only be answered 'YES' or 'NO'. When a time constraint exists, it is readily apparent.		5 - QR - Quality Requirement	
		4 - CR - Commitment Requirement	
		1 - LI - Leader Information	
		2 - ST - Problem Structure	
		2 - CP - Commitment Probability	
		5 - GC - Goal Congruence	
		3 - CO - Subordinate Conflict	
		4 - SI - Subordinate Information	
		- 1 - TC - Time Constraints	
		1 - MT - Motivation-Time	
		1 - MD - Motivation-Development	
		DECISION PROCESSES	
		AI - Autocratic Decision	
		AII - AI with Info. Collection	
		CI - One-on-One Consultation	
		GI - Joint Decision-Making	
		DI - Delegation	

PRESS A NUMBER OR 'H' FOR MORE HELP OR <ESC> TO QUIT

FIGURE 1-9   The manager scored Time Constraints as a value of 1 (No by definition). *Reproduced from* Managing Participation in Organizations—MPO *[Computer Program]. Copyright 1986, 1987 by Leadership Software, Inc. Used with permission. Decision processes adapted from Vroom, V.H., & Yetton, P.W. (1973).* Leadership and decision-making. *Pittsburgh: University of Pittsburgh Press.*

PROBLEM ATTRIBUTE: MOTIVATION-TIME (LIKERT SCALE 1-5)

(c) 1986, 1987 by Leadership Software, Inc.	ENTER PROBLEM ATTRIBUTES	PROBLEM ATTRIBUTES	
Decisions incur 'opportunity costs' reflected in the investment of human resources to solve the problem. This attribute refers to your motivation to reduce these costs by minimizing the time it takes to make effective decisions. Two considerations are relevant: (1) your overall managerial style, and (2) the press of work that currently exists in your organization. Your answer to this question will be relatively stable across situations (i.e., it should not change from one day to the next). In answering, do not let your responses to other questions affect you.		5 - QR - Quality Requirement	
		4 - CR - Commitment Requirement	
		1 - LI - Leader Information	
		2 - ST - Problem Structure	
		2 CP - Commitment Probability	
		5 - GC - Goal Congruence	
		3 - CO - Subordinate Conflict	
		4 - SI - Subordinate Information	
		1 - TC - Time Constraints	
		- 4 - MT - Motivation-Time	
		1 - MD - Motivation-Development	
		DECISION PROCESSES	
		AI - Autocratic Decision	
		AII - AI with Info. Collection	
		CI - One-on-One Consultation	
		GI - Joint Decision-Making	
		DI - Delegation	

PRESS A NUMBER OR 'H' FOR MORE HELP OR <ESC> TO QUIT

FIGURE 1-10   The manager scored Motivation–Time as a value of 4 (High Import). *Reproduced from* Managing Participation in Organizations – MPO *[Computer Program]. Copyright 1986, 1987 by Leadership Software, Inc. Used with permission. Decision processes adapted from Vroom, V.H., & Yetton, P.W. (1973).* Leadership and decision-making. *Pittsburgh: University of Pittsburgh Press.*

employee development, commitment by the employee, and the degree of factual information required to arrive at a solution (Figs. 1-12 through 1-15).

The manager gathered a complete summary of the predicted outcomes and the preferred choice of decision process suggested by the computerized model. It was important for the manager to have feedback that weighed the cost of time, individual development, and commitment. She knew the employee's behavior had significantly changed, yet she lacked knowledge of the cause for the change. The manager chose the suggested decision process GI (joint decision-making). She proceeded to contact the patient care coordinator and arranged a meeting within 24 hours. The manager explained the concern regarding the declining performance. She acknowledged the obvious positive past performance and hoped the open discussion of the events could help turn the present pattern back to a desired level of performance. The patient care coordinator appreciated the opportunity to consider possible reasons for the sudden decline in her performance. She admitted to the increased absenteeism and tardiness. She was not aware of the perception by her peers that she was irritable and not participating in work activities. The patient care coordinator knew that she had been very preoccupied the past weeks because of personal problems. She had tried to focus on her work responsibilities but felt that she could not adequately keep up with day-to-day problems. She explained that she had plans for the unit to expand accountability for quality review activities. At the time of her promotion, her husband had become very ill and she was trying to care for him and her three children. The tension of the home situation distracted her from putting into place some mechanisms to problem-solve unit patient care situations. She attributed the continued incidents of medication errors and procedural omissions to the lack of a unit staff mechanism to problem-solve day to day and to her own inability to focus on helping the staff design methods to resolve problems. The manager suggested that the patient care coordinator seek support and help through the organization's employee assistance program. The coordinator was very willing to follow this suggestion as a means to regain control over aspects of her personal life. The manager asked for her assistance in meeting with the 5-East unit staff and exploring the staff's perception of the declining unit performance. The manager agreed that the unit's problem-solving mechanisms did not need to depend solely on the individual work of the patient care coordinator. If the unit staff was approached to help participate in the design of a method, the patient care coordinator might find professional support. The manager explained to the patient care coordinator the decision-making model of Vroom and Jago and demonstrated on the computer the prescribed process for analyzing a group problem (Figures 1-16 through 1-20).

The manager and patient care coordinator considered the unit's problem and assigned values to the 12 group problem attributes (Table 1-1). Eleven of the 12 problem attributes and 3 of the 5 decision processes for a group problem are identical to those for an individual problem. Definitions of the 11 shared problem attributes appear in Figures 1-1 through 1-11. Table 1-2 compares the problem attributes and decision processes for individual and group problems as conceptualized in the decision-making model of Vroom and Jago.

Figure 1-16 shows the computer screen for the problem attribute GD, which is unique to a group problem.

When values had been assigned to each of the unit's problem attributes, the computer program predicted the most effective decision process according to five criteria, as illustrated in Figures 1-17. Figures 1-18, 1-19, and 1-20 show the suggested decision process, the relative overall effectiveness, and the subcriteria values of each of the five possible decision processes.

The manager and patient care coordinator agreed that the staff needed to be involved in determining a new design for day-to-day problem solving. The staff had grown accustomed to

Text continued on p. 16.

PROBLEM ATTRIBUTE: MOTIVATION-DEVELOPMENT (LIKERT SCALE 1-5)

(c) 1986, 1987 by Leadership Software, Inc.	ENTER PROBLEM ATTRIBUTES	PROBLEM ATTRIBUTES
Being involved in some types of decisions can further develop the managerial and technical skills of participants. It may also help develop teamwork, effective working relationships, and increase the understanding of, and commitment to, organizational goals. This question refers to the importance to YOU of such benefits. Your answer should be relatively stable across situations and reflect: (1) your managerial style, and (2) organizational needs for improved technical and managerial talent. Your answer should be unaffected by your other responses.		5 - QR - Quality Requirement 4 - CR - Commitment Requirement 1 - LI - Leader Information 2 - ST - Problem Structure 2 - CP - Commitment Probability 5 - GC - Goal Congruence 3 - CO - Subordinate Conflict 4 - SI - Subordinate Information 1 - TC - Time Constraints 4 - MT - Motivation-Time - 5 - MD - Motivation-Development ‖
		DECISION PROCESSES
		AI - Autocratic Decision AII - AI with Info. Collection CI - One-on-One Consultation GI - Joint Decision-Making DI - Delegation

PRESS A NUMBER OR 'H' FOR MORE HELP OR <ESC> TO QUIT

FIGURE 1-11   The manager scored Motivation–Development as a value of 5 (Critical). *Reproduced from* Managing Participation in Organizations — MPO *[Computer Program]. Copyright 1986, 1987 by Leadership Software, Inc. Used with permission. Decision processes adapted from Vroom, V.H., & Yetton, P.W. (1973).* Leadership and decision-making. *Pittsburgh: University of Pittsburgh Press.*

DECISION PROCESS OUTCOME AFTER COMPUTER CALCULATION OF VALUES

(c) 1986, 1987 by Leadership Software, Inc.	MPO ANALYSIS	PROBLEM ATTRIBUTES
GI — You share the problem with one of your subordinates and together you analyze the problem and arrive at a mutually satisfactory solution in an atmosphere of free and open exchange of information and ideas. You both contribute to the resolution of the problem with the relative contribution of each being dependent on knowledge rather than on formal authority.		5 - QR - Quality Requirement 4 - CR - Commitment Requirement 1 - LI - Leader Information 2 - ST - Problem Structure 2 - CP - Commitment Probability 5 - GC - Goal Congruence 3 - CO - Subordinate Conflict 4 - SI - Subordinate Information 1 - TC - Time Constraints 4 - MT - Motivation-Time 5 - MD - Motivation-Development
		DECISION PROCESSES
		AI - Autocratic Decision AII - AI with Info. Collection CI - One-on-One Consultation - GI - Joint Decision-Making ‖ DI - Delegation

PRESS ANY KEY OR 'H' FOR MORE HELP

FIGURE 1-12   The suggested decision process is Joint Decision Making (GI). *Reproduced from* Managing Participation in Organizations — MPO *[Computer Program]. Copyright 1986, 1987 by Leadership Software, Inc. Used with permission. Decision processes adapted from Vroom, V.H., & Yetton, P.W. (1973).* Leadership and decision-making. *Pittsburgh: University of Pittsburgh Press.*

PREDICTIONS OF OVERALL EFFECTIVENESS

(c) 1986, 1987 by Leadership Software, Inc.	MPO ANALYSIS	PROBLEM ATTRIBUTES
PREDICTIONS — CRITERION — Overall Effectiveness............ GI - Decision Quality .... GI - Decision Commitment .... DI - Decision Costs .... AI - Subordinate Development .... GI		5 - QR - Quality Requirement 4 - CR - Commitment Requirement 1 - LI - Leader Information 2 - ST - Problem Structure· 2 - CP - Commitment Probability 5 - GC - Goal Congruence 3 - CO - Subordinate Conflict 4 - SI - Subordinate Information 1 - TC - Time Constraints 4 - MT - Motivation-Time 5 - MD - Motivation-Development
		DECISION PROCESSES AI - Autocratic Decision AII - AI with Info. Collection CI - One-on-One Consultation - GI - Joint Decision-Making DI - Delegation

Press Any Key to Continue, 'H' for HELP, or <ESC> to Quit

FIGURE 1-13   The manager can weigh the effectiveness of subcriteria when specific decision processes are chosen for decision making. The style with the predicted best outcome is GI. Overall Effectiveness is a new addition in the Vroom and Jago model (1988). *Reproduced from* Managing Participation in Organizations — MPO *[Computer Program]. Copyright 1986, 1987 by Leadership Software, Inc. Used with permission. Decision processes adapted from Vroom, V.H., & Yetton, P.W. (1973).* Leadership and decision-making. *Pittsburgh: University of Pittsburgh Press.*

RELATED OVERALL EFFECTIVENESS

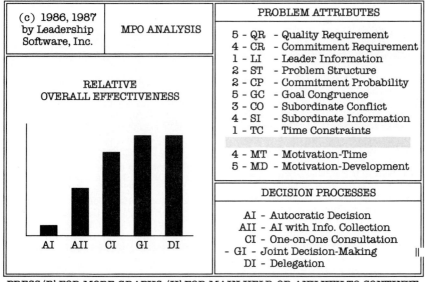

(c) 1986, 1987 by Leadership Software, Inc.	MPO ANALYSIS	PROBLEM ATTRIBUTES
RELATIVE OVERALL EFFECTIVENESS AI AII CI GI DI		5 - QR - Quality Requirement 4 - CR - Commitment Requirement 1 - LI - Leader Information 2 - ST - Problem Structure 2 - CP - Commitment Probability 5 - GC - Goal Congruence 3 - CO - Subordinate Conflict 4 - SI - Subordinate Information 1 - TC - Time Constraints 4 - MT - Motivation-Time 5 - MD - Motivation-Development
		DECISION PROCESSES AI - Autocratic Decision AII - AI with Info. Collection CI - One-on-One Consultation - GI - Joint Decision-Making DI - Delegation

PRESS 'B' FOR MORE GRAPHS, 'H' FOR MAIN HELP, OR ANY KEY TO CONTINUE

FIGURE 1-14   The potential strength of another choice is evaluated by this bar graph. *Reproduced from* Managing Participation in Organizations — MPO *[Computer Program]. Copyright 1986, 1987 by Leadership Software, Inc. Used with permission. Decision processes adapted from Vroom, V.H., & Yetton, P.W. (1973).* Leadership and decision-making. *Pittsburgh: University of Pittsburgh Press.*

SUBCRITERIA VALUES OF DECISION PROCESSES

(c) 1986, 1987 by Leadership Software, Inc.	MPO ANALYSIS	PROBLEM ATTRIBUTES
		5 - QR - Quality Requirement 4 - CR - Commitment Requirement 1 - LI - Leader Information 2 - ST - Problem Structure 2 - CP - Commitment Probability 5 - GC - Goal Congruence 3 - CO - Subordinate Conflict 4 - SI - Subordinate Information 1 - TC - Time Constraints 4 - MT - Motivation-Time 5 - MD - Motivation-Development

SUBCRITERIA VALUES

	QUAL	COMM	COST	DEVPT
AI	0.00	0.75	0.00	0.00
AII	2.25	0.98	0.44	0.07
CI	3.90	1.88	0.70	0.33
GI	4.00	2.55	1.13	0.87
DI	2.55	3.00	0.09	0.67

-Values in Remaining Bar Graphs-

DECISION PROCESSES

AI - Autocratic Decision
AII - AI with Info. Collection
CI - One-on-One Consultation
- GI - Joint Decision-Making   ‖
DI - Delegation

PRESS ANY KEY OR 'H' FOR MORE HELP

FIGURE 1-15 The manager can review the calculated values from the subcriteria of the model. This comparison can help support the choice of decision processes with projected outcome values in quality, commitment, cost, and development. *Reproduced from* Managing Participation in Organizations — MPO *[Computer Program]. Copyright 1986, 1987 by Leadership Software, Inc. Used with permission. Decision processes adapted from Vroom, V.H., & Yetton, P.W. (1973).* Leadership and decision-making. *Pittsburgh: University of Pittsburgh Press.*

PROBLEM ATTRIBUTE: GEOGRAPHICAL DISPERSION (YES OR NO)

(c) 1986, 1987 by Leadership Software, Inc.	ENTER PROBLEM ATTRIBUTES	PROBLEM ATTRIBUTES
Answer this question 'NO' if ANY of the following conditions exist: (1) subordinates are available at your location, (2) a scheduled meeting is to occur before the decision deadline, (3) teleconferencing is possible, or (4) the decision is important enough to warrant travel IF a meeting is deemed necessary. Answer this question 'YES' if NONE of these conditions exist. A 'MAYBE' is not allowed. If you are unsure about the costs of bringing together dispersed subordinates, further analyses are required to estimate the costs of travel or teleconferencing.		5 - QR - Quality Requirement 4 - CR - Commitment Requirement 1 - LI - Leader Information 1 - ST - Problem Structure 2 - CP - Commitment Probability 5 - GC - Goal Congruence 4 - CO - Subordinate Conflict 4 - SI - Subordinate Information 1 - TC - Time Constraints - 1 - GD - Geographical Dispersion ‖ 1 - MT - Motivation-Time 1 - MD - Motivation-Development
		DECISION PROCESSES AI - Autocratic Decision AII - AI with Info. Collection CI - One-on-One Consultation CII - Consultation in a Group GII - Group Decision (Consensus)

PRESS A NUMBER OR 'H' FOR MORE HELP OR <ESC> TO QUIT

FIGURE 1-16 The manager and patient care coordinator scored Geographical Dispersion as a value of 1 (no problem bringing group together). *Reproduced from* Managing Participation in Organizations — MPO *[Computer Program]. Copyright 1986, 1987 by Leadership Software, Inc. Used with permission. Decision processes adapted from Vroom, V.H., & Yetton, P.W. (1973).* Leadership and decision-making. *Pittsburgh: University of Pittsburgh Press.*

PREDICTIONS OF OVERALL EFFECTIVENESS

(c) 1986, 1987 by Leadership Software, Inc.	MPO ANALYSIS	PROBLEM ATTRIBUTES
PREDICTIONS — CRITERION — Overall Effectiveness........... GII -Decision Quality .... CII -Decision Commitment ...... GII -Decision Costs .... AI -Subordinate Development... GII		5 - QR - Quality Requirement 4 - CR - Commitment Requirement 1 - LI - Leader Information 1 - ST - Problem Structure 2 - CP - Commitment Probability 5 - GC - Goal Congruence 4 - CO - Subordinate Conflict 4 - SI - Subordinate Information 1 - TC - Time Constraints 1 - GD - Geographical Dispersion 4 - MT - Motivation-Time 4 - MD - Motivation-Development
		DECISION PROCESSES
		AI - Autocratic Decision AII - AI with Info. Collection CI - One-on-One Consultation CII - Consultation in a Group - GII - Group Decision (Consensus)‖

Press Any Key to Continue, 'H' for HELP, or < ESC> to Quit

FIGURE 1-17 The manager can weigh the effectiveness of subcriteria given the preferred decision-making process. These are complex mathematical functions. The style suggested is GII. Overall Effectivensss is a new addition in the Vroom and Jago model (1988). *Reproduced from* Managing Participation in Organizations—MPO *[Computer Program]. Copyright 1986, 1987 by Leadership Software, Inc. Used with permission. Decision processes adapted from Vroom, V.H., & Yetton, P.W. (1973).* Leadership and decision-making. *Pittsburgh: University of Pittsburgh Press.*

DECISION PROCESS OUTCOME AFTER COMPUTER CALCULATION OF VALUES

(c) 1986, 1987 by Leadership Software, Inc.	MPO ANALYSIS	PROBLEM ATTRIBUTES
GII — You share the problem with your subordinates as a group. Together you generate and evaluate alternatives and attempt to reach agreement (consensus) on a solution. Your role is that of chairperson, coordinating the discussion, keeping it focused on the problem and making sure that the critical issues are discussed. You can provide the group with information or ideas that you have but you do not try to press them to adopt 'your' solution and you are willing to accept and implement any solution that has the support of the entire group.		5 - QR - Quality Requirement 4 - CR - Commitment Requirement 1 - LI - Leader Information 1 - ST - Problem Structure 2 - CP - Commitment Probability 5 - GC - Goal Congruence 4 - CO - Subordinate Conflict 4 - SI - Subordinate Information 1 - TC - Time Constraints 1 - GD - Geographical Dispersion 4 - MT - Motivation-Time 4 - MD - Motivation-Development
		DECISION PROCESSES
		AI - Autocratic Decision AII - AI with Info. Collection CI - One-on-One Consultation CII - Consultation in a Group - GII - Group Decision (Consensus)‖

PRESS ANY KEY OR 'H' FOR MORE HELP

FIGURE 1-18 The suggested decision process is GII (Group Decision [Consensus]). *Reproduced from* Managing Participation in Organizations—MPO *[Computer Program]. Copyright 1986, 1987 by Leadership Software, Inc. Used with permission. Decision processes adapted from Vroom, V.H., & Yetton, P.W. (1973).* Leadership and decision-making. *Pittsburgh: University of Pittsburgh Press.*

RELATIVE OVERALL EFFECTIVENESS

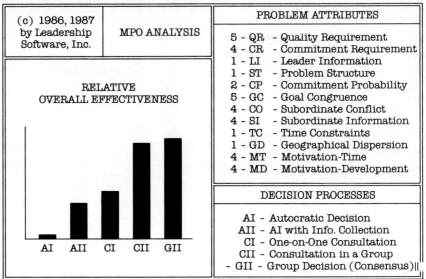

PRESS 'B' FOR MORE GRAPHS, 'H' FOR MAIN HELP, OR ANY KEY TO CONTINUE

FIGURE 1-19 The suggested decision process is measured against AI, AII, CI, and CII. The potential to choose another process can be evaluated by the bar graph. Consultation in the group demonstrates minimal difference in overall effectiveness. *Reproduced from* Managing Participation in Organizations—MPO *[Computer Program]. Copyright 1986, 1987 by Leadership Software, Inc. Used with permission. Decision processes adapted from Vroom, V.H., & Yetton, P.W. (1973).* Leadership and decision-making. *Pittsburgh: University of Pittsburgh Press.*

TABLE 1-1   Values Assigned to the Unit's Problem Attributes

Value	Problem attributes	
5	QR—	Quality Requirement
4	CR—	Commitment Requirement
1	LI—	Leader Information
1	ST—	Problem Structure
2	CP—	Commitment Probability
5	GC—	Goal Congruence
4	CO—	Subordinate Conflict
4	SI—	Subordinate Information
1	TC—	Time Constraints
1	GD—	Geographical Dispersion
4	MT—	Motivation-Time
4	MD—	Motivation-Development

SUBCRITERIA VALUES OF DECISION PROCESSES DEMONSTRATE
STRENGTH OF CHOICE

(c) 1986, 1987 by Leadership Software, Inc.	MPO ANALYSIS	PROBLEM ATTRIBUTES

SUBCRITERIA VALUES				PROBLEM ATTRIBUTES
	QUAL	COMM	COST	DEVPT
AI	-0.75	1.03	0.00	0.00
AII	1.33	1.14	0.10	0.05
CI	1.63	1.59	0.50	0.25
CII	3.85	2.35	0.99	0.59
GII	3.75	3.00	1.38	0.88

PROBLEM ATTRIBUTES

5 - QR - Quality Requirement
4 - CR - Commitment Requirement
1 - LI - Leader Information
1 - ST - Problem Structure
2 - CP - Commitment Probability
5 - GC - Goal Congruence
4 - CO - Subordinate Conflict
4 - SI - Subordinate Information
1 - TC - Time Constraints
1 - GD - Geographical Dispersion
4 - MT - Motivation-Time
4 - MD - Motivation-Development

-Values in Remaining Bar Graphs-

DECISION PROCESSES

AI - Autocratic Decision
AII - AI with Info. Collection
CI - One-on-One Consultation
CII - Consultation in a Group
- GII - Group Decision (Consensus)‖

PRESS ANY KEY OR 'H' FOR MORE HELP

FIGURE 1-20   Quality is ranked higher in CII than preferred choice GII. This demonstrates the value of using the full model and what values the manager chooses to set as priority in decision making. Cost is ranked higher in GII than in CII, illustrating the additional cost when more time is spent in group decision making. *Reproduced from* Managing Participation in Organizations — MPO *[Computer Program]. Copyright 1986, 1987 by Leadership Software, Inc. Used with permission. Decision processes adapted from Vroom, V.H., & Yetton, P.W. (1973).* Leadership and decision-making. *Pittsburgh: University of Pittsburgh Press.*

TABLE 1-2   **Comparison of Problem Attributes and Decision Processes for Individual and Group Problems**

	Individual	Group
Problem attributes	QR — Quality Requirement	QR — Quality Requirement
	CR — Commitment Requirement	CR — Commitment Requirement
	LI — Leader Information	LI — Leader Information
	ST — Problem Structure	ST — Problem Structure
	CP — Commitment Probability	CP — Commitment Probability
	GC — Goal Congruence	GC — Goal Congruence
	CO — Subordinate Conflict	CO — Subordinate Conflict
	SI — Subordinate Information	SI — Subordinate Information
	TC — Time Constraints	TC — Time Constraints
		GD — Geographical Dispersion
	MT — Motivation-Time	MT — Motivation-Time
	MD — Motivation-Development	MD — Motivation-Development
Decision processes	AI — Autocratic Decision	AI — Autocratic Decision
	AII — AI with Information Collection	AII — AI with Information Collection
	CI — One-on-One Consultation	CI — One-on-One Consultation
	GI — Joint Decision Making	CII — Consultation in a Group
	DI — Delegation	GII — Group Decision (Consensus)

the previous patient care coordinator, who handled problem resolution without staff input. The staff would need to adjust to different degrees of unit responsibility. The patient care coordinator believed that she could facilitate the group if they could verbalize some of their conflict with this change. The manager agreed to help cofacilitate the group because of the present stressors experienced by the patient care coordinator. The manager felt confident that commitment and staff development would be positive outcomes with the GII group decision process. She felt certain that the patient care coordinator would follow through with the employee assistance referral. The coordinator was able to separate her tensions and acknowledged support in the system. She thanked the manager for the opportunity to be involved in the problem-solving process demonstrated in the meeting. The manager commented that her approach had been highly influenced through the years by the development of the Vroom and Yetton decision-making model presented in 1973 and the revised model formulated by Vroom and Jago. The manager valued the situational problem-solving processes, the recognition of the situational variables that affect her style, and the efforts to validate the situational model by scientific research designs.

RESEARCH

> Decision making is the scientific problem-solving process. It involves identifying the problem, analyzing the situation, exploring alternatives and considering their consequences, choosing the most desirable alternative, implementing the decision, and evaluating the results. (Marriner-Tomey, 1988, p. 4)

The Vroom and Yetton model (1973) addressed the need for a normative decision-making model compliant with the scientific process. Vroom and Jago, when redesigning the model presented by Vroom and Yetton, retained the concepts of problem attribute and situational decision making. The 1988 model of Vroom and Jago improved utility in application and is an outcome of years of discussion, research, and continued revisions based on investigative findings.

Research in the social sciences (Vroom, 1967) did not have strong quantitative methodology. Vroom and Yetton recognized the difficulty in conducting research that would provide significant evidence of internal validity and reliability for the 1973 model. "Reliability and validity, in research, refer specifically to the measurement of data as they will be used to answer the research question" (Brink & Wood, 1983, p. 124). The initial multiple research studies by Vroom and Yetton (1973) were descriptive and demonstrated degrees of internal validity as the model developed in complexity. Their research question centered on the issue of leadership style (decision processes) as either a consistent phenomenon across situations or a change in style in response to situational factors (attributes) (Vroom & Yetton, 1973, p. 60). The research design focused on identification of attributes and the effort to measure variability in style and attributes while holding other variables constant. Methods commonly referred to in the literature used by Vroom and Yetton and Vroom and Jago were classified as recalled problems and standardized problems.

"Recalled problems" (Vroom & Yetton, 1973) was a research methodology used with 268 managers asked to recount an actual problem-solving situation. The managers described the leadership style used and the characteristics of the event that affected the decision process. Leadership styles corresponded to the taxonomy developed by Vroom and Yetton (1973) and ranged from autocratic to participative. Vroom and Yetton recognized that the recalled problem methodology did not measure in a controlled manner situational factors (attributes). It was evident that the reported data by managers did correspond to the situational factors described in the model. Multiple regression analysis was used as a statistical method. The outcome of multiple regression analysis demonstrated that "the location of information" (Vroom & Yetton, 1973, p. 91) influenced the degree of subordinate participation. The research findings suggested that leadership style does vary with the presence of certain situational attributes. The weakness of the research was the use of one case review (recall) by a manager. The design was vulnerable to manager perceptual bias in a retrospective situation.

Vroom and Yetton (1973) designed a standardized set of situational problems to overcome the weakness of the recalled problem methodology. The strength of the standard set design is its ability to emphasize a specific problem attribute in formulating a problem situation. The variables used in the standardized method were seven problem attributes. The attributes reflected the two consistent values of the model: quality and acceptance. The standardized cases (Vroom & Yetton, 1973) were obtained from management personnel employed in business, industry, and banking. The sets of cases obtained potentiated a weakness in design by threatening homogeneity in case descriptions (pp. 120, 121). The design was potentially vulnerable to the manager's choice of style if he or she had a past experience, similar to the standard case, influencing the decision process. "This feedback mechanism in which behavior or 'case n' influences the nature of 'case n + 1' was not built into the case studies, which were constant for all subjects" (Vroom & Yetton, 1973, p. 121). The results of the research study using standardized cases continued to support the premise that autocratic to participative situations should be considered as determinants of choice of leadership style.

The research studies conducted by Vroom and Yetton focused primarily on group situations. They concluded in the 1973 model presentation that the model influenced individual and group decision processes. Vroom and Jago (1974) conducted a research investigation for individual and group situations. The study supported revisions to the 1973 model. Vroom and Jago (1974) showed that managers discriminate between individual and group situations (p. 758). Decision processes used in individual versus group problems are based on differing roles of the problem attributes (Vroom & Jago, 1974, p. 768). This was a key finding in the research. Vroom and Jago (1988) account for this result in the design of the computerized model.

The research by Vroom and Jago (1974) continued to support the decision processes. The variable of homogeneity of a management group, strengthened by the research findings, demonstrated similar choice of a decision-making process (p. 769). This significant finding supports the argument against individual leadership trait (style) and supports an alternative theory. Vroom and Jago continued to provide internal validation for the decision-making model as demonstrated by reported research in 1978. The recalled situation method was used in the design. The investigation showed a predictive influence in the use of the model in the reported successful cases selected by the manager. A significant conclusion reached in the study encouraged development of a continuous scale to measure the problem attributes.

Jago (1981) conducted an investigation to measure the appropriateness of participation of subordinates as determined by the hierarchical level of a manager (p. 379). The human relations theory and human resources theory of participation are introduced by Jago (1981) as influencing the decision process. These theories are integrated into the decision-making model by suggesting that the degree of quality and the need to consider human resources (opportunity costs) or human relations (cooperation and development) partially determine the decision process. The investigations over the past 15 years significantly contributed to the 1988 model.

The revised decision-making model by Vroom and Jago (1988) was evaluated in an investigation for predictive validity. Jago, Ettling, and Vroom (1985) conducted the research study. It was reported by Vroom and Jago (1988) as the first significant study to support the new model's validity. The methodology involved a constant situational event described as a survival exercise. Four hundred subjects participated in the experiment. An expert panel was used to code the survival problem with the problem attributes. The analysis of variance statistical procedure was used to compare the decision outcomes. The results demonstrated the new model to be stronger in predictive power (Jago et al., 1985). The results cannot be generalized based on testing one situational problem. An additional significant outcome of the investigation was the obvious difference in the 1988 model's statistical results for decision effectiveness compared with those of the 1973 and 1978 models. "In terms of decision effectiveness, the new model accurately predicts decision success ($r = 0.75$) at a rate over two and one half times that of the former model ($r = 0.29$)" (Vroom & Jago 1988, p. 179). "The validity of the model hinges on its ability to correctly distinguish the relative effectiveness of different decision procedures when the attributes of problems vary" (Jago et al., 1985, p. 222).

The 1988 model requires further investigation to support its internal and external validity, but the research methodology will be greatly enhanced by the new format. The model's complexity contributes to the next research phase in the evolution of the decision-making model. Its mathematical formulas and computer-friendly format provide a new entry into social science investigation. The transfer of its utilization into nursing administration research is reasonable and inviting. The multiple roles of the nurse executive in the twenty-first century support a situational decision-making model that considers quality, opportunity cost, staff development, and commitment.

REFERENCES

Brink, P.T., & Wood, M.J. (1983). *Basic steps in planning nursing research, from question to proposal* (2nd ed.). Monterey, CA: Wadsworth Health Sciences Division.

Jago, A.G., & Vroom, V.H. (1978). Predicting leader behavior from a measure of behavioral intent. *Academy of Management Journal, 21*, 715-721.

Jago, A.G. (1981). An assessment of the deemed appropriateness of participative decision making for high and low hierarchical levels. *Human Relations, 34*(5), 379-396.

Jago, A.G., Ettling, J.T., & Vroom, V.H. (1985). Validating a revision to the Vroom/Yetton model: First evidence. *Proceedings of the 45th Annual Meeting of the Academy of Management,* 220-223. San Diego, CA: Academy of Management.

Managing participation in organizations — MPO [Computer program]. (1986, 1987). Houston: Leadership Software, Inc.

Marriner-Tomey, A. (1988). *Guide to nursing management* (3rd ed.). St. Louis: C.V. Mosby.

Tannenbaum, R., & Schmidt, W.H. (1973). How to choose a leadership pattern. *Harvard Business Review, 51*, 162-180.

Vroom, V.H. (1967). *Methods of organizational research.* Pittsburgh: University of Pittsburgh Press.

Vroom, V.H., & Jago, A.G. (1974). Decision making as a social process: Normative and descriptive models of leader behavior. *Decision Sciences, 5,* 743-769.

Vroom, V.H., & Jago, A.G. (1978). On the validity of the Vroom-Yetton model. *Journal of Applied Psychology, 63,* 151–162.

Vroom, V.H., & Jago, A.G. (1988). *The new leadership: Managing participation in organizations.* Englewood Cliffs, NJ: Prentice-Hall.

Vroom, V.H., & Yetton, P.W. (1973). *Leadership and decision-making.* Pittsburgh: University of Pittsburgh Press.

Chapter 2

Planned Change
Kurt Lewin

Carol S. Millay

CASE STUDY

General Hospital is a 300-bed hospital located in an active urban area. Because the community has a large university and several large industries, the hospital population is ever changing. The hospital is closely associated with a health maintenance organization (HMO) and clinic that supply 60% of the patient population. The hospital has historically been financially sound, benefiting from the capable direction of a future-minded chief executive officer (CEO). The hospital is a private, not-for-profit institution that offers a wide range of services and specialties to the community and surrounding areas.

One of the aspects of the institution that first attracts prospective employess is that General Hospital is a fast-paced, ever-growing organization that offers continual activity, growth opportunities, and professional challenges. In the past several years, clinical programs such as open heart surgery, trauma services, bone marrow transplantation, drug and alcohol rehabilitation, outpatient psychiatric care, and neonatal intensive care have been added. Many other programs are in the developmental or formal planning stages. Although this process has resulted in growth and additional market opportunities, the atmosphere can also invite a negative perspective or impact among employees, for activity is occurring at a constant, rapid pace that allows little time for processing and adjustment.

As are all other health care facilities, General Hospital is currently faced with a multitude of ominous factors that threaten its stability and, ultimately, its long-term survival. The nursing shortage is beginning to be felt, although the primary nursing care delivery system by an all-RN staff, along with the myriad of specialty areas, has always attracted more than a sufficient number of professional nurses.

The second major problem facing General Hospital is the financial environment in modern-day health care. There has been growing concern about and zealous attention paid to financial activity and control. A variety of occurrences underlies the changing fiscal situation. The changes in reimbursement from payers, Medicare in particular, have substantially decreased predicted income and are a major source of financial stress. Labor-intensive, high-acuity patient care has resulted in an increase in expenses per patient day. The competitive market forces attention to patient charges and routine services. Finally, small operating losses, previously balanced by other incomes, are beginning to be felt.

It has become imperative that definitive action be taken in order to keep the hospital in sound financial standing. To remain a leader in the patient service area and maintain a market share advantage, the hospital cannot discontinue any services currently offered or change plans for future services. Consequently, the CEO has formulated and announced a plan for solidifying the hospital from a fiscal perspective.

The overall goals of the plan are to increase efficiency of operations and to reduce expenditures in an effort to balance out or overcome the unpredicted shortfalls. The primary impetus for efficiency and expense reduction is a major budgetary cut, to be implemented in 15 days. The major component of the cut calls for each department to decrease operating expenses, inclusive of salaries, by 30%. Each manager is to create and use a departmental plan that will allow adherence to the given parameters. The demand for implementation of this plan most likely will require major operational changes for the employees.

Although managers are involved with change on a daily basis, the challenge to individual managers at General Hospital is enormous. Subsequently, to increase effectiveness in managing this change process, each manager must adopt an approach that includes formal application of the change process, working toward positive, productive outcomes.

| | | | | | | | | | | | | | | | | | | | | | | | | | | | | | | | | | | | | | | | | | | | | | | | | | | | | | | | | | | | | | | | | | | | |

PLANNED CHANGE

Classical change theory emanates from the work of Kurt Lewin, a German psychologist. His field theory is a means of analyzing causative relationships and thus providing a sound base for considering the process of planned change (Lewin, 1951). Lewin described change in terms of field and force. His force-field analysis is a basis for problem solving and decision making as major components of planned change, as well as a model for considering the effects of change on systems (Numerof, 1982).

Lewin outlines a process that results in effective change when implemented correctly. Change occurs when a group or system completes or moves entirely through the process. Very simply, Lewin suggests that change is an alteration or modification of an existing field of forces (Bennis, Benne, & Chin, 1969).

The most fundamental concept for Lewin is field. *Field* can be defined as life space. When considering a group, which is a main focus for change in an institutional context, life space is the group and its environment. Because factors that make up the life space include such things as needs, goals, values, and cognition, it is clear that many parts of the life space are interdependent. Lewin sees all behavior as some change in a field or life space at a given time. Behavior is a function of the life space, or of the group and the environment. Change can be viewed simply as a repatterning of behavior within a specific life space (Tappen, 1983). A system as a whole is also a field; subsequently change in one part of a system or in one subsystem must be considered in the context of the whole system or field.

An additional concept is that of force. Force can be defined as a directed entity. It is further defined through the characteristics of strength, direction, and focus (Burkman, 1988). Change can be seen as a transition to a different end or goal that is effected by force (Gillies, 1982). Change is a movement from the status quo. Lewin purports that the status quo is an equilibrium or balance of forces, and therefore movement from the status quo is a result of disequilibrium between opposing forces. Lewin identifies two kinds of forces involved in change. The first, *driving forces,* are the forces that facilitate movement toward a new goal or outcome. If they can be identified, these driving forces can be capitalized on to facilitate change. One tries to increase their strength. The second type, *restraining forces,* are forces of aversion or resistance and serve to impede goal attainment. One tries to decrease the strength of the restraining forces. These forces can be modified so that interference with change is minimized. Effective change is considered by Lewin to be a reaching of or return to equilibrium by a balancing of opposing forces. The strength of the sum of the driving and restraining forces is more important than the number of fields. Identification of the forces at play may help to predict or identify where and when change may be most successful (Numerof, 1982).

When the idea or issue of planned change is necessary, one considers what conditions must be altered in order to reach a desired outcome or new equilibrium. The prechange situation is maintained by a balance of equilibrium of the previously described driving and restraining forces. The structure of the group involved and the balancing forces active in the field or group environment must be evaluated. Lewin proposes that the group equilibrium maintenance process is based on well-established habits or standards or modes of operation. He suggests that influencing a group to make a transition from one point to another is accomplished by altering one or more of these habits by means of force. Although one could expect that the application of any new or additional force to a field would result in disequilibrium, change may not occur because of the strength of habit. The habit provides a "resistance to change" that requires additional force to break or "unfreeze."

The following assertions can be identified in Lewin's theory (1951, 1958):

1. All parts of a life space are interdependent.
2. Behavior is derived from a dynamic field or life space.
3. The point of application of force is the field.
4. The greater the value of the group standard (habit), the greater the resistance to change (restraining forces).
5. If a change occurs in group habits, a change will occur in the individuals who make up the group.
6. As driving forces increase, resistance to change decreases.
7. If strength of group habits is decreased, resistance to change decreases.

The change process and the above assertions can best be understood by breaking the process into three specific stages. The first stage, previously mentioned, is unfreezing. Lewin considers the stage of *unfreezing* as one of "breaking the habit." The process of developing an awareness of a problem or need area is initiated. This awareness may occur for a variety of reasons. Expectations may not be met. There may be concern about action taken, or about a lack of action. A former obstacle may be removed, allowing room for change (Brooten, 1984). Lewin labels these three reasons or mechanisms as the following:

1. *Lack of confirmation, or disconfirmation.* This is a realization that needs are not being met.
2. *Induction of guilt or anxiety.* This is a period of uncomfortableness about what is occurring or not occurring.
3. *Creation of psychological safety.* This occurs by removal of an obstacle to change.

In effect, what has occurred is a decrease in the restraining forces or an increase in the driving forces in order to force or cause a disequilibrium. Cognitively evaluated, the awareness of a problem or need for change results in motivation to seek an improvement or alternative. The ability to alter or improve the situation requires identification, definition, or clarification of the problem.

Once specification of the problem has occurred, the *moving* or second stage occurs. A response or solution becomes the aim of movement of the system. Welch (1979) defines a part of the second stage as selecting from among "possible avenues for solving the problem" (p. 308). Furthermore the change is planned in detail and then initiated. The actual change occurs.

The *refreezing* or third stage is the period during which the new behavior is consistently shown and acceptance is demonstrated by such behavior. This is followed by stabilization and integration of the change into the system. If the process is successfully implemented, the change is assumed to be an integral, inseparable part of the field value system.

Following completion of the change process, evaluation of the status of the field should occur. Success in meeting goals, effectiveness of interventions throughout the process, and cooperation and satisfaction of the target group are all areas for analysis. Unexpected results must also be assessed and acted on if necessary to maintain or realign a desired equilibrium.

In any organization change is synonymous with growth, and in the context of current health care, survival. However, any kind of change in the organization can create anxiety, communication disruptions, and a variety of other reactions that may result in resistance to change. Resistance to change is not inherently good or bad. Resistance may have a sound, logical basis, or it may not (Lawrence, 1969). What resistance provides is a sign or indication for further attention to management of the change process.

Resistance to change is a general term that encompasses all of Lewin's restraining forces. One of the strategies that must be used in facilitating effective change is the identification and neutralization of resistance. These issues or factors of resistance, or the restraining forces, are inherent in both the overall organization and the suborganizations. Some authors consider resistance as the most likely response to change, since any system will attempt to maintain equilibrium (Ward & Moran, 1984). According to Tappen (1983), resistance is the system's attempt to maintain integrity.

Potential causative factors for resistance to change could include self-interest of the group (suborganization) or organization. This self-interest may be prompted by the threat or fear of loss of something of value. The potential loss may be perceived as greater than the potential benefit. Role confusion or stress may be problematic. Lack of information or misunderstanding of the intent or implications of change may result in resistance. Equilibrium is preferred to delving into the unknown. An accompanying factor may be a lack of trust by the group in the change agent. Low tolerance and unresponsiveness of the group may be exhibited, particularly as they relate to change that may require acquisition of new skills or abilities by the group. Fear is a common factor of resistance (King, 1982; Kotter & Schlesinger, 1979). Resistance to change may be motivated purely by the fact that there is satisfaction with the present.

Mechanisms or strategies must be used to decrease some of the stresses or anxieties and resulting resistance related to change, for "the human system does not have infinite adaptive capacity" (Brennan & Weick, 1981, p. 18). Care must be taken to understand the nature of resistance. Many times it is based on social or human concerns (such as co-worker relations) rather than on technical or operational issues.

New and Couillard (1981) identify eight means of addressing resistance to change:

1. Participation of those affected by the change can be promoted. There are two criteria for this to be a successful mechanism. First, there must be a desire to participate. Second, an assumption must be made that those allowed to participate have a contribution to make, and the maturity to do so effectively.
2. Education or provision of a sufficient amount of information can facilitate change by increasing awareness and understanding of the group. Addressing specifically how the group will be affected can decrease anxiety related to fear of the unknown.
3. Supportive behavior is most helpful when general anxiety about the change is the major causative factor for resistance.
4. Coercion can effectively be used to induce change if the change agent has sufficient power to force change. Coercion may be necessary when changes are made within a short time frame.
5. Manipulation can be used to set up a specific context for change, which will increase the chance that the change will be accepted. Manipulation can be viewed negatively

since it is an intentionally underhanded approach, and therefore it must be used cautiously.

6. Use of a change agent who is outside the group or organization can be helpful if there is lack of a trusting relationship between the group and the original change agent or initiator.
7. Incentives can be used and can be anything on which the resisting party places value.
8. Gradual introduction of the change to those who will be affected by it may facilitate reduction in resistance to change.

Recognizing that resistance to change is an inevitable development allows managers to anticipate and plan for interventions to eliminate or minimize the negative or inhibitory effects that may result.

CASE ANALYSIS

In the ever-changing atmosphere of health care, managers in health care institutions are faced with the challenge of achieving organizational goals while dealing with major environmental or system changes. Many factors affect the manager's ability to guide the adaptation of a group to change. Alterations in organizational structure, the makeup of work groups, and laws and regulations are just a few of the factors that may have a strong impact on a manager's effectiveness. Alterations in any part of an organization are interwoven with changes in other parts of the organization. Analysis of mutual impacts initiated by change allows for a clearer understanding of interrelationships or causal relations and outcomes.

Change itself can be planned or unplanned. According to Burkman (1988), unplanned change can be random, unpredictable, unanticipated, and uncontrolled, and may therefore have negative results. Planned change, however, is a predictable and deliberate process that has a positive outcome as its purpose or goal (Brooten, Haymen, & Naylor, 1978). One mandatory managerial activity that assists in attaining productive outcomes, then, is the planning of change. Planned change is the idea of having a design for action (Dietrich, 1969). Marriner-Tomey (1988) indicates that development of a specific strategy for change is paramount to achieving positive outcomes.

The process of change is one of leadership and accountability, structure and management, adaptation and problem solving. The process includes the need to respond to and control some of the variables that influence change. Gaining control of force, or analyzing and decreasing resistance, is the key to effective change (Douglass & Bevis, 1983).

The application of Lewin's theory should occur in a step-by-step manner. The most important initial factor for the manager is to be cognizant of the content of the change to be implemented. Thought must be given in advance to possible solutions, alternative plans, available resources, personnel management, and potential response or reaction to the change process. In the case study presented the challenge and required overall change are clear, namely, budgetary reductions of 30% at General Hospital. The plan for specific nursing unit change, however, would include a multitude of issues. First and foremost, because the majority of a nursing service unit budget is related to labor costs, changes in staff utilization would have to occur. Other areas would need to be addressed as well, as secondary factors in the required budget reductions.

Specific, measurable objectives must be developed, along with activities that would provide means to meet the objectives. Objectives relating to the case study could be identified as:

1. Lessen expenditures on overtime by decreasing its occurrence by 50%.
2. Improve efficiency of staff utilization and flexibility.
3. Decrease outright salary expenditures.

Driving forces
(Actual)

Restraining forces
(Actual)

(Potential)

(Potential)

■| **FIGURE 2-1**   System elements.

4. Collect data to allow for measuring success of actions taken.
5. Efficiently control supply and equipment use.

Part of the plan to meet the objectives might include the following:

1. Implementation of a detailed procedure that requires formal approval of overtime before its occurrence.
2. Use of a mandatory on-call system to decrease the frequency of having extra staff hours when the daily patient volume decreases.
3. Initiation of a system of requiring staff to take unpaid days off when the unit/hospital is overstaffed for patient volume.
4. Required floating to other nursing units to increase flexibility in utilization of staff nurses.
5. Replacement of three vacant registered nurse (RN) positions with nursing assistant positions.
6. Maintenance of a daily log by the charge nurses detailing labor utilization, patient acuity, rationale for staffing decisions in the absence of the manager, and overtime justification.
7. Approval for opening new vacancies for interviews must be obtained from the assistant administrator of the hospital.

A second area for focus in the plan is stricter management of resources other than personnel, such as supplies and operating services. That portion of the plan might include:

1. All requisitions for routine supplies must be approved by the manager or designee.
2. Invoices for supplies provided from within the hospital must be reviewed at the end of each shift by the charge nurse to ensure accuracy of all charges.
3. Approval for replacement equipment purchased from outside the hospital is required from the assistant administrator of the hospital.
4. End-of-shift review of all patient charge processing to decrease the incidence of lost charges.

Each step of the plan must be reviewed by those affected by it at the appropriate point in the change process.

The next vitally important step is evaluation of the field or environment to identify forces that will work for and against change. Most imperative in this evaluation is knowledge of the overall system or organization, as well as the target subsystem. Potential and likely responses to the idea of major operational change should be identifiable. Projections should be made of how change will affect the target group. It may be helpful to map out the actual and potential forces and the system elements affected by the forces, as shown in Figure 2-1.

The forces that impact the change process can be internal or external. In the given case, external forces are economic (reimbursement), social (values, community responsibilities), and

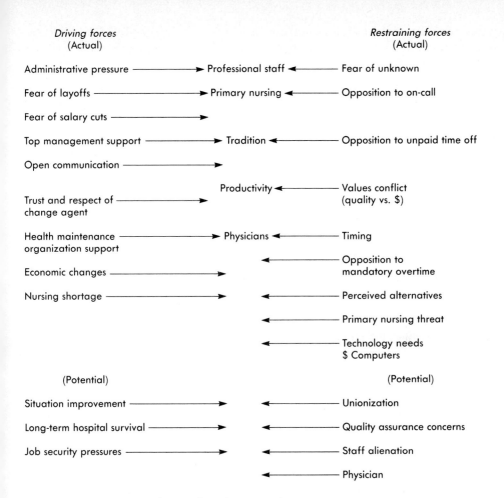

Driving forces (Actual)		Restraining forces (Actual)
Administrative pressure ⟶	Professional staff ◄───	Fear of unknown
Fear of layoffs ⟶	Primary nursing ◄───	Opposition to on-call
Fear of salary cuts ⟶		
Top management support ⟶	Tradition ◄───	Opposition to unpaid time off
Open communication ⟶		
	Productivity ◄───	Values conflict (quality vs. $)
Trust and respect of ⟶ change agent		
Health maintenance organization support ⟶	Physicians ◄───	Timing
	◄───	Opposition to mandatory overtime
Economic changes ⟶		
Nursing shortage ⟶	◄───	Perceived alternatives
	◄───	Primary nursing threat
	◄───	Technology needs $ Computers
(Potential)		(Potential)
Situation improvement ⟶	◄───	Unionization
Long-term hospital survival ⟶	◄───	Quality assurance concerns
Job security pressures ⟶	◄───	Staff alienation
	◄───	Physician

❚❘ FIGURE 2-2 System elements from the case study.

political (funding, labor laws). Potential and actual forces that are present at General Hospital can be mapped as shown in Figure 2-2.

After identification of forces, it is necessary to seek development of recognition of a need for change, while remaining aware of the forces at work. Unfreezing must be pursued by use of the three mechanisms previously discussed. An overall approach to the group should also be identified and employed. Staff meetings or small group sessions could be used to discuss the financial considerations and predicted revenue inadequacies.

First, disconfirmation may be achieved by a deliberate attempt to instill discontent or anxiety. Because many professional staff may be aware of the economic and political factors affecting health care, advantage may be taken of discussion of the fiscal fragility of hospitals relating to these factors. Since it is important to clearly demonstrate the need for the change, it may be helpful to share literature that addresses community issues or reports of hospital closures, for example. The issue of layoffs, particularly if that situation has been a reality in the geographical area, can be posed as a consequence of inactivity in the control of finances.

A second mechanism for unfreezing is to induce guilt and anxiety. The importance of the goals of the budget reduction, inefficiencies in the current system (such as payment of preventable overtime), and the existence of administrative support can all be demonstrated and promote unfreezing of the group. Examples of some of the problems being encountered in the hospital might also be presented. Insurance audits that result in disapproval of payments or utilization review summaries might be demonstrative of the need for change.

The third mechanism of unfreezing is the provision of psychological safety. It is very important to recognize the impact that individual needs and values have on response to change (Tappen, 1983). A helpful, supportive approach is to show attention to and appreciation of expressed concerns. A likely concern of professional nursing staff in the case study would be the threat to quality of care. The manager could offer examples of how certain areas would remain unaltered or how modifications would allow a continuation of current practice. For example, the introduction of nursing assistants should be clearly defined as to role, function, and tenure. Reassurance and supportive information could be provided that primary nursing would remain the mode of care delivery, for this would be a likely major concern. People by nature are frightened of the unknown, and displays of confidence in a group's ability to deal with changes are important. Allowing input and involvement of the group in idea development can invoke investment in the changes required. For example, staff members may be able to design an on-call system that would work for the group. Additional means of offering support can be used that are specific to the situation. Formal retention and recruitment activities may be a strong indicator that a high value is placed on the work group.

Throughout the change process, it is mandatory to consciously adhere to specific principles. Change should be built around a perceived need. The purpose of the unfreezing stage is to demonstrate that need. Effective communication and interpersonal relations are paramount to success. There should be no surprises for the target group. Opportunities for open communication and free exchange of ideas allow for questions to be answered and issues to be clarified. The change required in the case study is quite complex; therefore care should be taken not to overload the target group with information. A series of meetings could be used to provide the information and plan in phases.

Once there is a need perception, the moving stage begins. The specific plan is introduced and necessary information is provided. The ground rules are stated, as are the goals and objectives. Those areas of the plan in which a choice of alternatives or ideas are possible should be reviewed. Early involvement of the group can enhance commitment to the process and investment in reaching the desired outcomes.

Emphasis should be placed on problem solving and identification of contingency actions. A supportive, open climate must be maintained to lessen defensiveness of the group throughout the process. Behaviors supportive of the change (correct application of the overtime policy, for example) should be encouraged by positive feedback, updates on progress, and promotion of independence in the activities. Feedback can be facilitated in various ways including on-the-spot observations, written memos, or group meetings throughout the process. Individual discussion and group meetings also provide a forum for members of the group to vent feelings of anger, anxiety, conflict, and hostility as the change is implemented. Surfacing of these negative responses allows opportunity for dealing with issues that can thwart success of the change process. It is also a possibility that counseling and discipline may be necessary to deal with resistance to change.

Communications with other subsystems that may be affected by the change is necessary. Physicians are a primary group who may feel the effects of changes in staffing and resource availability. The potential impacts that alterations in resources may have on other groups should be addressed clearly and honestly. Progress reports on certain information such as hiring or the new use of nursing assistants may be helpful in minimizing problems or resistance.

A final but major activity for the manager during the moving stage is constant attention to possible resistance. Forces at work should be constantly identified and evaluated in terms of influence on the change process. Conflicts of values related to patient care concerns versus budget restrictions, increased demands for staff nurse financial accountability, and direction of loyalties are certainly potential areas for conflict or resistance at General Hospital.

The purpose of the final stage, refreezing, is to integrate the change so that it becomes normal behavior or regular functioning of the field. The manager's primary responsibility during the refreezing period is to continue to act as an energizer. Because change is often followed by attempts to return to previous behavior patterns or habits, maintenance of visibility and credibility of the change is important (Bennis et al., 1969). Guidance and follow-up must be consistent to ensure that the new behavior patterns persist. Policy reviews, monthly budget status reports, and routine sessions for solicitation of input are ways to apply significance to continued adherence to the change. Recognition of appropriate behavior should be given freely.

During the refreezing stage, some of the activities can be delegated to allow further independence of functioning. Various aspects of resource monitoring could be assigned. Quality control monitor completion can be rotated among staff members to allow the group firsthand access to quality-related data inclusive of problem areas. Follow-up procedures for problems identified can be developed by the staff group with guidance from the manager.

With the process of planning and implementing change, the manager undertakes a variety of risks. Mistakes, decreased efficiency, increased losses with staff dissatisfaction and turnover, and diminished staff morale are all potential reactions or results of the process applied to the case study. The manager must attempt to anticipate both the good and the bad effects of change, with the intention of lessening or eliminating the bad.

Change will always and should always occur. Successful, productive organizations are those that are dynamic and energetic, planning and dealing with change effectively. The key for the manager involved with change is control so that change occurs at the right time, the right speed, and the right place, with bad effects minimized and desired effects maximized. The means to achieve this outcome are being knowledgeable about and able to employ the formal planning of change.

RESEARCH

In considering the force-field approach to research as it relates to change, Lewin (1951) cited a study conducted at the Child Welfare Research Station of the State University of Iowa. The objective of the study was to find out why people eat what they eat, and what promotes change in their eating behaviors. The method used was an interview of sets of five groups of homemakers. The interviews addressed a multitude of food-related issues. Information gained from the study indicated the following:

1. The effect of forces toward a change of food habits is dependent on habit flexibility.
2. The lower the level of satisfaction with the current situation or behavior, the greater the chance for action toward change.
3. Lack of availability of a food source (driving force) resulted in change of behavior.
4. Change can be motivated by an alteration in the frame of reference (field).

The overall finding of the study was that a system of values forms the basis of forces that determines decisions regarding food.

A study by Bavelas (1942) presented findings that demonstrate group movement from one equilibrium to another following the introduction of force in the form of educational support aimed at improving production in a sewing factory. Procedures were used that decreased production restraints rather than using direct efforts at increasing production, but specific change occurred, as demonstrated by alterations in production levels.In the nursing literature, Breu and Dracup (1976) reported the use of force-field analysis as the basis for change. The planned change process outlined by Lewin was used to facilitate the application of research findings from a study by Hampe (1975), in a critical care unit.

Burkman (1988) presented an application of planned change in the introduction of sibling visitation in a neonatal intensive care unit. Evaluation of results or effectiveness of the change was made by positive feedback from parents.

The merger of two obstetrical units was accomplished based on the planned change process emanating from Lewin (Ellis, 1987). A descriptive analysis of the process was offered, indicating successful progression through unfreezing, moving, and partial achievement of the refreezing stage.

These and many other examples of the use of Lewin's model as a basis for institutional change or promotion of change can be found in the nursing literature. Little can be found, however, that reports specific research based on Lewin's theory. Part of the explanation for the lack of research studies related to change and to planned change specifically has to do with the difficulty involved with measuring change itself. This dilemma is addressed in a variety of sources such as Burckhardt, Goodwin, and Prescott (1982) and Harris (1963). The literature that addresses the measurement issue, as well as consideration of alternate mechanisms for effective measurement, is minimal.

Many studies relating to change, in fact, offer a measurement of something other than change, such as attitude, behavior, performance, or productivity. Although the conduct of a study may proceed according to Lewin's ideas, the theoretical basis is identified otherwise, such as cognitive dissonance, engagement-involvement, modeling, or any one of numerous other theories or models.

Kemp (1984) purported that change is a significant component of nursing theories relating to stress, adaptation, crisis, and other areas. These theories are used repeatedly in attempts to explain the concept of change. Bennis et al. (1969) indicate that planned change should include three steps: education, consultation, and research. Research on planned change based on Lewin's force-field analysis is needed. Conducting such studies may offer additional insight into facilitation of change, dealing with resistance to change, and maximizing effectiveness of all the managerial activities of planning, directing, facilitating, coordinating, and evaluating of nursing services.

REFERENCES

Bavelas, A. (1942). Morale and the training of leaders. In G. Watson (Ed.), *Civilian morale*. Boston: Houghton Mifflin.

Bennis, W.G., Benne, K.D., & Chin, R. (1969). *The planning of change*. New York: Holt, Rinehart, & Winston.

Brennan, E., & Weick, A. (1981). Theories of adult development. *Social Casework: The Journal of Contemporary Social Work, 62,* 13-19.

Breu, C., & Dracup, K. (1976). Implementing nursing research in a critical care setting. Journal of Nursing Administration, 6(10), 14-17.

Brooten, D.A. (1984). *Managerial leadership in nursing*. Philadelphia: J.B. Lippincott.

Brooten, D.A., Hayman, L., & Naylor, M. (1978). *Leadership for change: A guide for the frustrated nurse*. New York: J.B. Lippincott.

Burckhardt, C.S., Goodwin, L.D., & Prescott, P.A. (1982). The measurement of change in nursing research: Statistical considerations. *Nursing Research, 31*(1), 52-55.

Burkman, K.A. (1988). Effecting change: You can do it. *Neonatal Network, 6*(6), 41-45.

Dietrich, B. (1969). Effective change in nursing service is sometimes difficult to achieve because of a peculiar "two-headed" authority structure. *Hospital Management, 108*(6), 44-50.

Douglass, L.M., & Bevis E.O. (1983). *Nursing management and leadership in action*. St. Louis: C.V. Mosby.

Ellis, D.J. (1987). Change process: A case example. *Nursing Management, 18*(4), 14-19.

Gillies, D.A. (1982). *Nursing management: A systems approach.* Philadelphia: W.B. Saunders.

Harris, C.W. (1963). *Problems in measuring change.* Madison: University of Wisconsin.

Kemp, V.H. (1984). An overview of change and leadership. *Topics in Clinical Nursing, 6*(1), 1-9.

King, E. (1982, July). Coping with organizational change. *Topics in Clinical Nursing, 4,* 66-73.

Kotter, J., & Schlesinger, L. (1979, March-April). Choosing strategies for change. *Harvard Business Review, 57*(2), 107-114.

Lawrence, P.R. (1969). How to deal with resistance to change. *Harvard Business Review* [January–February Reprint] *47*(1), 4-10, 166-174.

Lewin, K. (1951). *Field theory in social science.* New York: Harper & Row.

Lewin, K. (1958). Group decision and social change. In E. Maccoby (Ed.), *Readings in social psychology* (p. 208). New York: Holt, Rinehart, & Winston.

Marriner-Tomey, A. (1988). *Guide to nursing management* (3rd ed.). St. Louis: C.V. Mosby.

New, J.R., & Couillard, N.A. (1981). Guidelines for introducing change. *Journal of Nursing Administration, 11*(3), 17-21.

Numerof, R. (1982). *The practice of management for health care professionals.* New York: Amacon.

Tappen, R.M. (1983). *Nursing leadership: Concepts and practice.* Philadelphia: F.A. Davis.

Ward, M., & Moran, S. (1984). Resistance to change. *Nursing Management, 15*(1), 30-33.

Welch, L. (1979). Planned change in nursing: The theory. *Nursing Clinics of North America, 14,* 307-321.

Chapter 3

Theories of Justice

M. Jan Keffer

❚❙ CASE STUDY

Two young women, both in full-term, active labor, are admitted to Generic General Hospital. Both pregnancies have been attended by competent health care professionals. Sally Sue, a 17-year-old single primigravida, has been followed at the hospital maternal health clinic by residents in family practice with backup from the hospital staff Ob-Gyn department. Becky Ann, a 19-year-old married primigravida, has been followed at a local physician's office (the same doctor who provides backup for the maternal health clinic). Her hospital costs are covered by the health insurance obstetrical policy from her husband's job.

Each woman's course of pregnancy has been similar in terms of number of visits, medication, teaching, and support by the clinic and physician's office personnel. The difference is in the form and amount of monetary payment to the hospital. Becky's care will be reimbursed by third-party payers. Sally's care has been absorbed within the educational budget of the hospital. The cost of running the maternal health clinic comes from private contributions and state and federal tax dollars (Medicaid funds) payable to the hospital. No reimbursement goes to the resident or the staff Ob-Gyn backup physician.

After Becky and Sally are settled in the labor room, the OB nurse enters with a large attractive diaper bag filled with personal care items, such as perineal pads, underpants, underpads, bath basin, and lotion. The diaper bag is free to each woman, compliments of the hospital. Along the course of the delivery of each woman's healthy baby other items, such as a yard sign proclaiming the birth of the baby at Generic General, a badge for the newborn with his or her footprint and name, and a monogrammed baby blanket are given to each woman. In addition, a grouping of photographs of the newborn and his or her new family and a videotape of the introduction of the baby into the family unit is given to the mother courtesy of the hospital.

The hospital administrator, Mr. Sam Jones, has met recently with the hospital board of directors and the vice president for nursing service, Dr. Mary Smith, concerning the continuing struggle to contain hospital costs. Reimbursement from Medicaid and third-party insurance payers has been decreasing each year for the past 2 years, and no change in the trend has been forecasted. The administrator mandates that Dr. Smith find ways, nonessential to direct care, to curtail the costs of labor and delivery for the 1800 deliveries done at the hospital each year.

What can she do to curtail costs that do not affect patient care? What items are

I gratefully acknowledge the assistance of Professor Gary J. Foulk, Department of Philosophy, Indiana State University, Terre Haute, Ind., for his thoughtful review of this manuscript.

nonessential to the care of the OB patient? She could eliminate the free public relations items given to each mother and baby. What would this do, though, to the community spirit the hospital is advocating? What are the reasons people come to have their babies at this hospital? How would this affect the hospital's competitive position? Would the elimination of the free items change the feelings of parents toward the hospital?

Dr. Smith has decided to forego giving the free items only to those women who receive care through the maternal health clinic. Her rationale is that their care is provided at no cost to them. Furthermore it seems unfair that the paying patients would not get full value for their money. Additionally the paying patients help keep the hospital solvent. Currently 15% of the hospital's deliveries originate from the maternal health clinic. No more maternal health clinic deliveries can be absorbed within the hospital's budgetary constraints.

When Dr. Smith tells the nursing staff of the change in policy, the staff express angry sentiments: How can I treat one differently than another? The indigent patient needs the free items more than the paying patient. The paying patient does not deserve special treatment any more than the poor patient. How can you ask me to treat people unequally?

| | | | | | | | | | | | | | | | | | | | | | | | | | | | | | | | | | | | | | | | | | | | | | | | | | | | | | | | | | | | | |

ETHICS

This case study points out how the allocation of medical resources, although resources that do not directly affect patient care, involves the hospital and its staff in making decisions that bear directly on the question of justice. To make such decisions in a rational manner, one needs a working knowledge of the definitions and theories of justice, not merely as a philosophical abstraction,* but in a pragmatic, practice-grounded manner.

This chapter first presents definitions that are needed to understand the ethical principles of justice. Following the definitions, the theories of justice are described. Finally, a discussion of how the theories apply to the allocation of resources is presented. The example used above pertains to decision making in an acute care hospital, but with slight modification it would be appropriate in any other situation in which a nurse administrator has to make a choice in allocating a product or service among conflicting demands.

The question of a just distribution of goods or services becomes more acute when a real or potential scarcity exists. Such a scarcity does exist within the health care industry. Because of societal decisions, health care reimbursement is limited to a smaller percentage of the total budget than that desired by participants needing the services and products of the industry. Competition for the remaining products and services elicits questions of what a person deserves, what constitutes a just distribution, and how a just distribution of resources may be effected. The ultimate question to be decided is what is justice?

Definitions

Beauchamp and Childress (1983) define *distributive justice* as "justified distribution of benefits and burdens in society" (p. 184). This distribution is a cooperative enterprise of a society. Two types of distributive justice exist. *Comparative justice* occurs "when what a person

---

* "It is a mistake to employ the rider that, when writing about medical ethics, one is not interested in philosophy just as a philosophical abstraction, although it is literally true. The problem is that the rider leads people to think that the difficult and involved abstractions do not have to be learned if one's interest is practical. One can hardly apply the abstractions intelligently to practice if one does not know them first *in the abstract*" (G.J. Foulk, personal communication, April 19, 1988).

deserves can be determined only by balancing the competing claims of other persons against his or her claims" (Beauchamp & Childress, 1983, p. 185). Here the question of allocation of medical resources, the question of who gets what and how much, is appropriate. *Noncomparative justice* occurs "when desert is judged by a standard independent of the claims of others" (Beauchamp & Childress, 1983, p. 185). The rule that an innocent person never deserves punishment is an example of noncomparative justice. This chapter deals wholly with comparative justice and the allocation of benefits and burdens.

Synonyms for "justice" are the words "fairness" and "getting what you deserve" (desert). If a person gets what he or she deserves, that person has been treated fairly. What the person deserves is also just. The concepts of fair and desert are often confused and can create differences in understanding a statement (Beauchamp & Childress, 1983).

Hospers (1982) made clear several distinctions about the concept of justice. First, "justice involves the treatment of human beings by other human beings." Second, "justice is past-looking." Justice requires that people be treated in accord with their deserts (giving to each his or her due or right), and their deserts depend on their past record. Third, "justice is individualistic." Each person deserves according to his or her own past record. Fourth, and last, comparative justice relates to injustice, having to do with the way one person is treated in relation to another (pp. 307-308).

Frankena (1973) recognized that a normative theory of moral obligation is a necessary component to a theory of ethical conduct. Frankena differentiated between *distributive justice* as "distribution of good and evil" and *retributive justice* as "punishment." An example of injustice would be where two similar persons are in similar circumstances and one is treated better or worse than the other (Frankena, 1973, p. 49). This example raises questions about how we are to tell if the persons are similar or if the treatment is dissimilar. Having answered these questions, we then have to decide on which rules of distribution or comparative treatment we are to act.

The concept of retributive justice refers primarily, but not exclusively, to the legal sense of justice, for example, the laws passed by a society to regulate the members of that society. *Law* may be defined as "a system of principles and rules of human conduct prescribed or recognized by the governing body" (Rakish, Longest, & Darr, 1985, p. 81). Justice as law differs from the principles of justice in ethics in that the laws of the society are generally enacted to benefit the greatest number of persons in the society (utilitarian view), whereas justice in ethics is the study of human conduct and moral judgment. Civil and criminal laws (even though they may have moral underpinnings) are made to control or direct the actions of a people. The law is "a minimum standard of performance, either positive or negative . . . , which is expected from members of society" (Rakish et al., 1985, p. 84).

A person might perceive that a direct relationship exists between law and ethics. It is not necessarily the case that anything that is lawful is ethical or vice versa. Rakish et al. give an example of a profession requiring higher standards of conduct than those required by compliance with the law of the land (Rakish et al., 1985, p. 84). Likewise, the law may not speak to a certain conduct or activity, but a profession's code of ethics may require the action. The activity would be legal, but not necessarily ethical (Rakish et al., 1985, p. 84).

The following definition of terms will help explain the interconnectedness of the theories of justice. The terms will also provide a basis for understanding the application of the theories.

Ethics is the philosophical study of morality. It is the study of human conduct and is concerned with such questions as, When is an act right or wrong? When is an act just? When is an act desirable? When is an act morally obligatory? (Hospers, 1982). A sentence is an *ethical statement* if it implies, entails, or contradicts any statement containing the ethical terms desirable, morally obligatory, or reprehensible (Brandt, 1959, pp. 2-3). Acts that are spoken of as "right or wrong" or we "ought" to do such and such are examples of ethical statements. When the principles of ethics are applied to a situation, we are asking the question, When is it right or wrong to do or not do an act? The study of the meaning of ethical terms has been called *metaethics*. The attempt to discover a rational criterion for determining the truth value of moral judgments has been termed *normative ethics*. The application of the ethical principles of justice in a situation is an example of the use of normative ethics. A *structured normative ethical theory* is a "system of principles by which to determine what ought and ought not to be done" (Beauchamp & Childress, 1983, p. 13). Normative ethical theory has been divided into *teleological* and *deontological* approaches. "The theories attempt to articulate and justify principles that can be utilized as guides for making moral decisions. . . . The ethical theories . . . offer a means to explain and justify actions" (Munson, 1988, p. 2).

Utilitarianism (one type of teleological normative theory) is an ethical theory formulated primarily by philosophers Jeremy Bentham (1748-1832) and John Stuart Mill (1806-1873). Numerous elaborations have evolved from the basic formulations (Munson, 1988, p. 3). Utilitarianism is grounded in the "thesis that an action or practice is right (when compared with any alternative action or practice) if it leads to the greatest possible balance of good consequences or the least possible balance of bad consequences in the world as a whole" (Beauchamp & Walters, 1982, p. 13). The most frequently cited objections to utilitarianism are that it appears to justify treating people as means and that the theory is lacking a principle of justice.

Deontology advocates argue that "moral standards exist independently of utilitarian ends." "An act or rule is right . . . insofar as it satisfies the demands of some overriding principle of duty" (Beauchamp & Walters, 1982, p. 19). The foremost author of deontology was the German philosopher Immanuel Kant (1724-1804) (Munson, 1988, p. 11). The main objection to deontology is that it leaves "unresolved how duty is to be determined when two or more duties are in conflict" (Beauchamp & Walters, 1982, p. 23).

For one to take a reasoned approach to understanding rules and problems, principles are needed that take a consistent approach to issues. Four moral principles are widely held to be the primary principles of biomedical ethics: autonomy, nonmaleficence, beneficence, and justice. Each of the principles is contained within the two ethical theories of utilitarianism and deontology (with the exception of justice). Nonmaleficence and beneficence are strongly integrated in utilitarianism. Autonomy and justice are inherent in deontology.

Principle of autonomy

Beauchamp and Walters (1982) formulated the principle as follows:

> Insofar as an autonomous agent's actions do not infringe on the autonomous actions of others, that person should be free to perform whatever action he or she wishes (presumably even if it involves considerable risk to himself or herself and even if others consider the action to be foolish. (p. 27)

Autonomy is considered to be the primary moral principle and takes precedence over all other moral considerations.

Principle of beneficence

Munson's formulation of the principle of beneficence is:

> We should act in ways that promote the welfare of other people. (1988, p. 35)

Principle of nonmaleficence

Munson's formulation of the principle of nonmaleficence is:

> We ought to act in ways that do not cause needless harm or injury to others. (1988, p. 33)

Principle of justice

There have been different analyses of justice, but fundamentally the term *justice* has come to represent fairness and desert. In Beauchamp and Walters's formulation

> A person has been treated justly when he [sic, she] has been given what he or she is due or owed, what he or she deserves or can legitimately claim. (1982, p. 30)

Common to all theories of justice is the minimalist principle of justice: equals ought to be treated equally and unequals may be treated unequally. This principle is referred to as a *formal* principle of justice and is attributed to Aristotle (Gillon, 1985a, p. 201). The reason that the principle is called formal is because it "states no particular respects in which equals ought to be treated the same" (Beauchamp & Childress, 1983, p. 186). Philosophers are quoted as stating that the principle lacks substance and does not define who is considered equal. As an answer to this supposed lack in Aristotle's minimal principle of justice, other philosophers have specified the relevant differences between the individual's claim for justice by defining the *material* principles of justice (Beauchamp & Childress, 1983, p. 186).

The theories of justice have been developed around the relevant differences between individuals and the criterion of desert. Principles that specify these relevant differences concerning how people are to be treated are said to be *material* principles, because they put material content into a theory of justice (Beauchamp & Childress, 1983, p. 187). Each of the material principles identifies a property whereby burdens and benefits may be distributed. Beauchamp and Childress (1983), Brandt (1959), Engelhardt (1986), and Hospers (1982) give a similar listing of material principles of distributive justice:

1. To each person an equal share
2. To each person according to individual need
3. To each person according to individual effort
4. To each person according to societal contribution
5. To each person according to merit

Summary

The ethical theories of utilitarianism and deontology have been briefly defined, the principles of biomedical ethics have been presented, and the material principles of justice enumerated. The reason given by philosophers for the need of additional conceptions of justice is that the formal principle lacks substance and is not adequately represented in the basic normative ethical theories of utilitarianism and deontology.

THEORIES OF JUSTICE

In the following section the foremost theories of justice are sketched. Each theory is defined, its assumptions presented, and its possible strengths and limitations discussed.

"Most theories of justice attempt to systematize and simplify moral intuitions by selecting and emphasizing one or more of the . . . material principles of distributive justice." (Beauchamp & Childress, 1983, p. 189). It is with this understanding that the theories of justice are presented.

> *Egalitarian* theories emphasize equal access to the goods in life that every rational person desires. *Marxist* theories emphasize need. *Libertarian* theories emphasize rights to social and economic liberty (implicity invoking the criteria of contribution and merit). *Utilitarian* theories emphasize a mixture of criteria so public and private utility [usefulness] is maximized. (Beauchamp & Childress, 1983, p. 189).

These aforementioned theories of justice are an attempt to introduce principles to order our diverse judgments about right and wrong. Each theory emphasizes a material principle and its rational strength makes reason the chief arbiter in whether it is or is not accepted by the philosophical community. I do not purport to argue the logic of each theory, but merely to present the consensus of a few learned sources about each of these four theories of justice.

Egalitarian Theories

In these theories individuals are to be treated equally and burdens and benefits are to be distributed on an equal basis — everyone is to be treated the same in all respects. John Rawls, in 1971, produced an outstanding and far-reaching discussion in his book, *A Theory of Justice*. Rawls's treatise received considerable attention when published and continues to be a major source of discussion among philosophers. His central contention is that all vital economic goods and services should be distributed equally, unless an unequal distribution would work to everyone's advantage (Rawls, 1971, p. 62). He used the hypothetical device called the "original position." A group of people who make up a normal society (range of intelligence, talents, ambitions, social advantage, sex, and races) are placed behind a "veil of ignorance." Being ignorant of his or her sex, race, social and economic position, this group of people agree on two principles that maximize the minimum level of primary goods in order to protect vital interests in uncertain, but perhaps disastrous contexts. Each member of society, irrespective of wealth or position, would be provided with equal access to an adequate (although not maximal) level of health care for all available types of services (Beauchamp & Childress, 1983, p. 191).

Rawls's two principles of justice are as follows (1971, p. 302):

> *First principle.* Each person is to have an equal right to the most extensive total system of equal basic liberties compatible with a similar system of liberty for all.
> *Second principle.* Social and economic inequalities are to be arranged so that they are both:
> (a) To the greatest benefit of the least advantaged, consistent with the just savings principle, and
> (b) Attached to offices and positions open to all under conditions of fair equality of opportunity.

The two principles and the veil of ignorance represent major assumptions in Rawlsian theory. Another assumption is that primary goods are not preowned and therefore do not come to the public for distribution with a history. In other words, Rawls's theory is based on an *ahistorical* foundation for the allocation of resources. Likewise, an assumption inherent in the theory is that equal distribution will in fact benefit the least well-off segment of society.

Strengths of the theory lie in the fairness doctrine that allocations or distributions, if equal, will therefore be fair. Consequently, the society will be just. Engelhardt (1986) referred to Rawls's theory as a "goals-based justice which is concerned with the achievement of the good of individuals in society, and where the pursuit of beneficence is not constrained by a strong principle of autonomy" (p. 353).

In goals-based justice, a limitation, as noted by Engelhardt (1986), is that justice will vary as

> one attempts to (a) give each person an equal share; (b) give each person what that person needs; and (c) give each person a distribution as a part of a system designed to achieve the greatest balance of benefits over harms for the greatest number of persons; and (d) give each person a distribution as a part of a system designed to maximize the advantage of the least-well-off class within conditions of equal liberty for all and of fair opportunity. (p. 353)

A major limitation of Rawls's theory of justice is the assumption that the primary goods of a society do, in fact, include health care (Daniels, 1981; Engelhardt, 1986; Hospers, 1982;

Munson, 1988). A second limitation is that Rawls's theory of justice might not "apply to a society ... that has among its members people with serious disabilities and severe chronic diseases" (Munson, 1988, p. 25). It is well that discussion continues so that Ralsian theory and other theories can be utilized as was intended by their authors, rather than as hybridized by well-meaning, but invalid formulations.

Marxist Theories

This theory of justice is attributed to the early twentieth century social reformer, Karl Marx (1818-1883). The people who deserve social goods are those who need them the most. The primary assumption is "from each according to his ability, to each according to his need" (Gillon, 1985a, p. 201; Hospers, 1982, p. 323). The material principles of ability and need are of foremost concern in this formulation. The principle of beneficence is the primary criterion that transposes the theory. Nozick (1974) referred to the theory as one form of "the productive resources theory of value" (p. 256). The theory asserted that the "value (V) of a thing (X) is equal to the sum total of a society's production (Y) of that thing." Additionally the "ratio of the value of two things [V(X)/V(Y)] is equal to the ratio of the amount of productive resources embodied in them (M)" (Nozick, 1974, p. 256). The resulting formula is:

$$\frac{V(X)}{V(Y)} = \frac{M \text{ (resources in X)}}{M \text{ (resources in Y)}}$$

Therefore, the theory of need is based on labor and the value of resources. Assumptions are that the society has similar needs and that all things are commonly owned. Strengths are that all persons in the society have their minimal needs met by the society. Limitations are found in defining needs and in providing capital to move the society forward. A major question in Marxist theory is how to resolve the situation in which two people have equal need for a commodity and only one commodity exists. The theories of justice based on need have been widely refuted among philosophers for the lack of the definition of "need" (Beauchamp & Childress, 1983; Hospers, 1982; Nozick, 1974; Rawls, 1971).

Libertarian Theories

This theory of justice was developed by Robert Nozick in his book *Anarchy, State, and Utopia,* published in 1974. He emphasized that the right act should not be coerced for the distribution of economic benefits and burdens. This formulation emphasizes rights to social and economic liberty. The theory invokes the material principles of contribution and merit. The theory's foundations are the autonomous actions on the part of rational persons. "Libertarian theories of justice concentrate on the individual rights of persons to enter and withdraw freely from arrangements in accordance with their perceptions of their own interests" (Beauchamp & Childress, 1983, p. 190).

Nozick gave a historical account for the allocation of resources. He assumed that "(a) the condition for morality is mutual respect, and (b) people already own things prior to any particular society" (Nozick, quoted in Engelhardt, 1986, p. 351). Nozick's axiom became: From each as they choose, to each as they are chosen (Nozick, 1974, p. 160).

> For Nozick, moral agents are not obligated out of considerations of fairness to attempt to blunt the consequences of the natural lottery through which some are born healthy and others with serious illness. In addition . . . the adverse outcomes of the social lottery, through which some are wealthy through gifts, inheritance, or cooperation of others . . . are simply unfortunate." (Engelhardt, 1986, p. 352)

In Nozick's theory of justice, beneficence is constrained by the principle of autonomy. Allocation of goods within this freedom-based theory of justice will operate within the respect of the free wishes of persons (Engelhardt, 1986, p. 354). A freedom-based approach to health care "holds that justice is first and foremost giving to each the right to be respected as a free individual in the disposition of personal services and private goods: that is what is due *(jus)* each individual" (Engelhardt, 1986, p. 354).

Both the strengths and the limitations of the libertarian theories pertain to the principle of autonomy for the individual. The individual can decide what he or she values enough to allocate resources for. However, if everyone allocates without consideration of future mishaps, the society would falter. A major assumption remains that the persons in Nozick's society would be moral agents, who would protect both their and others' needs for the benefit of the society. The libertarian formulation continues to be debated in philosophical, economic, and political circles.

Utilitarian Theories

As has been said previously (see earlier section on definitions), the theory of utility suffers from a lack of a conception of justice. It would seem obvious that an act that increases the general happiness of many at the expense of increasing the unhappiness of the few could not be considered a right or just act. Some mechanism must be found to distribute happiness and unhappiness under this theory while avoiding exploitation of the few. It is for this reason that application of utilitarianism usually results in usage of mixed material criteria (Munson, 1988, p. 3).

Summary

The major theories of justice have been defined, their assumptions described, and their major strengths and limitations identified. The theory of Rawls with emphasis on justice as fairness was proposed to represent an egalitarian theory. Marxist theory stressed the material principle of need. Libertarian theories stressed autonomy and the material considerations of merit and ability. Utilitarian theories stressed societal and private usefulness and emphasized a mixture of material principles depending on the situation of interest.

FORMULATIONS OF JUSTICE WITHIN THE HEALTH CARE INDUSTRY

Aristotle's minimalist theory is implicitly accepted by all theorists of justice. Aristotle required that resource allocational decisions be made on moral grounds (Gillon, 1985b, p. 266). Having considered various theories, a person will intuit that the solution to any allocational problem will be different depending on which theory is chosen. The appropriate solution will probably involve consideration of several theories. Gillon warned us that "justice is not achieved simply by basing a scheme for resource allocation on a good theory of justice. Its decisions must be implemented" (1985b, p. 266). Equally important as an appeal to normative theories is the process of deciding how to define moral terms.

Major theories of justice are capable of allocation of good and evil in society, not merely the allocation of health care resources. Since allocation within the health care industry is the prime focus of nurse administrators, it would be well to mention three major approaches that have been devised to deal with microallocationary decisions. *Microallocation* represents allocation of available health care dollars to specific patients—deciding which patients should receive what form of treatment. Selection of which patients receiving which service could be viewed as a higher level microallocational choice (Engelhardt, 1986, p. 346).

How a decision maker views justice in health care determines what delivery system will be acceptable. How a person understands the principle of justice will indicate how he or she strikes a balance among the four goals of a health care system (Engelhardt, 1986):

1. The provision of the best possible care for all
2. The provision of equal care for all
3. Freedom of choice on the part of the health care provider and the consumer
4. Containment of health care costs (p. 354)

If a freedom-based view of justice is endorsed, the person will support freedom of choice by an individual. If a goals-based view of justice is endorsed, the person will be more likely to support the goal of the best possible care and equal care for all (Engelhardt, 1986, . p. 354).

It is well to remember that health care systems are fashioned by a society to "blunt" the outcome of the forces of nature (the *natural lottery*). The health care system is likewise an attempt to "blunt" the responses of the *social lottery* (the uncaring choices by others who will not respond with sympathy to those in need). "Health care systems function as a societally fashioned web of caring, support, and aid" (Engelhardt, 1986, p. 355).

Engelhardt (1986) classified systems of health care under three rubrics:

1. Those that rely on the market alone and provide no social safety net for those who lose in the natural and social lotteries.
2. Those that attempt to provide an equal level of health care for all.
3. Those that allow for two tiers of health care, one provided through a social safety net, and a second tier that can be purchased by private resources. (p. 355)

In an excellent argument Engelhardt supported the two classes of health care as a compromise between egalitarian and libertarian theories. The principles of autonomy and beneficence are supported in the two-tiered system. The task is to create a "decent minimum" as a support for all members of society" (Engelhardt, 1986, p. 362).

Engelhardt measured a two-tiered system against the four goals for health care systems and decided that although some minor substitutions were needed, the system essentially fulfilled the criteria. A notion of minimal health care is substituted for the goal of equal health care. The goal of best possible care for all would be realizable only insofar as the society wished to invest ample resources. Free choice (1) would be supported by defending individual providers and (2) would include positive right of access to health care to those who have not been advantaged by the social lottery. The goal of containment of health care costs would exist primarily in the tier of health care provided through communal resources (Engelhardt, 1986, p. 364). Advancement of the health care system would come from private and donated funds, the second tier of the system.

Another system of allocation of health care resources is based on chance or randomness (first come, first served) or an artificial lottery allocation. This allocation methodology was proposed by Childress (1970) in an article, "Who Shall Live When Not All Can Live?" The proposal supported the principle of autonomy, but perhaps was limited in beneficence. The argument would have difficulty proving fairness or justice. It was based on equality, since everyone theoretically would have an equal chance to be picked in the lottery (Childress, 1970).

A particular health care system as a *fair* compromise, will be *just,* in a sense of being the result of a *fair* procedure, one that respects the freedom of the participants in the compromise. However, it may still be regarded as inadequate from the point of view of particular understandings of beneficence" (Engelhardt, 1986, p. 367). Engelhardt suggested that the pattern of a compromise, as well as justification and history, will need to be attended to in "order to give a meaning to the language of rights to health care" (Engelhardt, 1986, p. 368).

Gillon urged that practical systems be set up to allocate scarce medical resources. Systems should take into account fundamental moral values of respect for autonomy, beneficence, and nonmaleficence. Systems should incorporate Aristotle's formal principle of justice with its demands of formal equity, impartiality, and fairness. If practice systems used these principles they "would be just systems and their deliberations could be expected to yield just results despite . . . the conflict within them" (Gillon, 1985b, p. 268).

Summary

We have looked at three possible formulations for allocating health care resources. The two-tiered system was proposed by Engelhardt. A lottery or chance system was proposed by Childress. Gillon suggested that Aristotle's formal principle of justice is indeed implicitly accepted by theorists and should be merged into a practical system of allocation.

CASE ANALYSIS

In this section, the case study presented at the beginning of the chapter is analyzed according to the various theories of justice: egalitarian, Marxist, libertarian, and utilitarian. The case study is then applied to the two-tiered system and the lottery formulations.

Egalitarian: Within this theory Rawls's concept of fairness is paramount. Beneficence is the biomedical ethical principle of concern. The material principle would be equality for all. To be fair and just, the free items presented in the case study would be given to all or none.

Marxist: In this formulation persons deserve to have their needs met. The Marxist corollary of "from each according to his ability, to each according to his needs" would entail giving the first items only to those patients who had the greatest need. Since need is usually defined in health care situations as those unable to provide monetary payment, the free items would be given only to those patients unable to pay for them.

Libertarian: Theories of justice using this formulation emphasize that people should be accorded maximal respect for their personal liberty (Gillon, 1985b). Nozick (1974) argued against any taxation that would benefit the disadvantaged, but instead relied on the largess of the affluent to create a just society. Under this formulation, if the paying patient in the case study wanted the items that originally were supplied she (or a significant other) could purchase them. Likewise she could purchase them to be donated to those unable or unwilling to pay for them. All people are able to choose what is valued for purchase. Perhaps the maternal health clinic patient would value the photos, diaper bag, or blanket to the extent that she would give up a less valued item.

Utilitarian: Theories of justice that utilize this formulation emphasize that people deserve to have their welfare maximized. Likewise, the principle of beneficence and the material criteria of need, merit, and equality could all be applied if the utility of the individual is to be respected. If the hospital deems the public relations value to be higher than the cost to the facility, the free items will be provided. If the nurse administrator could hire a full-time employee and thus provide direct care for many with the saved cost from the items, she would be potentially doing good for a greater number of patients. The overriding concern in this formulation is helping the greatest number within the restrictive allocationary environment.

Each specific formulation for allocating scarce health care resources (the two-tiered system, the lottery, and Aristotle's formal principle) would provide the items with respect to the assumption of the model. The two-tiered system would provide the basic obstetrical care to the maternal health clinic patient and newborn care for her infant. If the insurance company paid for the "free" items or if the family of the paying patient paid for the items, the private patient could receive the items and not the clinic patient, since her basic care needs were being met. The autonomy of the paying patient is upheld. Likewise, the beneficence (doing good) of care is provided for the clinic patient.

Under the auspices of the random or chance model, each patient would be given an equal opportunity to receive the items, irrespective of needs. Every so many patients, at random, would be chosen to receive the free items from the hospital. The public relations value would be intact for the hospital while reducing some monetary cost. The items could still be available for purchase by anyone.

Within the formulation of the Aristotelian model (equals must be treated equally, but unequals unequally in proportion to the relevant inequalities), the equality of justice has to be understood as meaning fair or proportionate treatment (Gillon, 1985b). Accordingly the clients who needed more deserved more. This would not disallow paying patients from receiving the free items if the criteria for need so justified the allocation. This would not disallow any patients from paying for the items if they so wished.

Summary

The nurse administrator must know her or his institution's philosophy of care intimately. She or he must know the community demographics, and her or his own philosophical moral understandings, as well as those of nursing staff of the unit. The particular theory of justice the nurse administrator embraces could vary with the change in the budget or what the hospital defined as important. The important consideration is that the nurse administrator know what possibilities exist and how to justify the action taken.

RESEARCH

Research is necessary into the types of decisions that most frequently create ethical dilemmas in nursing administration (indeed, all nursing practice) (Sietsema & Spradley, 1987). Research is needed to test the effectiveness of different approaches to moral resolution (Huckabay, 1986) and to devise how the field of philosophy can apply to the practice-grounded field of nursing.

To date no research studies were found in the literature that empirically tested the theories of justice as applied to nursing administrative roles. Philosophical analysis* continues in the philosophical field concerning the logic of the theories, and findings should be followed by the nursing profession.

Mayberry (1986) suggested that one role of the nurse administrator is to "provide a setting that will give nurses the opportunity to think through the consequences of alternative courses of action" (p. 80). Providing in-service education so that nurses are aware of the various theories of justice and alternative choices would include unit nurses in the decision process.

---

* Research on theories of justice is ongoing and is composed mainly of critical papers supporting or criticizing the major theorists. There are relevant empirical aspects of philosophical investigation. "Testing of philosophical claims, as opposed to the empirical sciences, consists mainly in intellectual reflection about their meaning, consistency, and the evidence for and against them and their competition." Crucially important is the method of formulating counterexamples to general claims that force their revision (G.J. Foulk, personal communication, April 19, 1988).

Nurse executives must consider the important moral dimensions of their decisions as they represent nursing's chief moral agent in the institution (Fry, 1986; Silva, 1984). Nursing administration should actively seek a role for nursing on the hospital ethics committee or work to establish a committee for the hospital (Grillot & Davis, 1986).

Ethical decision-making models have been developed and are becoming increasingly important in the nursing repertoire of knowledge (Goertzen, 1980; Kaluzny, 1988; Young & Hayne, 1988). If the nurse administrator has a workable method of dilemma identification and can apply her or his knowledge of the theories of justice and the biomedical principles of autonomy, beneficence, nonmaleficence, and justice, the task of allocating scarce medical resources within a moral environment will be made easier.

This brief presentation of the theories of justice and their applications would seem at first glance to raise more questions than it answers. Essential and critical to the resolution of allocational problems in health care is the realization that ethical theories and principles do not provide "cookbook" solutions to such problems. Rather, they provide a logical method of arriving at conclusions that will be rational, consistent, and moral. It is only with careful attention to this concept that the nurse administrator can formulate policies that will provide justice for the patient.

REFERENCES

Beauchamp, T.L., & Childress, J.F. (1983). *Principles of biomedical ethics* (2nd ed.). New York: Oxford Press.
Beauchamp, T.L., & Walters, L. (1982). *Contemporary issues in bioethics* (2nd ed.). Belmont, CA: Wadsworth.
Bentham, J. (1984). An introduction to the principles of morals and legislation. In O.A. Johnson (Ed.), *Ethics: Selections from classical and contemporary writers* (5th ed., pp. 210-222). New York: Holt, Rinehart & Winston.
Brandt, R.B. (1959). *Ethical theory.* Englewood Cliffs, NJ: Prentice-Hall.
Childress, J.F. (1970). Who shall live when not all can live? *Soundings, 53,* 339-355.
Daniels, N. (1981). Health-care needs and distributive justice. *Philosophy and Public Affairs, 10*(2), 146–179.
Engelhardt, H.T., Jr. (1986). *The foundations of bioethics.* New York: Oxford.
Frankena, W.K. (1973). *Ethics* (2nd ed.). Englewood Cliffs, NJ: Prentice-Hall.
Fry, S.T. (1986). Moral values and ethical decisions in a constrained economic environment. *Nursing Economics, 4*(4), 160-163.
Gillon, R. (1985a, July 20). Justice and medical ethics. *British Medical Journal, 291,* 201-202.
Gillon, R. (1985b, July 27). Justice and allocation of medical resources. *British Medical Journal, 291,* 266-268.
Goertzen, I. (1980). A nursing administrator's view of ethics in practice. In American Nurses' Association Committee on Ethics (Ed.). *Nursing: A social policy statement.* Kansas City, MO: ANA.
Grillot, A., & Davis, A.J. (1986). Facing ethical dilemmas. *Nursing Success Today, 3*(5), 4–7.
Hospers, J. (1982). *Human conduct* (2nd ed.). San Diego: Harcourt Brace Jovanovich.
Huckabay, L.M.D. (1986). Ethical-moral issues in nursing practice and decision making. *Nursing Administration Quarterly, 10*(3), 61-67.
Kaluzny, M.A. (1988). An ethical decision-making model for the nurse administrator. In M.K. Stull & S.E. Pinkerton (Eds.), *Common strategies for nurse administrators* (pp. 107-114). Rockville, MD: Aspen.
Kant, I. (1984). Foundations of the metaphysics of morals (from Sections 1 and 2). In O.A. Johnson (Ed.), *Ethics* (5th ed., pp. 190-209). New York: Holt, Rinehart & Winston.
Mayberry, M.A. (1986). Ethical decision making: A response of hospital nurses. *Nursing Administration Quarterly, 10*(3), 75-81.
Mill, J.S. (1984). Utilitarianism (Chapters 1, 2, and 4). In O.A. Johnson (Ed.). *Ethics* (5th ed., pp. 259-283). New York: Holt, Rinehart & Winston.
Munson, R. (1988). *Intervention and reflection: Basic issues in medical ethics* (3rd ed.). Belmont, CA: Wadsworth.
Nozick, R. (1974). *Anarchy, state, and utopia.* New York: Basic Books.
Rakish, J.S., Longest, B.B., & Darr, K. (1985). *Managing health service organizations.* Philadelphia, W.B. Saunders.
Rawls, J. (1971). *A theory of justice.* Cambridge, MA: Harvard University Press.
Sietsema, M.R., & Spradley, B.W. (1987). Ethics and administrative decision making. *Journal of Nursing Administration, 17*(4), 28-32.
Silva, M.C. (1984). Ethics, scarce resources, and the nurse executive. *Nursing Economics, 2*(1), 11-18.
Young, L.C., & Hayne, A.N. (1988). *Nursing administration from concepts to practice.* Philadelphia: W.B. Saunders.

Chapter 4

Language in Organizations
Louis R. Pondy

Kay Ann Jackson-Frankl

‖ CASE STUDY

Pierce Memorial Hospital is a 240-bed community-based organization. It is located in a rural community where most of the residents have worked, shopped, and socialized for the majority of their adult lives. Recently the area has seen an upsurge of "outsiders" settling in the community and either joining the community work force or commuting to the nearby city. Mindy Hollaron, RN, BSN, recently moved into the area to accept the position of Unit Manager/Surgical Unit at Pierce Memorial. This position simultaneously represents two distinct firsts: it is Mindy's first management/leadership position, and it is the first time that the hospital has filled a unit manager position from the outside.

The demographics of Mindy's unit are as follows: There are 30 inpatient general surgical beds and 10 same-day surgery beds. Patients range in age from 3 years to 90+ years. The staff consists of 8 registered nurses (RNs), 7 licensed practical nurses (LPNs), and 3 nurse assistants (NAs). The resignation and retirement of the previous unit manager, Mrs. Anderson, represents the first staff turnover in more than 5 years. She had held that position for more than 18 years. She was proud of her "girls" and felt that they were excellent nurses.

Mrs. Anderson was quite traditional in her beliefs and values, and did not believe that nurses, even at the unit manager level, needed basic management skills such as human relations and budgeting. She gave an order and it was followed. She kept track of supplies in a notebook. Unfortunately, as acuity and census kept rising she had had a difficult time keeping both human and material resources under control. Tardiness and complaints began rising, and the unit was losing money. Mrs. Anderson decided that it was time to retire.

The Director of Nursing decided to use the opening as an opportunity to introduce new ideas. He selected Mindy because of her fresh and progressive ideas and her willingness to be part of an organization about to undergo several changes, including additions to the physical structure, expansion of services, and a more participative philosophy. He assured Mindy of his support with her decisions.

As Mindy prepared for her first unit meeting, she tried to picture where she wanted her unit to be next year. How could she get the staff to see and want a compatible picture?

| | | | | | | | | | | | | | | | | | | | | | | | | | | | | | | | | | | | | | | | | | | | | | | | | | | | | | | | | | | | | | | | | |

LANGUAGE IN ORGANIZATIONS

The paradigm or world view of Pondy's theory is the social definition paradigm. This paradigm has a process orientation to action rather than a stimulus-response focus. The process orientation focuses on how individuals interpret and develop meanings related to their situations. An individual ascribing to this view sees a human being as actively creating his or her own definition of a particular situation. In other words, humans are responsible for creating their own social reality (Pondy & Boje, 1980, p. 85).

The social definition paradigm can be included within the interpretative-interactionist perspective. This perspective assumes that individuals interpret experiences through the lens that is created by the already existing base of knowledge and meanings, which includes all lived experiences already encountered and often taken for granted (tacit). Pondy's focus on the role of interaction between self and situation further emphasizes the theory's placement within this perspective. A person who chooses the interpretative-interactionist perspective sees each event as being knowable only through the person experiencing the event. All action is emergent, or unexpected, and is situationally defined as the person attempts to create meaning for and attribute meaning to the experiences within the given event. The influence of the interpretative-interactionist perspective on Pondy's work is significant. Although a complete discussion of Pondy's theory base is beyond the scope of this chapter, it is important to note the influence of Herbert Blumer's theory (1969) of symbolic interactionism (SI) on Pondy and to delineate the essential components of Blumer's SI theory.

According to Blumer (1969), SI has three premises. In the first premise, Blumer stated that "human beings act towards things on the basis of the meanings things have for them" (p. 2). Within the second premise, Blumer elaborated the concept of meaning by stating, "Meanings are social products that develop as a person acts towards a thing in the presence of another" (p. 2). In other words, a person's interaction with self or others facilitates the formation of the meaning for the "thing." The object, the event, begins to make sense as the person interacts and gathers information about the experience. The gathered information establishes relationships about the experience, and how these relationships interact with the context *and the relationships already known by the person* establishes the conditions for meaning development. This concurs with Blumer's final premise. In this premise Blumer stated, "The meaning of things is formed in the context of social interaction and is derived by the person from that interaction" (p. 3).

The SI process is interpretative and requires the person to make a decision about which of the various "things" to act toward and to then transform the meaning for the "thing" based on the situation or context and the necessary action. For example, when a nurse enters a patient's room a variety of "things" are readily observable — the appearance of the patient, the room, the patient's voice, and various odors. The action that the nurse first takes depends on the meaning that these various "things" hold for the nurse. If the particular odors mean that the patient has been incontinent, the first action taken is to confirm the suspicion and then cleanse the patient. However, if the patient has also fallen, the primary action changes to one of safety. The decisions made were based on meanings formed from social interactions that took place within the particular context.

Blumer's three premises form the base for four central ideas or beliefs about the development of meaning within organizations and individuals. These beliefs are:

1. People, individually and collectively, are prepared to act on the basis of the meanings of the objects that comprise their world.
2. It is through the interaction with self and others that meanings are created and modified through interpretation and then exchanged and reinterpreted by both.

3. Social acts are created through an interpretative process where the individual, as a singular entity or as a collective, assesses the situation, interprets the events, and establishes meaning.
4. The interlinkages of acts between organizations, institutions, divisions of labor, and networks of interdependency are moving and not static affairs (1969, p. 59).

These premises and central conceptions make up the core components of Blumer's SI. They are also central in understanding the concepts found within Pondy's theory.

Pondy's theory is concerned with the use of language by leaders and specifically those leaders within organizations. Pondy applied several concepts within his theory; however, many were not explicitly defined. Those with explicit definitions are presented first and those with implied definitions are presented last.

According to Pondy (1978), language is a technology that a person uses to process or develop information and meanings (p. 25). Language enables persons to absorb stimuli (things) and then classify, categorize, and utilize the knowledge in various situations. As the person processes the stimuli, meaning is developed or transformed for that particular experience. However, a person's interpretation and construction of meaning, which is his or her social reality, is predefined by the person's language. Language imposes certain classifications and categories that shape a person's reality. For example, when most people see and experience snow they utilize one word, or one word with adjectives, to express what they mean about the situation. However, the Eskimos have *25 different words* for snow (Nordland, 1985, p. 54). They see and experience 25 different categories or realities of snow, whereas others see and experience only one. If one wished to communicate with an Eskimo about snow, one would have to learn their snow language.

Organizations also have specialized languages. Pondy (1979) defined organizations as "collections of jargon groups, within each of which specialized sublanguages grow up that set it apart from the other jargon groups in the organization" (p. 26). Jargon can be conceptualized as specialized and/or technical language. For example, both a surgical department and a maternal-child department may be located within one hospital but this does not mean that they speak the same language. Both departments have developed jargon that enables them to communicate with greater effectiveness and efficiency. Someone who wishes to transfer into one of these units must learn the language so that appropriate actions are taken and accurate information reported.

Language permits the organization to move toward two different achievement levels. The first level of achievement is the functional level. It is at this level that jargon and procedures (language) become a type of routine or ritual. These routines can then become metaphors or other symbols that facilitate the sharing of language and task completion. For example, the name of a physician can serve as a metaphor, for it conjures up images of past encounters, while at the same time it can symbolize a set of routines and actions, for example, Dr. M. always uses DeLee forceps.

Achievement of the functional level of operation permits the organization to advance toward higher language use. At this level, language enhances change and evolution of an organization. Those within the organization grow as they experience the change. As the language within the organization broadens, the categories and classification used by each person expand. The expansion offers the person opportunities to transform his or her own reality and ultimately the organization. This higher level of language use is reified when leaders construct and share meaning with followers.

Pondy (1978) defined leadership as a "form of social influence; . . . we mean social (i.e., interpersonal) influence exercised by a person in some position of superior authority (leaving aside for the time being the source of the authority) over some subordinate" (p. 87). Leaders can be described as effective or good if they are able to get subordinates to do something

(p. 94). To achieve this end, leaders must first make sense (interpret) of what needs to be done and then translate the interpretation into words that are important to the subordinates. By using words important to the subordinates, leaders facilitate subordinates' creation of meaning for their work. Once subordinates establish a meaning for their work, they are then able to transform the meanings, through further social interactions, so that changes in their environment continue to make sense. As an illustration, consider these interpretations. Nursing homes are now long-term care facilities. "Old folks' homes" and "rest homes" are now retirement centers. Outpatient areas are now titled "ambulatory care." Leaders in the respective areas interpreted their environments and then translated these interpretations into words commonly used by those who worked in the area. By so doing, they provided the workers with a language for gathering information about their work, which then established the base for meaning development. According to Morris (cited in Pondy, 1978), "Sharing a language provides the subtlest and most powerful tools for controlling the behaviors of these other persons to one's advantage" (p. 92). Obviously, social influence is directly related to Pondy's conceptualization of a leader and the practice of leadership.

At this point, it should be evident that the ability to socially interact with self or others is of vital importance to Pondy's theory. Hence, the definition of a person, the actor of the theory, involves the process of interaction. According to Pondy, a person is someone who has "different programs for learning" and who is able to "select and execute" a program based on his or her "image" of the situation (1977, p. 65). Implied within this definition is the belief that people are cognitive processors of information. People develop knowledge and meaning for events as they socially interact with self or with others. A person is not born with a set of knowledge and meanings. Instead knowledge and meanings develop as the child interacts with others. These interactions expand the child's language, which further increases his or her ability to interact. The process continues throughout life. Language, the increase in knowledge and the creation of meaning, are inexorably intertwined within Pondy's theory.

There is not an explicit definition for the concept of meaning as it is used within Pondy's theory. However, Blumer's (1969) definition of meaning is congruent with the theory. Blumer defines meaning as a definition of a thing or object that develops through a social process. Meanings are not inherent within an object; rather, a person establishes meaning for something based on how others act around him or her (p. 4). Thus, the context, the language, all previous experiences and all meanings already formed come into play when a person interprets a situation and creates a reality. As an illustration, consider the varied subjective experiences of pain. The context of the pain experience, and past encounters with painful stimuli and/or people in pain all interact to create the reality for a current painful encounter. Meaning, sense making, and interpreting are all synonyms for the most basic act performed by humans everyday—that of creating and defining an order for the various interactions encountered and the person's place within the interaction.

In sum, these five concepts of language, leadership, organization, person, and meaning compose the core phenomena of Pondy's theory concerning language in organizations. These concepts share 11 assumptions. Seven of these assumptions are from symbolic interactionism. These were presented earlier. The remaining four assumptions were explicitly developed within the theory and are now presented.

The first assumption is that an object or a situation does not exist if the person has not had the opportunity to interpret it and establish a meaning. As an example, consider yourself in a room full of odd-looking tools. Someone tells you to bring them a "¾-inch drill bit and the Phillips head." Now unless you have had the opportunity to experience those words before, and to then place in relationship the words with the tools, the person's statement will not have any meaning for you—it will not make sense.

The need to have words and objects in relationship forms the basis for Pondy's second assumption. In this assumption, Pondy (1978) stated that language helps to define the meaning of our experiences because it permits the "categorization of streams of events" (p. 24). It is through language that a person is able to cognitively structure relationships, which facilitates the grouping of common objects and actors without losing any distinctive features. The more interactions we have with an object or actor, the broader and more expansive the category. Thus the more tools you have interpreted, the broader the category.

In his third assumption, Pondy (1978) stated that language influences the ease of communication; one cannot exchange ideas, information, or meanings except as shared language permits (p. 24). In order for communication to be effective, the language in use must be familiar to those involved in the interaction. I cannot pass a tool to you if I do not understand what the name of the tool signifies. We cannot discuss theory, unless we understand each other's language. The greater the amount of shared language, the more successful the interaction. It is the relationship between shared language and successful interactions that forms the basis for Pondy's final assumption.

Within his final assumption, Pondy (1978) stated that "language provides a channel of social influence" (p. 24). According to Pondy (1979) the possession of a common language "facilitates the exercise of social control" (p. 26) and improves the leader's ability to provide feedback, make corrections, reduce conflict, and absorb uncertainty. Leaders must be able to translate the uncertainty and ambiguity associated with changing technologies into a language that will provide subordinates with the framework necessary for meaning construction.

In spite of the well-described and defined concepts and the presentation of several assumptions, Pondy's theory does not provide any explicit theoretical assertions or relationship statements. However, these can be deduced. For example, one relationship statement is "the greater the amount of language overlap between the leader and the workers, the greater the leader's potential effectiveness other things being equal." Another assertion is that "the amount of cohesiveness within a unit depends on the amount of language overlap among all the unit's employees." As another example, the relationship between an organization's jargon groups and its size, age, technology, and amount of employee turnover might be tested. Theoretically, the older, more structured organization, with less employee turnover would have more jargon groups. These assertions are not an exhaustive group but they do represent the possibilities inherent within the theory.

The final component concerning the theory presentation is a brief discussion of its logical form. Pondy's theory used both inductive and deductive logic. Deductive reasoning, or logic, is moving from the general to the specific. Pondy used deductive logic in his movement from the assumptions of symbolic interactionism to the assumptions of his theory. For example, Blumer's third assumption (1969) stated, "Social acts, whether individual or collective, are constructed through a process in which the actors note, interpret, and assess the situations confronting them" (p. 50). From this Pondy deduced that leadership occurs through the development of an evocative language that is widely shared in the organization, and that assists people in making sense of their activities by using symbols (words) that are meaningful to most of the participants (1978, p. 94).

Inductive reasoning is moving from a set of specific instances to a generalization. There are several instances of inductive logic within Pondy's theory. The first, and perhaps most obvious, is the statement that a leader is more effective if the language used overlaps that of the workers. This statement has an inherent "ring of truth" that may or may not hold. Another example is Pondy's statement (1978) that critical resources are defined through the process of shared language, which establishes the reality of the organization. Again, there is that feeling of inherent "rightness." Will it hold for every organization? Is there ever a time when structure or technology predominate? Pondy has provided the researchers with some provocative questions.

In sum, this section has provided the reader with an overview to Pondy's theory. Specifically, the world view and phenomena of interest were presented and the underpinning assumptions described. Examples of possible theoretical assertions were provided. The final component was a brief discussion of the logic represented within the theory. The next section applies the theory to the case study.

CASE ANALYSIS

The purpose of this section is to apply Pondy's theory concerning language in organizations to the case study. It is anticipated that this application "sketch" will provide the user with a framework for future implementation.

As previously described, Mindy is preparing for her first unit meeting with her new staff. She is contemplating how she can best present her vision of the unit so that the vision will be shared by all the staff members. While no one theory is best in all situations and with all people, if Mindy focuses on the concepts and relationships found within Pondy's theory she will have an excellent chance of communicating her vision by shared language. To facilitate the analysis, each of the five concepts are individually applied to the case and discussed. Examples of actions and responses congruent with the theory and the case are provided.

Language

Language is the core element of Pondy's theory and it represents an essential component in the human process of sense making. In order for Mindy to create a compatible picture with her staff, she must first understand the current picture as it is drawn by the staff. Mindy's ability to understand the staff's current reality depends on her knowledge of the staff's language, particularly any jargon. Therefore Mindy's first step is to schedule frequent interactions with all her staff members. This is above and beyond the unit meeting, since there are always staff members who are unable to attend because of shift conflicts. It requires Mindy to work the various shifts so that maximal interaction opportunities are created. These interactions will provide Mindy with data concerning the language used by the staff in creating their subjective experiences.

As Mindy interacts with her staff, it is important that she does not assume that their subjective experiences will be the same or even similar. A person structures a unique reality by his or her language in use. Thus Mindy must carefully listen to the words chosen by the staff to describe their work and their expectations of it, of themselves, and of the unit manager. This groundwork will provide Mindy with valuable information for structuring the language of her vision. This is a crucial step! For if Mindy were to language her vision in a manner different from the staff's language in use, the vision would not meet with success.

As an example, consider the following. Suppose that Mindy has decided that one way to reduce her unit's budget deficit is to halt the use of agency nurses. This change will require the nurses to practice a more unit-based staffing pattern. Unfortunately this also means that the nurses will have to provide their own "cover" for illness, vacations, and periods of high census. Perhaps Mindy has had the opportunity to do some limited interacting before this first staff meeting. She knows that the staff highly value their off-duty time. To mention that they may need to come to work on their off day will most likely be met with opposition. However, Mindy is also aware that the staff values several things at work: continuity of care, patient contact, and teamwork. One of their major complaints about agency nurses is that they do not always "fit in," which then impacts on the "team feeling" and amount of available time for patient contact. Mindy now has some valuable information for structuring this part of her vision.

If Mindy decides to communicate her vision at this initial meeting, she will need to keep in mind what her staff has shared. The language and meaning need to reach all her staff; otherwise the vision will not be shared. After much consideration, Mindy decides to verbally communicate the vision during a future staff meeting. The vision will be languaged in the following manner:

"For the past month, I have had the opportunity to meet and talk with all of you about your work—what you like about it and what you don't like about it. I have really enjoyed our talks and I have learned a lot from you. One thing that came up more than once was the use of agency nurses. Although you all agreed that agency nurses tried hard, you often felt that they detracted from the team feeling—and your patient contact. I appreciate your strong feelings on these areas and I would like to strengthen these feelings through a process called unit-based staffing."

Mindy will then outline her plan, taking care to highlight the measures taken to preserve the staff's off-duty time. This is also when she will discuss how the staff will be reimbursed for their on-call time. Perhaps some would prefer time off rather than money. These issues are placed into words that are important to the staff.

What all this means for Mindy's first unit meeting is that it should not be too much of a formal meeting. Instead Mindy should use this as her first opportunity to interact with her staff and to listen to their words.

Leadership

When Mindy structured her vision in a way compatible with the staff's, she was executing a necessary condition of leadership. A leader must be able to make sense of (interpret) what needs to be done and then translate the interpretation into words understood and valued by the workers. Mindy knows that her unit has to bring the budget under control. Yet to how many staff nurses is the budget really important?

Most staff nurses, of any level, are not concerned with bringing and keeping the budget under control. They see (interpret) this as part of the unit manager's responsibilities. Instead, staff nurses see (interpret) their job as patient care. If Mindy had used the budget to structure her vision, she would have been trying to impose her interpretation on the nurses. Since this is not how they see (interpret) the vision, the probability of success is low. It is not possible to lead if people do not understand what you are saying. Since people use their own language in use to structure reality, if a word is not understood, and therefore not valued, it does not become part of the person's subjective experience.

Through the process of sense making, leaders assist workers to find meaning in their work. Consider the following. Instead of verbally communicating, in the staff's language, the move to unit-based staffing, Mindy hangs a memo stating, "Effective immediately, agency nurses will no longer be used. All personnel must find their own coverage. Failure to do so will result in a written warning." How effective would Mindy be in creating a shared meaning for the staff's actions? Not very. The complaints will be shared, but the meaning behind actions necessary for unit-based staffing will not be shared. This omission deprives the staff of the opportunity to share and unite behind a "common cause." One only needs to remember Dr. Martin Luther King's "I have a dream" speech to recognize the power behind leaders and followers who share a meaning.

People

If Mindy truly believes and practices the processes of interpretation and translation to the language in use, then she also believes that people are cognitive processors of information. This belief places a high value on lifelong learning through social interaction with self and others.

Consequently Mindy emphasizes staff interaction in her unit manager role. She plans on visiting all the shifts on a routine basis and keeping communication by memo at a minimum. Mindy plans to encourage the staff to share their ideas — and to share in the implementation of the vision. In addition, Mindy will encourage her staff to go to workshops and to participate in other forms of both formal and informal learning. Mindy is aware that the more exposure her staff has to other ideas, the more they have to offer to each other and the patients. The exposure broadens their language and expands their personal reality. Mindy plans on sharing these values at the unit meetings but will emphasize how these elements will help the nurses with patient care.

Meaning

Mindy's belief that people are cognitive processors, who thereby create their own reality, focuses her attention on the individual as a way to the whole unit and not vice versa. Her unit consists of individuals who may have different meanings for events and objects. To assume that everyone shares the same understanding because "they all work together" is not valid for Mindy. This is why she is going to take the time during this first unit meeting to talk with them about their work. Meaning is not inherent within the object; it is within the person. This is also why Mindy values interacting with the staff about various changes in policies and procedures; she needs to know how the staff have integrated these things into their meaning structure and hence their reality.

Organization

Mindy visualizes her unit as a mini organization. The unit has its own jargon concerning the care of the inpatient and outpatient surgical patient. However, because the previous unit manager had a different philosophy, the "organization" has not advanced. Mindy believes that as the individual grows, so will the organization. This is why she values frequent and varied interactions. Mindy intends to begin the process of sharing this meaning of the unit at the unit meeting. One of the things that she plans on discussing with the staff is their feeling on attending workshops and sitting for certification.

Summary

Mindy definitely has much work ahead of her. As anyone in administration knows, it is after the honeymoon that the real work sets in. Since the staff were exhibiting signs of frustration with the previous manager, Mindy's outsider status may not be an initial issue. This will enable her to develop rapport and history with the staff before this happens. Eventually the fact that Mindy is not of the community will become an issue. History with a company and community form an important component of an organization's culture and has impact on an individual's language. The fact that Mindy has the interactionist-interpretative perspective will assist her in resolving this issue.

RESEARCH

The purpose of this section is to provide the reader with examples of current research related to language in organizations and specifically within nursing organizations. Unfortunately, a very extensive literature review did not uncover any studies researching language in nursing organizations. There are several instances in which communication and communication patterns were analyzed, but the study of language and the study of communication are not the same. The study of language focuses on words, symbols, and meaning, while the study of communication tends to probe how language is transmitted. What follows is a synopsis of some current research in the general area of language in organizations. This includes Pondy's frequently quoted works. The section concludes with a review of those nursing articles that represent the profession's initial attempt to address the issue of language in organizations.

It is ironic that the topic of language, which has been addressed as important since the time of Aristotle, has received very little attention by researchers. It is only within this most recent decade that inquiry into the topic has become a more common phenomenon. Most of the literature and research related to language in organizations is located within the topical areas of organizational symbolism and organizational cultures. The two areas are tightly integrated.

Organizational symbolism is the study of language, metaphors, and other symbols within organizations. According to Staw (1985), research on organizational symbolism has two fundamental tasks: (1) "awakening scholars to the importance of symbolic acts by pointing out new patterns of behavior or non-obvious implications of everyday events;" and (2) "to use symbolism in theoretical networks so that our understanding of organizational life is substantially increased" (p. 117). A core premise of organizational symbolism is that organizations do not function on the traditional mechanistic model. Instead, the ontological commitment of organizational symbolism places the focus of the organizational model onto the individual's creation of a subjective experience for his or her work. The fact that organizational symbolism is counter to the dominant paradigm, which values the rational structuring of human beings and organizations, must also be remembered when considering research within the area of language in organizations. Organizational symbolism represents an alternative to the dominant paradigm and creates a "crisis at the level of theory" (Benson, 1983, p. 35).

The result of this "crisis" has been the development of creative and innovative methods for seeing and understanding organizations. The book *Organizational Symbolism* (1983), edited by L. Pondy, P. Frost, G. Morgan, and T. Dandridge, represents a collection of alternative ways for making sense of organizations. The majority of researchers interested in inquiry into the phenomenon of language in organizations use approaches similar to those found within anthropology, such as ethnographic research and interview analysis. These techniques represent a point of departure away from quantitative methodologies and toward qualitative methods — a departure that is also counter to the dominant paradigm. However, since language is a creation of the mind, the study of language provides the researcher an opportunity for gaining insight into how a person has framed and understood an event.

Unfortunately, Pondy's most frequently cited works tend to be theoretical in content. In "Organizational Conflict: Concepts and Models," Pondy (1967) offered an in-depth presentation and discussion of the phenomenon of conflict within organizations. Pondy developed a working definition of conflict and applied the definition to the establishment and maintenance of organizational equilibrium. The basis for his theory concerning organizational conflict were the following conceptual models: the Bargaining model, the Bureaucratic model, and the Systems model. The applicability of the theory to an organization was not taken beyond the point of hypothesis formation.

Hypothesis formation is also the core component of Pondy's (1978) article, "Leadership Is a Language Game." In this article, Pondy elucidated his ontological and epistemological commitments concerning his definition of leadership. Pondy argued for diversity in leadership through language. To structure his stance, Pondy developed an analogy between linguistics and leadership. Briefly the analogy stated that since leadership is a form of social influence, and because language is a key tool for social influence, then the process of leadership has the capacity for great diversity and creativity since "virtually all utterances are novel — never before spoken" (p. 90). It is our brain that produces the finite characteristics of language and the possibilities of leadership.

Pondy and Mitroff's (1979) article "Beyond Open Systems Models of Organization" is a classic example of Pondy's ability to synthesize diverse perspectives into a congruent segment of theorizing. Using Boulding's hierarchy of system complexity, Pondy and Mitroff described organizations, and various models of organizations, in an attempt to clarify the state of organizational theory and potential possible directions for it. In this article Pondy developed the role of language in organizations. According to Pondy, the consideration of language in organizations places the complexity of the organization in Boulding's system at 7, "symbol processing systems," which has greater complexity than the prevailing mode of "open systems," which rates only a 4. According to Pondy and Mitroff, as complexity increases, finding "correctional models of causation" becomes inappropriate because it interferes with understanding the organization. Instead, understanding the organization requires looking beyond the obvious and seeking the rituals, myths, sagas, and metaphors expressed within the organizational community.

Pondy's "sequel" to "Beyond Open Systems Models of Organization" was "Bringing Mind Back In" (Pondy & Boje, 1980). Within this article, Pondy and Boje explored paradigmatic and multiparadigmatic organizational "frontier" issues. The argument was made that the major paradigms for inquiry into organizational theory were the social facts paradigm and the social behavior paradigm and that these paradigms "have served as well in the insights and understanding they have generated, and probably will continue to be productive ways of going about our craft" (p. 83). However, the authors then introduced the paradigm of social definition and stated that this paradigm could "provide fresh insight into organizational behavior and should be developed to a parity with the two reigning paradigms" (p. 84). The authors applied the paradigms in isolation and in unison (multiparadigm) to organizations citing both the benefits and the problems with such inquiries. However, the authors showed their bias for the definitionist paradigm when they stated that the "best strategy for introducing multiparadigm inquiry into organization theory is by using a definitionist formulation . . . as a fulcrum for 'trans-specting' into and back from the factist and behaviorist paradigms" (p. 97).

The one exception to the "theory" articles is Pondy's (1977) article, "The Other Hand Clapping: An Information-Processing Approach to Organizational Power." In this article, Pondy follows much the same attack as was present in the article dealing with conflict. The traditional definitions of power are presented and critiqued. The presentation of the traditional forms the backdrop for Pondy's presentation of power. Pondy's assumptions concerning humans, language, and context are made explicit and integrated into his theory concerning power. Pondy then applied the power concept to four settings or questions (p. 66). The fourth question, the one concerning jargon groups, offers the most research-based application. One of the assumptions stemming from his mode is that "centralized power is associated with a small number of jargon groups and decentralized or fragmented power with a large number" (p. 82). The findings from all four questions illuminated several structural variables important to the concept of power. These are behavior of self and others, preprogrammed behavior repertoires, socialization process, language and natural jargon groups, formal structure of communication patterns, and evoking mechanisms (including interruptions, power attributions, and lay theories of power) (p. 86). These structural variables and their relationships formed a model for conceptualizing Pondy's theory concerning an information-processing approach to power.

There are at least two nursing theories compatible with Pondy's theory—the Riehl Interaction model and Parse's Man-Living-Health model. The Riehl Interaction model (Riehl, 1980) is based on symbolic interactionism. The assumptions of the model are consistent with those found within the symbolic interaction perspective. The model places a high value on the process of interaction and specifically the process of role taking by the nurse. Role taking by the nurse enables her or him to see the situation as it is seen by the patient. This facilitates the study and understanding of a patient's problem. For example, a patient is admitted to the labor and delivery unit. Upon assessment, the nurse discovers that although the patient values "being in control," in this situation she currently feels helpless and without control. Through role taking, the nurse can develop some understanding for the problem as it is seen by the patient. As the nurse communicates with the patient, an understanding for the other roles that the patient has played is established. From this assessment, the nurse is able to use words and environmental manipulations as tools for assisting the woman to assume her "control" role.

The connection to Parse is simultaneously complex yet clear. Parse's theory is grounded in the human sciences and values the human being's creation of meaning through subjective experience. A core component of the assumptions and concepts is human beings' ability to interact with the environment, with self, and with others. "Man is an open being, freely choosing meaning in situation, bearing responsibility for decisions" (Parse, 1981, p. 25). The concept of languaging is one of three concepts related to "structuring meaning." People develop their own unique languaging as they experience human-environment interrelationships. "It is through the process of languaging that each individual symbolizes unique realities" (Parse, 1981, p. 47).

It is only recently that nursing has become interested in furthering the development of the concept of language. In the Fall 1985 edition of *Image,* Pridham and Schutz discussed the need for nursing to develop a language consistent with the task and goals of the profession. According to the authors, "a language for nursing must be formulated in terms that are meaningful to and stated from the perspective of the individuals who present health-related problems to nurses" (p. 122).

Pincus (1986) in the *Journal of Nursing Administration* looked at organizational communication, job satisfaction, and job performance among hospital nurses. He found that communication with the supervisor, communication climate, and personal feedback were strongly correlated with job satisfaction. In addition, he found that communication and satisfaction with the supervisor formed the basis of the superior-subordinate relationship. The major implication is that "positively perceived communication activities can substantially affect nurses' attitudes towards their work environment and to a lesser degree, their performance on the job" (p. 24). In essence, in order to excel, organizations must be able to take their message to their people in a positive and meaningful manner.

Language was also the focus of Donna Diers's (1986) editorial in *Image.* In this editorial, Diers described her reaction to a manuscript that had the phrase "they had a knowledge deficit." She stated that the manuscript no longer had the phrase because "it doesn't mean anything very precise." What exactly is a knowledge deficit? "Does the phrase mean that those in question did not have the information? The information was wrong? They could not understand it? They were ignorant? Stupid? Deluded? Untutored? Brain damaged? (p. 30). Obviously, the phrase offers several interpretations even for those who are within the profession and who are assumed to share a common language.

Another editorial focusing on the importance of language and jargon was Leah L. Curtin's (1987) editorial opinion, "Watch Your Language." In the editorial, Ms. Curtin focused on the role that language plays in image shaping. "In short, powerful words create a powerful image. Wimpy words convey a wimpy image. And this is my chief reason for worrying about the wimpy language nurses use" (p. 9). The words chosen influence how you are understood and how you are visualized by others. "Language — simple, clear, direct, concise, and forceful — is the tool for powerful communication" (p. 10).

"Language, Leadership and Power" (Henry & LeClair, 1987) is perhaps nursing's premier article concerning the significance of language in organizations. According to the authors, "administrative effectiveness may well be contingent on being in the vanguard of change — seeing, labeling, talking about new phenomena and establishing shared understanding that strengthens commitment; . . . we think attention in nursing to the use and subtleties of language is an essential endeavor" (p. 19). The article provided a theoretical overview of the topic of language in organizations and sketched an initial integration of the various perspectives into nursing administration. The article concluded with a strong call for further research, and the authors provided the willing and interested researcher with several potential research questions. For example, "What jargon do nurses use that administrators, physicians and consumers find foreign and mystifying?" "How many and what kind of languages do nurse executives use?" "What are the nonverbal, natural, and special purpose languages used in health care organizations?" Researchers are limited only by the language that they may not yet have.

REFERENCES

Benson, J.K. (1983). Paradigm and praxis in organizational analysis. *Research in Organizational Behavior, 5,* 33-56.

Blumer, H. (1969). *Symbolic interactionism.* Englewood Cliffs, NJ: Prentice-Hall.

Clark, B. (1972). The organizational saga in higher education. *Administrative Science Quarterly, 17,* 178-184.

Curtin, L. (1987). Watch your language. *Nursing Management, 17,* 9-10.

Diers, D. (1986). On words. *Image: The Journal of Nursing Scholarship, 18,* 30.

Henry, B., & LeClair, H. (1987). Language, leadership, and power. *Journal of Nursing Administration, 17,* 19-24.

Nordland, R. (1988). How to speak basic Baksheesh. In M. Ziegler (Ed.) (Spring, 1988). *Trips* (1), 53.

Parse, R.R. (1981). *Man-living-health.* New York: John Wiley & Sons.

Pfeffer, J. (1982). *Organizations and organization theory.* Cambridge, MA: Ballinger.

Pincus, J.D. (1986). Communication: Key contributor to effectiveness — the research. *Journal of Nursing Administration, 16,* 19-25.

Pondy, L.R. (1967). Organizational conflict: Concepts and models. *Administrative Science Quarterly, 12,* 296-320.

Pondy, L.R. (1977). The other hand clapping: An information-processing approach to organizational power. In T.H. Hammer & S.B. Bacharach (Eds.), *Reward systems and power distribution in organizations: Searching for solutions* (pp. 56-91). Ithaca, NY: Cornell University, New York School of Industrial and Labor Relations.

Pondy, L.R. (1978). Leadership is a language game. In Pondy, L.R., *Leadership: Where else can we go?* Durham, NC: Duke University Press.

Pondy, L.R., & Boje, D.M. (1980). Bringing mind back in. In W.E. Evan (Ed.), *Frontiers in organization and management* (pp. 83-101). New York: Praeger Scientific.

Pondy, L., Frost, P., Morgan, G., & Dandridge, T. (1983). *Organizational symbolism.* Greenwich, CT: J.A.I. Press.

Pondy, L.R., & Mitroff, I.I. (1979). Beyond open systems models of organizations. In B. Staw & G. Salancik (Eds.), *Research in organizational behavior,* (Vol. 1, pp. 3-39). Greenwich, CT: J.A.I. Press.

Pridham, K., & Schutz, M. (1985). Rationale for a language for naming problems from a nursing perspective. *Image: The Journal of Nursing Scholarship, 17,* 122-127.

Riehl, J. (1980). Implementing the Riehl interaction model in nursing administration. In J. Riehl & C. Roy (Eds.), *Conceptual models for nursing practice* (2nd ed.). New York: Appleton-Century-Crofts.

Staw, B. (1985). Spinning on symbolism: A brief note on the future of symbolism in organizational research. *Journal of Management, 11,* 117-118.

Chapter 5

Symbolic Interactionism
Herbert Blumer

Kathleen Kay Clevenger
Mary C. Alderson

‖ CASE STUDY

The surgical intensive care unit (SICU) has 14 beds, with the north and south ends each having seven beds. Mary Clayton is the evening shift patient care coordinator (PCC) of the SICU. A PCC's responsibilities include being charge on her shift, assigning staff to the north or south end of the units, assigning a charge nurse for the oncoming shift (in the absence of that shift's PCC), being on 24-hour call at times, scheduling, counseling, and developing staff. Mary has been a PCC on the evening shift for 1 year and has previously worked 3 years in SICU as a student nurse and staff nurse. Patty Dodson has been a staff nurse in SICU for 1 year on the night shift and has previous critical care experience. Recently Patty was the only applicant for the other night shift PCC position and did not receive the promotion.

Patty arrived for a 12-hour night shift at 7 PM and became very upset after looking at the assignment board. Mary had assigned Patty charge responsibilities because Sue Martin, the night shift PCC, was ill. Sue has frequently been ill and Patty, being a senior nurse on nights, has often been assigned charge responsibilities. However, Patty seemed to enjoy the role, had requested to be charge in the past, had recently applied for the PCC position, and had not expressed a need for relief from the charge role.

When Patty looked at the assignment board, she went to the north side of the unit where Mary was delivering patient care. Patty approached her, outside a patient's room near the nurse's station, and hostilely screamed, "You've put me in charge again and I'm not going to do it tonight! Sue is always sick!" Mary responded defensively, "Then leave. If you can't do what I need you to do, just go home."

Patty did not leave but took a bedside report on her patient assignment and began patient care. She continued to display much hostility with her nonverbal behavior of slamming cabinet doors and throwing around charts and supplies. She was short-tempered with other staff and patients.

Mary observed Patty's behavior but was very busy with her own patient assignment, which included a fresh postoperative patient. When she felt she was able to take a few minutes from her patient care, Mary asked another nurse to watch her patients. She then approached Patty and said, "Let's go into this empty patient room. I really need to talk with you, but I can't leave the unit with my patient assignment." Patty begrudgingly followed Mary. Mary closed the door and stated, "Patty, I know you're upset about having to be charge nurse so much recently, and I realize Sue has been ill a lot. The unit has been extremely busy this evening, and it really took me by surprise when you said you weren't going to be charge tonight. The type of behavior you have been displaying, along with raising your voice in front of patients and staff, is nonprofessional and not acceptable. If you're going to continue with this type of attitude, you'd be doing yourself and the unit a favor by leaving. This unit is in an uproar and your patients obviously know you're upset. If you can't do what I need you to do, I would like for you to go home." Patty listened, and by the end of the conversation, both nurses were in tears. Patty responded, "I'm not getting paid to be charge this frequently. I'm tired of acting like the PCC but not having the position. Sue is never here." By this time, it was close to 10 PM and Mary felt that the unit would be all right if Patty left. Patty gave a report on her patients to Mary and left. Mary worked a double shift to cover the charge role.

| | | | | | | | | | | | | | | | | | | | | | | | | | | | | | | | | | | | | | | | | | | | | | | | | | | | | | | | | | | | | | | | | | | | | | | | | | | | | | | |

SYMBOLIC INTERACTIONISM

According to the symbolic interactionist (SI) theorists, communication's main objective is to find meaning and understanding (Duldt & Giffin, 1985). Language is used by people to reveal reality. People create meaning out of routine experiences through collaboration within personal relationships in order to give these experiences more meaning.

Herbert Blumer defines symbolic interactionism as "a label for a relatively distinctive approach to the study of human group life and human conduct" (1969, p. 1). The concept is built around three simple premises. First, human beings act toward things or objects on the basis of the meaning that the thing or object has for them. An example in the category of human beings would be how a person views his or her friend or enemy. Second, the meaning of such things is derived from social interaction that one has with others. Third, the person has an interpretative process that is used in dealing with things (Blumer, 1969). The unique meanings that things have for each person is central in the position of SI. The interpretative process of each person involves two steps. The person communicates with himself or herself regarding how things have a certain meaning. Then the interpretation becomes a matter of handling meanings.

SI is grounded in a number of basic ideas or root images. These include human groups or societies, social interaction, objects, the human being as an actor, human action, and interconnection of lines of action. These root images represent how human society and conduct are viewed by SI.

Human groups are human beings engaging in action. The action consists of one's activities when encountering another person and dealing with situations. SI recognizes social interaction to be of vital importance because it is a process that forms human conduct (Blumer, 1969). Society consists of individuals interacting with each other, with the activities of its members occurring in response to one another. SI involves interpretation of the action. "Mutual role-taking is the sine qua non of communication and effective SI" (Blumer, 1969, p. 10). In other words, people interacting must take on each other's roles to understand one another.

The nature of objects is anything that can be indicated or pointed to, such as physical (chairs, bicycles), social (students, president), or abstract (moral principles) objects. The nature of the object consists of the meaning it has for each person. The human being is seen as an acting organism that makes indications to others and interprets their indications (Blumer, 1969). Blumer explains how Mead defined role taking as one places oneself in the position of others and views oneself from that position.

In the nature of human action, a person has to cope with certain situations, ascertaining the meaning of the actions of others, and mapping out one's own line of action in light of such interpretation (Blumer, 1969). In the interlinkage of action, participants in a network or organization engage in actions on the basis of given sets of meanings. The way in which people respond is the result of how they define the situation in which they need to act.

CASE ANALYSIS

The concepts of people, association, and social acts, as well as SI's three premises, reflect the development of certain interactions in the case study. Both Mary and Patty are nurses (social objects: people) in the SICU and have frequently assumed more than one role. Both consider the role of charge nurse to carry additional responsibilities, and both are capable of acting accordingly (premise 1).

Association has to do with how the two nurses relate to each other. Patty approached Mary with a very hostile attitude, and Mary responded in a curt, defensive manner. Through this interaction, Patty associated the role of charge nurse with a type of punishment (premise 2).

Social acts relate to how Patty dealt with being assigned charge and how Mary had to deal with Patty's open hostility. Mary interpreted Patty's hostility and was initially unable to respond in a professional, caring manner (premise 3).

RESEARCH

Research concerning interactionism is heavily concentrated in the social sciences (Rose, 1962). Early pioneers such as Mead (see Mead, 1934) and Blumer have provided much stimulus for today's researchers. SI's impact is also felt in nursing.

Riehl's interaction model was first presented to the nursing profession in 1980. She followed one of SI's basic beliefs that the self-concept is the key element between behavior and the social organization to which the individual belongs. The self-concept is therefore necessary for us to behave as humans. Her model adapts other concepts described by Blumer, including people, association, social acts, and interlinkages.

The concept people in Riehl's model is used to refer to the nurse, patient, family, and disciplinary team members. Association is the process of how these people relate to one another and interpret each other. An example is the nurse-patient relationship. Social acts occur when people note, interpret, and assess the situations confronting them. An example is a process recording that occurs when the nurse assesses and responds to a patient's behavior (Riehl, 1980). The complex interlinkages of acts are moving and not static affairs.

Riehl also examines the "me" and "I" developed by Mead. "Me" is equivalent to the role taker. Riehl advocated role taking by nurses and others to better understand the cause of a patient's behavior. Through this activity, the self-concept, or "I," can be analyzed (Riehl, 1980). The "I" is the summation of one's roles and reflects a person's total behavioral perceptions (Gochnauer & Miller, 1986). Riehl cites two examples of the concept role: role reversal and the sick role. Role reversal is a potential interaction in which the patient becomes the therapeutic agent and the nurse becomes the care recipient. The sick role is not completely defined; simply stated, it occurs when the patient is reluctant to give up being sick (Riehl, 1980).

Bonnie Weaver Duldt proposed humanistic nursing communication in 1985. The model evolved over a 5-year period and draws heavily from SI (Duldt & Giffin, 1985). Duldt began work on the model when she realized that the future of health care delivery would be more complex and difficult. She proposed that nurses change their perspectives since it is unlikely that the context in which they practice will change. Duldt believes that the study of humanizing, meaningful interpersonal communications can lead to a more positive feeling of self-worth among nurses (Duldt & Giffin, 1985). As a result of this, patients will feel better about their care.

Research related to the above models is sparse but does exist. Both Riehl and Duldt have conducted studies on their own models. Duldt has expanded her focus to include alienating communication patterns such as verbal abuse (Duldt & Giffin, 1985). She continues to work on a more descriptive definition of humanizing communication.

Riehl's doctoral dissertation addressed elements of her model. The study examined autistic children's ability to role take as compared with their siblings' ability (Riehl, 1980). More recent research on Riehl's model has illustrated its wide applicability. Since Riehl's model conceptualizes nursing action as the nurse taking the role of the other in client relationships, its use is not limited to specific patient settings (Kim, 1983). Also, being a middle range theory (versus a grand theory such as Rogers's theory of unitary man), Riehl's theory is more realistic and testable (Kim, 1983).

Because of its major focus on roles, Riehl's interaction model is very appropriate for nursing administration. One of the keys to good management is the ability to understand the actions of other people. This can be accomplished through role taking. Marilynn Wood (1980) suggests using the Riehl interaction model for nursing administration because of its focus on roles.

REFERENCES

Blumer, H. (1969). *Symbolic interactionism: Perspective and method.* Englewood Cliffs, NJ: Prentice-Hall.

Duldt, B.W., & Giffin, K. (1985). *Theoretical perspectives for nursing.* Boston: Little, Brown.

Gochnauer, A., & Miller, K. (1986). Symbolic interactionism. In Marriner, A. (Ed.), *Nursing theorists and their work.* St. Louis: C.V. Mosby.

Kim, H.S. (1983). *The nature of theoretical thinking in nursing.* Norwalk, CT: Appleton-Century-Crofts.

Mead, G.H. (1934). Mind, self, and society. Chicago: University of Chicago Press.

Riehl, J. (1980). The Riehl interaction model. In J. Riehl & C. Roy (Eds.), *Conceptual models for nursing practice* (2nd ed.). New York: Appleton-Century-Crofts.

Rose, A.M. (1962). *Human behavior and social processes: An interactionist approach.* Boston: Houghton Mifflin.

Thibodeau, J. (1983). *Nursing models: Analysis and evaluation.* Monterey, CA: Wadsworth.

Travelbee, J. (1976). *Interpersonal aspects of nursing* (3rd ed.). Philadelphia: F.A. Davis.

Wood, M.J. (1980). Implementing the Riehl interaction model in nursing administration. In J. Riehl & C. Roy (Eds.), *Conceptual models for nursing practice* (2nd ed.). New York: Appleton-Century-Crofts.

Chapter 6

Attribution Theory
Fritz Heider

Jan Austin
Kathleen A. Holmes

❙❙   CASE STUDY

The personnel in the obstetrical department of a small community hospital are beginning to perform cesarean sections. Before this, all planned and emergency cesarean sections were performed by the operating room (OR) personnel in the surgery department. Training for the obstetrical (OB) personnel is being done by the operating room personnel.

The training of the obstetrical personnel has presented a problem. Several of the operating room nurses have been uncooperative, refusing to allow the obstetrical nurses and technicians to perform under their supervision. This situation has caused resentment by both staffs. Neither staff had any choice or voice in the arrangement, which was coordinated by the director of nursing for the hospital. To compound the problem, the operating room nurses receive specialty pay for working in surgery, which the obstetrical nurses do not receive and will not receive in the future.

❘❘

ATTRIBUTION THEORY

The rationale people have for their own behavior and the behavior of others has a powerful effect on their feelings, plans, hopes, and well-being. These explanations and the ensuing consequences are the basis for one important motivation theory called attribution theory. Attribution theory is concerned with the perceptions people have about the causes of their own and others' behavior and the effect that these perceptions have on their subsequent behavior (Bardwell, 1986, p. 122).

Attribution theory was originated by Fritz Heider in the 1940s and was concerned with understanding an individual's naive perceptions about the cause of an event. Heider used the term *naive* because it was based on a layperson's knowledge. Heider was more concerned with events that occur in everyday life on a conscious level rather than an unconscious level as presented in other theories of personality. Heider describes the attribution process as the ordering and classifying of stimuli perceived in a situation. Individuals respond to the meaning of another's behavior, not to the overt behavior (Harvey, Ickes, & Kidd, 1976).

Heider believed that if you could understand the cause of a behavior you could predict the behavior and emotional responses of people to a situation. By predicting the response of an individual or group you could better control the environment (Frieze, Bar Tal, & Carroll, 1979).

Heider believed that individuals reacted to what they thought the other person was perceiving, feeling, and thinking in addition to what he or she was doing. Heider proposed that the perceiver of behavior was more inclined to attribute actions to stable causes, such as personality traits, rather than unstable or variable causes, such as moods (Harvey & Weary, 1985). Valle and Frieze proposed a mathematical representation of the importance of stable or unstable traits, $P = E + O [f(S)]$, where P is the prediction for the future, E is the individual's expectation before the outcome, O is the most recent outcome, and S is the amount to which the outcome is attributed to stable factors (1976, p. 581). The more an outcome is attributed to stable causes, the more predictive power it has.

Kelley (1979) elaborated on Heider's theory and postulated that three factors influenced a person's assumptions about other people or objects. The first factor is consistency, which is the extent the person feels that the other person would manifest the same behavior to the object in other situations. The next factor is distinctiveness, which is the extent to which a person would demonstrate the same behavior to the object or person under similar situations. The final factor is consensus, which is the way people other than the person involved would behave under similar circumstances (Wyer & Carlston, 1979).

Heider views human beings as in a constant process of attempting to make sense of the environment and using attribution to infer causality. The more a person or object is seen as causing an action, the less influence the environment is seen as an exerting force, and vice versa (Harvey & Weary, 1985, p. 284).

A distinction is made between "factors within the person" (internal locus of causality) and "factors within the environment" (external locus of causality) as perceived determinants (Heider, 1958). Heider further distinguishes between positive and negative experiences and states that they affect the attribution of an event to internal or external sources (Feldman, 1986, p. 77).

The assumption underlying attribution theory is that people engage in a causal search in order to make sense of their lives, especially in important life events (Lowery, Jacobsen, & McCauley, 1987, p. 92).

CASE ANALYSIS

Peterson (1984) uses attribution theory in her work in crisis intervention. She encourages workers in crisis intervention to have the client use the reattribution process to discover other possible causes for the crises that are less distressing to the client. It should be noted that while Peterson's work, in its purest form, involves crisis intervention on a one-to-one basis, the ease with which nurse managers can adapt these theories for effective problem solving with staff is illustrated here.

Caplan describes a crisis as a period of threat that severely challenges the continuation of the individual's present way of organizing living (Peterson, 1984, p. 133). During a crisis situation the person experiences shock, disbelief, and denial. He or she begins to ask, Why did this have to happen to me? The answers lay the groundwork for reorganization, which leads either to a positive resolution (functioning is resumed at the same or higher level than before the crisis) or to a negative resolution (functioning is resumed at a lower level). It is at this point, when the person is struggling to make sense out of what happened, that intervention can play a crucial role in facilitating the person's reorganization toward positive resolution (Peterson, 1984, p. 133).

Managers must view this case study as a crisis and focus on a strategy that will facilitate the two nursing staffs to resolve their differences and be motivated to strive for cohesiveness and professional growth. This strategy will be the application of attribution theory and the utilization of the nursing process.

The initial phase for resolution would be for the manager to make an adequate assessment of the problem and of individual behaviors. The planning phase elicits from all staff members heightened perceptions of their own behavior, as well as defines the motive for the behaviors of others. An "attribution" is the inference that an observer makes about either the causes of his or her own behavior or that of another person (Davidhizar & McBride, 1985, p. 284). During the intervention phase, the manager must initiate the reattribution process. According to Peterson, the reattribution process facilitates and explores other causes or reasons for the behavior elicited by individuals. In doing so the manager motivates the person toward more appropriate problem solving. The attribution approach treats people as constructive thinkers searching for causes of the events confronting them and acting on their imperfect knowledge of causal structure in ways that they consider appropriate (Davidhizar & McBride, 1985).

For example, internal causes of behavior by the OR staff could be loss of power and authority, inability to provide instruction to the OB staff, lack of trust, and loss of job. External causes could be the autocratic decision of higher management, change of job requirements without monetary reward, and the reduction in the OR budget along with staff layoffs.

If one would examine the internal causes of behavior by the OB staff it could include more responsibility, inability to perform cesarean sections, and the sense of resentment by the OR staff. External causes could be the autocratic decision by higher management, change of environment, increase in budget and staff, and no increase in pay.

By assisting with this process, the manager would be able to promote reorganization toward successful resolution. Resolution, reinforcement, and support is the final phase.

Because attribution theory assumes that individuals are interested in understanding their own behavior, the reasoning behind the nurses' actions is considered (Harvey et al., 1976). First, the OR staff behavior, as seen by themselves, was attributed to change in their job requirements and a change in dispositional properties. The OR staff nurse, in addition to her regular duties, had the job of instructor thrust on her with no preparation or compensation for the duty. The dispositional properties according to Heider are properties that "dispose objects and events to manifest themselves in certain ways under certain conditions" (Heider, 1958, p. 80). The dispositional property in this case is that the hospital has limited funds and each department must compete with the other departments for available money. The operating room budget is based on the number of cases performed. If the obstetrical department performs their own cesarean sections, the operating room budget may be reduced. The OR staff realizes that the training of the obstetrical staff could actually reduce the OR budget and possibly lead to staff cuts.

The obstetrical nurses view their behavior as a necessary evil. They do not particularly want to care for women who had cesarean sections. This will lead to more responsibility and more work with no additional pay. They resent the treatment they are receiving from the OR staff because it is not a change they wanted either. Although not happy with the addition of the cesarean sections, the obstetrical staff realizes that their budget will be increased and extra help may be hired.

The obstetrical nurses resent the action of the OR staff because they see the action of the OR staff as representative of their sentiments toward the obstetrical staff as individuals instead of looking at the cause for their behavior. According to Heider, the sentiments of the operating room nurses were displayed to the obstetrical nurses because "in some cases all the negative feelings of a person were focused on the person who is closest" (Heider, 1958, p. 190). Since the director of nursing was not close enough, the obstetrical nurses were the target of the behavior.

RESEARCH

Currently there is limited nursing research involving attribution theory. Much of the research is being done in the field of social psychology. The research is based on the original model of attribution theorist Bernard Weiner (1972, 1974, 1979). "The model focuses on attributional analysis of achievement-related behavior in terms of ability, effort, the difficulty of the task and/or good or bad luck" (Frieze et al., 1979).

Most of the nursing research using attribution dealt with patient reactions to their illnesses such as viewing their illness or accident as blaming themselves for the illness or seeing it as chance. A study by Lowery and Jacobsen (1985) asked patients to determine causes for their perceived failures or successes in dealing with their chronic illness. The results of this study indicated that patients having difficulty with their illnesses were more likely to deny any reason for their illnesses. Chronically ill persons attributed success to internal causes and effort, and failure to external causes and task difficulty (Lowery, 1981).

Studies by Buhlman and Wortman (1977), Rudy (1980), and Keane and Ducette (1981) are also health related and not focused on nursing management research.

It is imperative that nurse managers are aware of individual perceptions of environment and behavior. A responsibility of the manager is to direct individuals to improve their problem solving, thus making the environment and individual behaviors less threatening.

Future research needs to be conducted on attribution theory in relation to behavior in the workplace. Attribution theory has relevance for nurse managers in dealing with individual behavior.

REFERENCES

Bardwell, R. (1986). Attribution theory and behavior change: Ideas for nursing settings. *Journal of Nursing Education, 25,* 122-124.

Barron, C. (1987). Succeeding in a man's world: Women's expectations for success and perceptions of ability. *Journal of Nursing Education, 26,* 310-315.

Buhlman, R., & Wortman, C. (1977). Attributions of blame and coping in the "real world": Severe accident victims react to their lot. *Journal of Personality and Social Psychology, 35*:351-363.

Cronenwett, L. (1982). Helping and nursing models. *Nursing Research, 32,* 342-346.

Davidhizar, R., & McBride, A. (1985). How nursing students explain their success and failure in clinical experiences. *Journal of Nursing Education, 24,* 284-290.

Donnan, H., & Pipes, R. (1985). Counselor trainees' explanations of behavior: Attributions to traits, situations, and interactions. *Journal of Clinical Psychology, 41,* 729-733.

Einhorn, H., & Hogarth, R. (1986). Judging probable cause. *Psychological Bulletin, 99*(1), 3-19.

Feldman, H. (1986). Self-esteem, types of attributional style and sensation and distress pain ratings in males. *Journal of Advances in Nursing, 2,* 76-86.

Felton, G., & Parsons, M. (1987). The impact of nursing education on ethical/moral decision making. *Journal of Nursing Education, 26,* 7-10.

Frieze, I., Bar Tal, D., & Carroll, J. (Eds.). (1979). *New approaches to social problems.* Washington, D.C.: Jossey-Bass.

Harvey, J., Ickes, W., & Kidd, R. (1976). *New directions in attribution research,* Vol. I. Hillsdale, NJ: Lawrence Erlbaum Associates.

Harvey, J., & Weary, G. (1985). *Attribution: Basic issues and applications.* New York, Academic Press.

Heider, J. (1958). *Psychology of interpersonal relations.* New York: John Wiley & Sons.

Keane, A., & Ducette, J. (1981). *An attributional analysis of surgical care outcomes.* Manuscript in preparation.

Kelley, H. (1979). *Personal relationships: Their structures and processes.* New York: Lawrence Erlbaum Associates.

Lowery, B. (1981). Misconceptions and limitations of locus of control and I.E. scale. *Nursing Research, 34,* 82-88.

Lowery, B., & Jacobson, B. (1985). Attributional analysis of chronic illness outcomes. *Nursing Research, 34,* 82-88.

Lowery, B., Jacobsen, B., & McCauley, K. (1987). On the prevalence of causal search in illness situations. *Nursing Research, 36,* 88-93.

Peterson, L. (1984). Attribution theory and its application in crisis intervention. *Perspectives in Psychiatric Care, 22,* 133-136.

Rudy, E.B. (1980). Patients' and spouses' causal explanations of a myocardial infarction. *Nursing Research, 29,* 352-356.

Strickland, L. (1958). Surveillance and trust. *Journal of Personality, 26,* 200-215.

Thibaut, J., & Reichen, H. (1955). Perception of social causality. *Journal of Personality, 24,* 133.

Valle, V., & Frieze, I. (1976). Stability of causal attributions as a mediator in changing expectations for success. *Journal of Personality and Social Psychology, 33,* 579-587.

Weiner, B. (1972). *Theories of motivation: From mechanism to cognition.* Rand McNally, 1972.

Weiner, B. (1974). Achievement motivation as conceptualized by an attribution theorist. In B. Weiner (Ed.), *Achievement motivation and attribution theory.* Morristown, NJ: General Learning Press.

Weiner, B. (1979). Theory of motivation for some classroom experiences. *Journal of Educational Psychology, 71,* 3-25.

Wyer, R., & Carlston, D.E. (1979). *Social cognition, inference, and attribution.* New York: Lawrence Erlbaum Associates.

Chapter 7

Group Process
Bruce W. Tuckman

Diana Boyer

❙❙ CASE STUDY

Working in a group composed of personally selected, amiable, intelligent, rational, and competent individuals can be a most rewarding experience — one that occurs only in the dreams of many nursing managers. In reality, managers belong to various groups whose members are set by the position a person holds and not by his or her unique abilities to contribute to the group process.

Janice White knows this truism all too well. Janice is the Division Director for Surgical Services at Eternal Hope Hospital (EHH), a 500-bed facility. The Surgical Services area includes the Surgery Department (OR), Ambulatory Surgery (AS), and the Post-Anesthesia Care Unit (PACU). The Surgical Services Committee, which Janice chairs, includes the managers of the three areas, the Director of Nursing (DON), the Chief of Surgery, the Chief of Anesthesia, and the Chief Operating Officer (COO).

The functions of this administrative committee are to establish policies, problem-solve, and facilitate smooth operation of the surgical services with the outcome of cost-effective, quality patient care.

The committee has been cohesive and effective for the past 2 years. The heads of surgery and anesthesia have been open-minded, cooperative, and supportive of the nursing staff. The nursing managers are very capable, self-directed, and effective in their positions. The DON has been supportive of the managers and Janice. The COO is supportive and attends the meetings when possible. The Chiefs of Surgery and Anesthesia have taken much criticism from their colleagues over the perceived "selling out" to nursing because of their support of the nursing managers and hospital administration.

The physicians are upset and threatened by the current economic climate and the increased regulation of their practices. Any further regulations or changes proposed by the hospital administration would be met with strong resistance.

It is now November, and Janice is contemplating the future of the Surgical Services Committee, for its composition changes in January with the election of the new Chiefs of Surgery and of Anesthesia. The two physicians joining the committee have much to offer. The new Chief of Surgery, however, has been openly critical of nursing services in the past. The Chief of Anesthesia is generally supportive of nursing. The other committee members will remain the same.

How does Janice facilitate the re-formation of the group, and what can she expect? Janice decided to review the models and theories that might help her with a framework on which to build her strategy. She finds Bruce Tuckman's developmental model to be most beneficial as a basis for her plan.

| | | | | | | | | | | | | | | | | | | | | | | | | | | | | | | | | | | | | | | | | | | | | | | | | | | | | | | | | | | | | | | | | | | | | | | | | | | | |

TUCKMAN'S MODEL

Tuckman's inductive model was presented in 1965 after an extensive review of the literature relating to small-group development and function. He cited many shortcomings of the research methodologies: (1) the focus on group therapy settings and human relations training groups; (2) the lack of experimental control and manipulation of independent variables; (3) the lack of consideration of the changes occurring over time in a group; (4) the lack of research to test already proposed models—most studies were observational in nature and concerned with postulating new stages or variations in stages of group development; and (5) the paucity of research with natural or laboratory groups.

Tuckman reviewed the existing studies of therapy groups, natural and laboratory task groups, and human relations training groups from the perspectives of social and task-oriented behaviors. He proposed interpersonal stages of (1) testing and dependence, (2) intragroup conflict, (3) development of group cohesion, and (4) functional role relatedness. The task-activity stages were (1) orientation to task, (2) emotional response to task demands, (3) open exchanges of relevant interpretations, and (4) emergence of solution. Tuckman fused these stages to form his developmental stages of (1) forming, (2) storming, (3) norming, and (4) performing.

The *forming stage* is a time of identifying the rules, standards, and boundaries of the group structure. There is a concurrent testing of interpersonal relationships.

Much conflict and emotion characterizes the *storming stage*. These interpersonal issues impede task-related activities.

Group roles are assumed during the *norming stage* as members move toward cohesiveness and develop a feeling of belonging. The members are now free to express themselves openly.

In the *performing stage,* the interpersonal structure is set and functional. The members have assumed flexible roles and can concentrate on task performance (Tuckman, 1965).

In 1977 Tuckman and Mary Ann Jensen examined the research published since Tuckman's original model was formulated. Runkel, Lawrence, Oldfield, Rider, and Clark (1971) published the only attempt at empirical testing of Tuckman's hypothesis. Their findings supported the hypothesis. However, the methodology used introduces serious questions of observer bias. The observers were given descriptions of Tuckman's four stages and were instructed to relate their observations in terms of the model's stages.

The research review also revealed the parsimony of Tuckman's model with the more recent findings, with one exception. Lacoursiere (1974) observed a final stage of "termination." Spitz and Sadock (1973) categorized the last stage as "disengagement." Braaten (1974-1975), Mann (1967), and Yalom (1970) also listed "termination" as a final stage. These researchers were reflecting the life cycle model (Gibbard & Hartman, 1973; Mills, 1964).

After Tuckman and Jensen completed this review, Tuckman's model was modified to include a fifth stage of *adjourning* (Tuckman & Jensen, 1977). This stage is a time of closure for group members. See Table 7-1 for a review of Tuckman's stages.

TABLE 7-1   Tuckman's Group Process Model

Stage	Activity
1. Forming	Identify the rules and standards
2. Storming	Deal with conflict and power struggles
3. Norming	Assume group roles
4. Performing	Accomplish tasks
5. Adjourning	Complete closure

CASE ANALYSIS

Janice's circumstances deviate from the developmental sequence in that a mature, functioning group already exists. The loss of two members of the current group and the incorporation of two new members complicate the group process, but Tuckman's model is still applicable.

Janice has already observed the beginning of the disengagement of the outgoing physicians from the group. This began during the October meeting after the nominations for the new chiefs had been made. The retiring chiefs became uncommunicative, withdrawn, and reluctant to pursue any new programs. It seemed to be more than the "lame duck" syndrome to Janice.

Janice's review of Tuckman's model led to the recognition that the physicians were entering the adjourning phase. Looking back at the managers' behaviors she became aware that the whole group had come to the realization that the end of the present group was imminent. A quietness and melancholy, not unlike that of mourning, characterized the meeting.

To facilitate the adjourning phase, Janice met with the group members (excluding the physicians). They discussed the upcoming changes and their feelings concerning these changes. As a group, they decided to send personal notes of appreciation to the physicians for their support. Janice plans to initiate an open discussion during the November meeting about the end of the terms for the two chiefs. The two incoming chiefs will be named and invited to attend the December meeting.

Janice will use the December meeting to complete the adjourning process for this year's group and begin the forming process for next year's group. Included will be the group's recognition of the accomplishments and cooperation of the retiring chiefs. Then the new chiefs will be introduced and Janice will state the expectations of group cooperation, positive interactions, and accomplishments for the new group.

This forming stage will continue in the January meeting as Janice reviews the committee's procedures, functions, and desired outcomes. This will clarify the expected interpersonal and task behaviors. Janice will introduce a relatively uncontroversial problem and let the group work through it to allow testing of the rules, boundaries, and interpersonal relationships.

Janice anticipates the initiation of the storming stage at the February meeting when she will introduce the controversial topic of regulation of the surgery scheduling system. This topic evokes strong emotional responses from all committee members because the outcome affects the profitability of the physicians' practices, of the involved units, and of the entire hospital. The control of the schedule has been an issue for many years at EHH. Janice must consider Lewin's force field analysis (1951) when broaching this topic. Each member has a number of forces influencing his or her particular stand. The group must be persuaded to look at the overall outcome of the scheduling process in terms of physician accommodation, patient services, staff availability, quality of care, and hospital profitability.

This conflict should promote rapid progression of the storming stage to the norming stage. The number of interactions is expected to be high. With continued interactions comes the evolution of roles by the group members and a standard pattern of behaviors. Janice, as the leader, must monitor the interactions and promote appropriate self-expressions and problem-solving behaviors.

Because of time restraints related to the programming of the computerized scheduling system, Janice needs to facilitate positive interactions to move the group to the performing stage by April. She must exert diplomacy to assure functional conflicts. Janice realizes that additional meetings may be necessary to resolve the structural issues and role conflicts. Only after resolution of these issues will the group be able to focus on task performance.

Once the performing stage is achieved, the group can expend energies on task accomplishment and problem resolution. Barring the unexpected addition or replacement of members, Janice can anticipate a cohesive, functioning Surgical Services Committee for the next 18 months until the new chiefs will be nominated for the next 2-year term.

RESEARCH

A search of the literature on group process reveals a wealth of articles and studies published in the years between 1964 and 1980. Sociologists, psychologists, psychotherapists, and social psychologists were most prolific in this area of study.

Nursing professionals published some studies in this area in the 1970s and 1980s. Psychiatric nurses and nurse educators conducted studies of group process. Psychiatric nurses focused on group therapy and patient outcomes, whereas educators concentrated efforts on student learning processes in group situations.

There were no studies found in the area of nursing management. *Nursing Administration Quarterly* carried an article in its Forum column that discussed "process management" from a consultant's point of view (Vogel, 1986). The *Journal of Advanced Nursing* featured a study by two nurses leading a counseling group for physically disabled adults (O'Hagan & Lobb, 1982). The *Journal of Nursing Education* printed the article, "A Group Experience to Combat Burnout and Learn Group Process Skills" (Lammert, 1981). The information gained from this study could be useful to managers.

The early literature in all disciplines was primarily descriptive and observational in nature. Most of the authors observed group behavior and proposed their own models of group development. These same authors called for further research for verification of their hypotheses (Tuckman & Jensen, 1977). Thus nursing managers are not unique in neglecting such research.

The current economic climate illustrates more clearly than ever that hospital and nursing administrators must keep current with management theories and group process models. Group process is a continual activity for an administrator—whether he or she is part of a group or the leader of a group.

Nursing needs empirical data to establish a knowledge base for all areas of nursing practice. Nursing administrators are no exception. Many models have been proposed by other disciplines. Research needs to be conducted to determine the validity and generalizability of these models in nursing management. There is a great need for nursing researchers to put forth new models or theory applications specific to nursing.

REFERENCES

Braaten, L.J. (1974-1975). Developmental phases of encounter groups and related intensive groups: A critical review of models and a new proposal. *Interpersonal Development, 5,* 112-129.

Gibbard, G., & Hartman, J. (1973). The oedipal paradigm in group development: A clinical and empirical study. *Small Group Behavior, 4,* 305-349.

Lacoursiere, R. (1974). A group method to facilitate learning during the stages of a psychiatric affiliation. *International Journal of Group Psycotherapy, 24,* 342-351.

Lammert, M. (1981). A group experience to combat burnout and learn group process skills. *Journal of Nursing Education, 20*(6), 41-46.   .

Lewin, K. (1951). *Field theory in social science.* New York: Harper & Row.

Mann, R.D. (1967). *Interpersonal styles and group development.* New York: John Wiley & Sons.

Mills, T.M. (1964). *Group transformation.* Englewood Cliffs, NJ: Prentice-Hall.

O'Hagan Lobb, M. (1982). Seating arrangement as a predictor of small group interaction. *Journal of Advanced Nursing, 7,* 163-166.   ;

Runkel, P.J., Lawrence, M., Oldfield, S., Rider, M., & Clark, C. (1971). Stages of group development: An empirical test of Tuckman's hypothesis. *Journal of Applied Behavioral Science, 7,* 180-193.

Spitz, H., & Sadock, B. (1973). Psychiatric training of graduate nursing students. *New York State Journal of Medicine, 6,* 1334-1338.

Tuckman, B.W. (1965). Developmental sequence in small groups. *Psychological Bulletin, 6,* 384-399.

Tuckman, B.W., & Jensen, M.A. (1977). Stages of small group development revisited. *Group and Organizational Studies, 2,* 419-427.

Vogel, G. (1986). Consulting focus: Process management. *Nursing Administration Quarterly, 10,* 69-72.

Yalom, I. (1970). *The theory and practice of group psychotherapy.* New York: Basic Books.

SUGGESTED READINGS

Bednar, R.L., & Kaul, T.J. (1979). Experimental group research: What never happened! *Journal of Applied Behavioral Science, 15,* 311-319.

Hare, A.P., Borgatta, E.F., & Bales, R.F. (1965). *Small groups: Studies in social interaction.* New York, Alfred A. Knopf.

Lewin, K. (1935). *Dynamic theory of personality.* New York: McGraw-Hill.

Llewelyn, S., & Fielding, G. (1982). Group dynamics 2: Under the influence. *Nursing Mirror, 155*(4), 37-39.

Luft, J. (1984). *Group processes: An introduction to group dynamics.* San Francisco: Mayfield.

Napier, R.W., & Gershenfeld, M.K. (1981). *Groups, theory and experience.* Boston: Houghton Mifflin.

Sampson, E.E., & Marthas, M.K. (1977). *Group process for the health professions.* New York: John Wiley & Sons.

Stogill, R.M. (1959). *Individual behavior and group achievement.* New York: Oxford University Press.

Tischler, N.G., Morrison, T.L., Greene, L.R., & Steward, M.S. (1986). Work and defensive processes in small groups: Effects of leader gender and authority position. *Psychiatry, 49,* 241-252.

Zander, A. (1986). *Making groups effective.* San Francisco: Jossey-Bass.

Chapter 8

Economic Theories

Robert M. Saywell, Jr.
Andrea L. Ziegert

❙❙   CASE STUDY*

During the past two decades, there has been increasing pressure to contain the rapid increase in the cost of health care. One cost-containment strategy is to develop lower-cost alternatives to acute-care inpatient hospitalization. For patients requiring hospitalization, strategies have been developed to reduce the cost of the inpatient stay. For example, intermediate or step-down care has been proposed for the patient who does not require the services of an intensive care unit but is unable to be placed on a regular nursing unit. For patients well enough to leave the regular nursing unit but too sick to go home, the creation of cooperative care units has been suggested. The cooperative care unit is designed to teach patients and their care partners how to handle the care themselves and ultimately to better prepare them for home discharge.

Metropolitan Hospital, a 1100-bed tertiary teaching hospital located in a large midwestern city, is affiliated with a state-owned university medical school and serves as a major neonatal referral center. As part of a rigorous cost-containment strategy, Metropolitan opened a 19-bed cooperative care program for medical and surgical patients. The majority of the patients using the unit were obstetrical patients, but other patients could use the unit as well. The unit was located in an adjoining hotel connected with the hospital facility by a skywalk. The Obstetrics-Gynecology Department, a strong supporter of the unit, believed the unit resulted in considerable cost savings since patients stayed in a hotel room and relied on care partners for most of their routine care. However, following the opening of a new hospital building, the average daily census in the cooperative care unit declined from 18 to 3 patients. The hospital viewed the unit as a source of savings although no one was sure of the amount saved for the recipient (the patient or the third-party payer). The hospital also realized that the cooperative care unit was a viable albeit partial remedy to the nursing shortage faced by the hospital, because care partners were substituted for nurses on the unit. The hospital received many letters of support from patients who had been on the unit, and the staff felt that the unit contributed positively to the patient's recovery phase. Both patient satisfaction and quality of care indicators were high for the unit.

Before implementing strategies to encourage increased use of the unit, Metropolitan sought answers to two crucial questions: Was the cooperative care unit cost-effective? and What was the primary reason for the decline in use?

* This case study has been adapted from Woods, J.R., Saywell, R.M. & Benson, J.T. (1988). Comparative costs of a cooperative care program versus inpatient hospital care for obstetric patients. *Medical Care, 26,* 596-601.

The decline in admissions to the unit led to an increase in cost per patient and seemed to coincide with the opening of the new hospital building. If the unit was cost-effective, then strategies to increase patient use should be implemented. The administrator of Metropolitan Hospital requested a study to determine the cost-effectiveness of the cooperative care unit.

Before progressing with the study, we need to develop a thorough understanding of the situation in order to answer the following questions:

What information do we need to determine the cost-effectiveness of the unit?

What information is available and how do we access it?

What assumptions do we need to make regarding the design of the study?

What are the inherent limitations of the study design and how can we best address them?

What are the future implications and possible strategies that might result from the results of the study?

The next section introduces some basic economic theories that will be useful to further examine the issue presented in this case study.

| | | | | | | | | | | | | | | | | | | | | | | | | | | | | | | | | | | | | | | | | | | | | | | | | | | | | | | | | | | | | | | | | | | |

ECONOMIC THEORY

As a health care management professional, you will be faced with many questions in the course of your daily work: How best to allocate scarce nursing time among various patients? What is the best way to achieve individual patient health goals, given a variety of possible treatment plans? What is the best way, for you as an individual, to balance the demands of your patients and/or staff, the demands of other health care professionals, and your own personal career goals? Similarly, the health care organization where you work, whether it is a hospital, visiting nurse association, or other health care provider, must answer other important questions: How many and what types of health care professionals should be hired to best provide high-quality patient services? What patient mix should our facility be serving? In what type of health care technology should we invest? How much does it cost to provide various services? How should we pay for these services? How much should we charge patients for the health care we provide?

All these questions, whether asked by an individual health care provider or a facility, are important as we strive to provide the best possible health care. But how do we begin to answer these questions? How do we start to balance out the competing claims for our time and our resources? Traditional economic analysis has offered some guidelines to answer these questions. This section will allow you to consider some of these issues in a different way.

The study of economics is about more than just dollars and cents. It is about common sense too. At its simplest, economics is the study of society's choices regarding scarce resources. The study of economics exists because of one fundamental characteristic of human nature—more is preferred to less. We as human beings seem to have an unlimited set of "wants"; just ask any 4-year-old or any government bureaucrat. There always seems to be an unlimited number of things we would like to have. On the other hand, our society is limited by finite resources to meet those unlimited wants; just ask the 4-year-old's parent, or consult the bureaucrat's budget. What becomes important is how we use these scarce resources to best satisfy our unlimited wants. This involves choices: we must choose among competing wants when we use our resources. Here is where economics comes in; economics does not make the choices, but instead helps to clarify the choices involved and aids decision makers in ranking these choices. Economics will not tell us what to do; on the contrary, it only provides us with information to make better decisions.

Traditional economic analysis has dealt with a number of important questions in trying to best allocate society's scarce resources:

1. What types of goods and services should society produce; for example, how much should we devote to acute treatment versus preventive health care?
2. Who should produce these goods and services; for example, how should we use allied health professionals in the delivery of health care?
3. How and where should we produce these goods and services; for example, what health care services should be provided as inpatient versus outpatient services?
4. How many goods and services should we produce; for example, what percentage of our gross national product should go to health care, to education, and to national defense?
5. For whom do we produce these goods and services; for example, how do we distribute health care to the young, the old, the rich, the poor?

In reality these are questions you will face in your career. Economics can help you decide how to allocate scarce resources among different patients in your facility or decide which method of care is preferred. To best understand how the study of economics can aid you in your decision making, we need to consider two basic tools of economic analysis: supply and demand theory, and production theory and cost analysis.

SUPPLY AND DEMAND THEORY

Any economic analysis involves two basic types of players: *consumers,* those individuals who want certain goods and services, and *producers,* those individuals who provide those goods and services. In the area of health care, the consumers are the people who use health care services in preventive, acute, or chronic care. Nurses, physicians, dentists, respiratory therapists, and other allied health professionals are examples of the producers of health care services. For health care services to actually be provided, these two groups, consumers and producers, have to "get together" and agree on the type and amount of service provided and the price of that service. A *market* is the area where consumers and producers "come together" to decide the quantity and price of a particular service. Markets can be thought of as any number of physical places, such as Wall Street, a physician's office, or a hospital. Market transactions can also involve consumers and producers who are physically located in different locations.

To understand the workings of a market, economists often use a simple diagram (Figure 8-1) to summarize the interaction of consumers and producers (demanders and suppliers). The vertical axis measures the price of a good; the farther we move up the axis, away from the origin, the higher the price of the good. The horizontal axis measures the quantity of a good; the farther we move to the right, away from the origin, the greater the quantity of the good. The points within the axes represent various combinations of price and quantity. For example, point A in Figure 8-1 represents a price of $4 and a quantity of 2 units, while point B represents a price of $6 and a quantity of 5 units. We can measure price in dollars and cents, yen, drachmas, or any monetary unit, and we can measure quantity in units, hundreds of units, pounds, ounces, or whatever is more appropriate for the good or service in question. Figure 8-1 is a simple representation of a market. To find out which price-quantity combination we will end up with in our market, we have to add our economic players, the consumers and the producers. The *demand curve* for goods and services represents the wants of our consumers and the *supply curve* represents the quantity of goods and services that producers are able to provide. Let us take a look at demand and supply curves in detail.

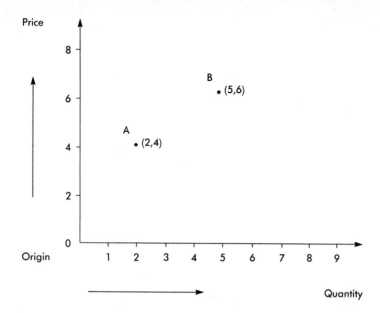

FIGURE 8-1 The vertical axis measures the price of the good. The horizontal axis measures the quantity of the good. Points between the axes represent various price-quantity combinations.

Demand

What is demand? Demand is a relationship between various amounts of a particular good and various prices for that good. In particular, the law of demand postulates an inverse or negative relationship between the price and quantity of a good that a consumer is both willing and able to purchase per unit of time. Therefore, according to the law of demand, the lower the price charged for a product, resource, or service, the greater will be the quantity demanded per unit of time. Conversely, the higher the price charged, the smaller will be the quantity demanded per unit of time. With a little bit of thought, you should be able to find examples of the law of demand from your own experience. For example, all things being otherwise equal, the lower the price of an aspirin tablet, the greater the quantity of aspirin demanded. There are several points worth noting in the definition of the law of demand. First, emphasis is on the amount of a good that a consumer is "able and willing" to purchase. A consumer's ability and willingness to pay are the important components of demand. Economics is interested in explaining actual behavior in the marketplace. At any point in time, there are many things we as consumers wish we could have but, for whatever reason, are unable to obtain. These wishes remain wishes or dreams and are not demand. Demand represents a consumer's desire for a good that can be effectively followed through with a purchase. A second point to note is that demand is measured for a specific period of time, such as a day, a month, a quarter, or a year. As we will see shortly, a consumer's desire to purchase a certain good can change, either increase or decrease, as other important factors change. So when we talk about demand, we are assuming a time period when these factors stay the same. Economists often refer to the assumption that all other factors stay the same by using a Latin phrase, *ceteris paribus,* which means literally "all other things remaining the same." Thus the law of demand postulates an inverse relationship between the price of a good and the quantity demanded, *ceteris paribus.*

There are several ways to illustrate the law of demand. Consider the demand data for aspirin, as shown in Table 8-1.

TABLE 8-1   An Individual's Demand for Aspirin*

Price per bottle ($)	Quantity demanded (bottles/month)
2	18
4	15
6	12
8	9
10	6

*Hypothetical data.

We can easily summarize the data in Table 8-1 by plotting and connecting these price-quantity combinations on a diagram with axes such as those found in Figure 8-1. The result, Figure 8-2, is called the demand curve for aspirin, line segment DD. Notice that our demand curve is consistent with the law of demand: as price falls from $10 to $6, the quantity of aspirin demanded doubles from 6 to 12 bottles; that is, there is an inverse relationship between the price and quantity of aspirin demanded. When we draw the demand curve, we are focusing solely on the relationship between price and quantity demanded; when we move along a demand curve, for example, from point V to point X, we are assuming that only the price and quantity demanded of a good change and that everything else remains the same. What are these other factors, assumed to remain constant? They are (1) prices of other goods, (2) consumer income, (3) consumer tastes or preferences for a good, and (4) consumer expectations about the future. If one of more of these factors change, the relationship of price and quantity demanded in Table 8-1 or Figure 8-2 could change. We shall examine each of these factors in detail.

Price of other goods

When we are considering the demand curve for a particular good, for example, aspirin, it is often useful to classify other goods on the basis of their relationship to the studied good, aspirin. Basically other goods can be classified in one of three ways: as *substitutes* for aspirin, as *complements* to aspirin, or as goods entirely *unrelated* to aspirin. Let us consider each of these relationships.

Good Y is a substitute for good X, if good Y can satisfy similar needs or uses as does good X. Acetaminophen may be considered a substitute for aspirin. Substitute goods vary in their ability to satisfy the same needs or uses as other goods, and to some extent, the classification of a good as a substitute for another good depends on each consumer's tastes. But how does the price of a substitute good, acetaminophen, affect the demand for aspirin? When the price of good Y, a substitute good for good X, rises, the demand for good X will increase. This can be easily illustrated in Figure 8-3. As the price of acetaminophen rises, consumers will purchase less acetaminophen, and some consumers will switch to the substitute good, aspirin. This leads to an increase in the demand for aspirin as shown by a rightward shift of the entire demand curve, DD to D'D'. This means that at any given price of aspirin (as measured on the vertical axis), the quantity of aspirin demanded (as measured on the horizontal axis) will now be larger as a result of the increase in the price of acetaminophen.

The fall in the price of a substitute good will have the opposite effect: when the price of good Y, a substitute good for good X, falls, the demand for X will decrease. Again we can illustrate this with a demand curve diagram (Figure 8-4). As the price of acetaminophen falls, some consumers of aspirin will decrease their consumption of aspirin and switch to

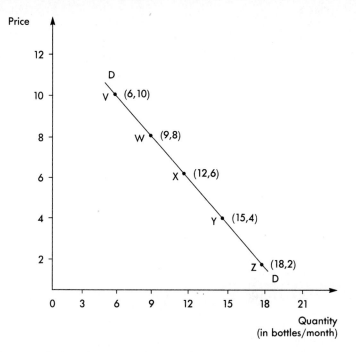

FIGURE 8-2   The law of demand postulates an inverse relationship between price and quantity demanded. Graphically, this implies that demand curves are downward sloping: as price increases (decreases), quantity demanded decreases (increases).

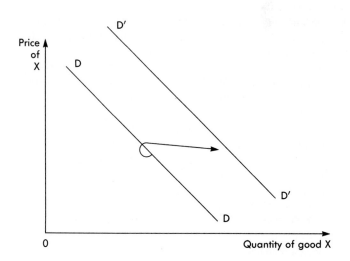

FIGURE 8-3   An increase in demand implies that at each and every price, consumers are willing to purchase more of the good or service. Graphically, an increase in demand is illustrated by a rightward shift of the demand curve. Demand for good X, a normal good, will increase if the price of a substitute good increases, the price of a complementary good decreases, or income increases.

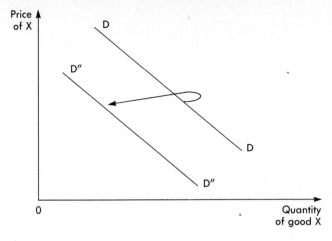

FIGURE 8-4 A decrease in demand implies that at each and every price, consumers are willing to purchase less of a good or service. Graphically, a decrease in demand is illustrated by a leftward shift of the demand curve. Demand for good X, a normal good, will decrease if the price of a substitute good decreases, the price of a complementary good increases, or income decreases.

acetaminophen. This leads to a decrease in demand for aspirin as illustrated by a leftward shift of the demand curve, from DD to D″D″. At any given price of aspirin (as measured on the vertical axis), the quantity of aspirin demanded (as measured on the horizontal axis) will be decreased, as the price of a substitute good, acetaminophen, falls.

We can summarize the impact of a change in the price of a substitute good as follows: an increase (decrease) in the price of good Y, a substitute good for good X, will lead to an increase (decrease) in the demand for good X and a rightward (leftward) shift of the demand curve for X.

A good can also be classified as a complementary good. A good, Z, is a complement to good X, if good Z can be used jointly with good X. For example, x-ray film is considered a complement to x-ray procedures. How would a change in the price of x-ray procedures affect the demand curve for x-ray film? An increase in the price of a complementary good will lead to a decrease in the demand for the good to which it is a complement. An increase in the price of an x-ray procedure might lead to a decrease in the quantity of x-ray procedures demanded and in turn, a decreased demand for x-ray film. The decrease in the demand for x-ray film is seen as a leftward shift of the demand curve, as illustrated in Figure 8-4. The opposite is also true. A decrease in the price of a complementary good will lead to an increase in the demand for the good to which it is a complement. As the price of an x-ray procedure falls, an increase in the quantity of procedures demanded will occur. This will result in an increase in the demand for x-ray film. Therefore, a decrease in the price of x-ray procedures will lead to an increase in the demand for x-ray film, and a rightward shift of the demand curve, as shown in Figure 8-3.

To summarize, an increase (decrease) in the price of a complementary good will lead to a decrease (increase) in the demand for the good to which it is a complement, and a leftward (rightward) shift of the demand curve.

Finally, it is difficult to classify some goods as either complements or substitutes to good X. These goods are basically unrelated to good X. It is difficult, for example, to find a particular relationship between x-ray procedures and calculators or aspirin and garden shears. Changes in the price of unrelated goods will leave the demand for good X unchanged.

Consumer income

There are other things that may affect the demand for good X besides the price of other goods. When we draw a demand curve, we also assume that consumers' money income is held constant. How would an increase or decrease in consumer money income affect the demand curve for a particular good? The answer depends on the characteristics of the good in question. When discussing changes in income, we are interested in two types of goods: *normal* goods and *inferior* goods.

A normal good is a good that consumers typically want more of as their income increases. Examples of normal goods include food, clothing, and education. An increase in income will lead to an increase in the demand for a normal good, and a rightward shift of the demand curve (Figure 8-3). Conversely, a decrease in income will lead to a decrease in the demand for a normal good, and a leftward shift of the demand curve (Figure 8-4). For example, if annual physical examinations are normal goods, an increase in consumer income will lead to an increase in the demand for annual physical examinations.

An inferior good, on the other hand, is a good that consumers typically want less of as their income increases or want more of as their income decreases. For example, hamburger may be considered an inferior good to many people. An increase in consumer income will lead to a decrease in the demand for hamburger as consumers increase their consumption of other, more tasty sources of protein such as tenderloin steak. Inferior good status, like beauty, is in the "eye of the beholder"; that is, one person's inferior good may be another person's normal good, and vice versa. An increase in income will lead to a decrease in the demand for an inferior good and a leftward shift of the inferior good demand curve. Conversely, a decrease in income will lead to an increase in demand for an inferior good and a rightward shift of the demand curve.

In sum, when considering the impact of income on the demand for a particular good, we need two pieces of information: the direction of the change in income (either increase or decrease) and the nature of the good in question (either a normal or an inferior good).

Consumer expectations

Another factor assumed constant when we draw an individual's demand curve for good X is his or her expectations regarding the economic future. Suppose a consumer expects the price of aspirin to increase dramatically in the future because of an expected shortage in the components used in making aspirin. This may impact the consumer's demand for aspirin today. All things remaining equal *(ceteris paribus)*, a consumer may increase his or her demand for aspirin today to avoid paying the future higher prices. Conversely, if a consumer expects prices to be lower tomorrow, he or she may decrease demand today in anticipation of future lower prices. Consumer expectations regarding income may also affect the demand for good X.

Consumer tastes

The last factor assumed constant as we move along a demand curve is consumer tastes. Over time, a consumer's taste or preference for particular goods will change. This change will in turn impact on a consumer's demand for these goods. For example, if a person becomes more health conscious, his or her preferences for fish may increase and the preference for red meat decrease. This change in consumer taste will lead to an increase in the demand for fish and a decrease in the demand for red meat.

• • •

Thus there are several factors we assume constant when we consider a consumer's demand curve: prices of other goods, income, tastes, and expectations. An important distinction is worth noting—make sure you know the difference between a change in quantity demanded

TABLE 8-2   Individual Producers' Supply for Aspirin*

Price per bottle ($)	Quantity demanded (bottles/month)
2	4
4	8
6	12
8	16
10	20

*Hypothetical data.

and a change in demand. We say a change in quantity demanded occurs when the price of the good in question (as measured on the vertical axis) changes. A change in quantity demanded is depicted graphically as a movement along a demand curve, for example, from point V to point W in Figure 8-2. On the other hand, a change in any of the other factors (prices of other goods, income, consumer tastes and expectations) will lead to a change in demand. Graphically, a change in demand is represented by a shift in the demand curve, for example, from DD to D'D' in Figure 8-3 and DD to D"D" in Figure 8-4.

Supply

So far we have focused our attention on the consumer's role in the marketplace, the demanders of goods and services. However, for markets to work, and transactions to be completed, we need to consider producers, the suppliers of goods and services. Supply may be defined as the relationship between quantities of a good that suppliers are able and willing to supply at various prices. Again, what concerns us is "effective supply," what producers can actually back up with a delivery of a product. The law of supply defines this relationship more precisely. The law of supply postulates a positive relationship between the price and quantity supplied of a product: the higher the price, the greater is the quantity supplied. Hypothetical information on aspirin production is located in Table 8-2. We can easily illustrate the concept of supply graphically by plotting this information.

If we plot the data in Table 8-2, we form the supply curve SS in Figure 8-5. Our supply curve indicates the quantities that suppliers are able and willing to supply at different prices. Notice that our diagram conforms with the law of supply: as price increases from $8 to $10, quantity supplied increases from 16 to 20 bottles. When we draw a supply curve, we assume that everything except the price of the good remains unchanged. In particular, we assume the prices that suppliers pay for inputs stay the same. If prices of inputs remain constant and the price of the product increases, producers will clearly earn increased profits per unit sold. These profits encourage producers to increase their output. This is one rationale for upward-sloping supply curves. What are the factors that remain constant when we draw a supply curve? They are (1) prices of inputs, (2) technology, (3) number of suppliers, and (4) supplier expectations. As might be expected, if one or more of these factors change, the supply of the good in question will change. Let us look at each of these factors in more detail.

Prices of inputs

The production of goods and services requires the purchase of various inputs or "factors of production." Typically, these factors of production include raw materials, fuel, labor services of individuals, machinery and equipment, and other resources. A supplier purchases these inputs to create an output of goods or services. For example, our aspirin manufacturer might

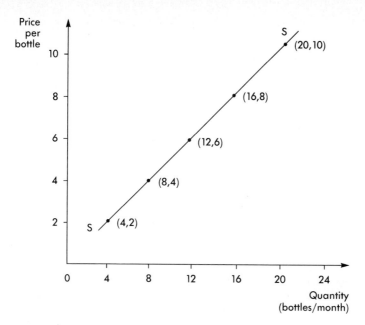

FIGURE 8-5 The law of supply postulates a direct relationship between price and quantity supplied. Graphically, this implies that supply curves are upward sloping: as price increases (decreases), quantity supplied increases (decreases).

buy machines and hire laborers to produce aspirin. If the price of machinery or labor increases, the manufacturer may not be able to buy as many of these inputs and the production of aspirin might decline; that is, an increase in input prices leads to a decrease in the quantity demanded of those inputs, and a resultant decline in the supply of the product. Graphically, this can be illustrated by a leftward shift of the supply curve from SS to S'S' as seen in Figure 8-6.

Given an increase in input prices, aspirin producers will find it profitable to reduce their output at each and every price level. Conversely, a fall in input prices can lead to the purchase of additional inputs and an increase in the production of aspirin. This will lead to a rightward shift of the supply curve from SS to S"S" as seen in Figure 8-7. As input prices fall, *ceteris paribus,* profits increase and aspirin producers are willing to supply more aspirin at each and every price.

In sum, an increase in input prices will lead to a decrease in the supply of the product that makes use of those inputs, while a decrease in input prices will result in an increase in the supply of the product.

Technology

A second factor assumed constant when we draw supply curves is technology. Technology refers to the production processes and know-how used to combine inputs to produce outputs. It is a recipe for the manufacturing firm. Technology is important because it often determines the productivity of an input. Productivity in turn refers to the output achieved per unit of input. Productivity is often measured as output per labor hour. Because an advance in technology increases productivity, it lowers the cost of producing goods and services, and suppliers will be willing to supply more output. For example, suppose our manufacturer discovers a new, less wasteful way to combine aspirin's chemical components. This new technique may increase the firm's output of aspirin even though the number of inputs stays the same.

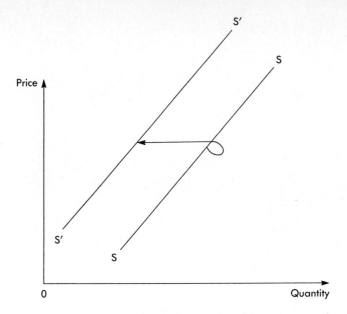

FIGURE 8-6 A decrease in supply implies that at each and every price, suppliers are willing to supply less of the good or service. Graphically, a decrease in supply is illustrated by a leftward shift of the supply curve. Supply of a good may decrease if the price of inputs used to make the good increase, the number of suppliers decrease, technology changes, or supplier expectations change.

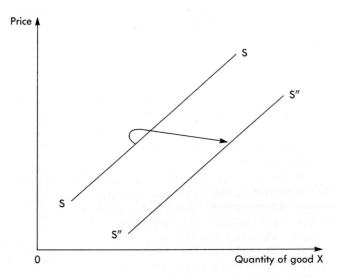

FIGURE 8-7 An increase in supply implies that at each and every price, suppliers are willing to supply more of the good or service. Graphically, an increase in supply is illustrated by a rightward shift of the supply curve. Supply of a good may increase if the price of inputs used to make the good decrease, the number of suppliers increase, technology changes, or supplier expectations change.

Number of suppliers

Another factor assumed constant when we draw a supply curve is the number of suppliers in the market. The impact of the number of suppliers on market supply is straightforward: as additional producers enter the industry, the supply of the good will increase and the supply curve will shift rightward from SS to S"S", as seen in Figure 8-7. When producers leave the industry, the market supply will decrease and the supply curve will shift from SS to S'S', as shown in Figure 8-6.

Supplier expectations

Supplier expectations about the future economic situation will affect their decisions regarding product supply today. These expectations cover a wide variety of issues, including what suppliers think will happen to future input and product prices, future consumer demand for their product, and future actions of their competitors. How these expectations will shift the supply curve depends on the particular situation. However, any movement *along* a supply curve assumes supplier expectations remain unchanged.

• • •

To summarize, supply curves reflect a direct, or positive, relationship between product price and quantity supplied. A *change in quantity supplied* refers to a *movement along* a supply curve. This occurs whenever the price of the product in question changes. A *change in supply,* on the other hand, results in a *shift* of the supply curve. A change in supply occurs whenever input prices, technology, the number of suppliers, or supplier expectations change.

MARKET EQUILIBRIUM

Now that we have discussed in detail how various consumer actions can be summarized and demonstrated in demand curves, and various producer actions can be summarized and demonstrated in supply curves, what happens if we analyze the actions of consumers and suppliers concurrently? Can we use our techniques of supply and demand to understand how markets work? You bet we can! We can use our supply and demand curves to illustrate how suppliers and consumers interact to determine the amount of a good sold in the market, and the price at which that amount will be sold. Once this price and quantity are determined, the market is said to be in *equilibrium.* Once market equilibrium is achieved, there is no tendency for price, quantity supplied, or quantity demanded to change.

Equilibrium Price and Quantity

To understand the mechanics of equilibrium price and quantity determination, one combines *market* supply and demand data, as seen in Table 8-3. Columns 1 and 2 are similar to the data used to construct the demand curve in Figure 8-2; columns 1 and 3 are similar to the data used to construct the supply curve in Figure 8-5. The important difference between Tables 8-1, 8-2, and 8-3 is worth noting: Table 8-3 contains *market* data for all consumers and all producers, while the previous tables contain information for an *individual* consumer and producer.

To understand how our producers and consumers arrive at an equilibrium price and quantity, suppose an imaginary auctioneer starts the bidding in the market at a price of $2. At that price, consumers in the market would be willing to purchase 18,000 bottles of aspirin per month, while suppliers are only willing to supply 4000 bottles of aspirin at that price. Some consumers will be unable to buy the aspirin they want, and a shortage will develop. A shortage exists whenever the quantity demanded by consumers in a market exceeds the quantity supplied

TABLE 8-3 Market Supply and Demand Data for Aspirin*

(1) Price per bottle ($)	(2) Quantity demanded (bottles/ month)	(3) Quantity supplied (bottles/ month)	(4) Shortage (−) or surplus (+)	(5) Price change required to establish equilibrium
2	18,000	4,000	14,000 (−)	Increase
4	15,000	8,000	7,000 (−)	Increase
6	12,000	12,000	0	No change
8	9,000	16,000	7,000 (+)	Decrease
10	6,000	20,000	14,000 (+)	Decrease

*Hypothetical data.

by producers in the market. A similar situation exists at a price of $4: consumers demand 15,000 bottles of aspirin, producers supply only 8000 bottles, and a shortage of 7000 bottles develops. To eliminate these shortages, the price of aspirin must increase. As the price of aspirin increases, the quantity of aspirin demanded by consumers falls and the quantity of aspirin supplied by producers increases; that is, the increase in price reduces and eventually eliminates the shortage. Suppose price increases to $8: consumers demand only 9000 bottles of aspirin, while suppliers are willing to sell 16,000 bottles of aspirin. Producers are unable to sell all their aspirin, and a surplus of 7000 bottles develops. A surplus exists whenever the quantity supplied in a market exceeds the quantity demanded in the market. At higher prices, the situation only gets worse: when the price is $10, quantity demanded is 6000, quantity supplied is 20,000, and a surplus of 14,000 bottles exists. To eliminate these surpluses, producers must reduce prices. As price decreases, the quantity supplied by producers decreases and the quantity demanded by consumers increases; that is, the decrease in price reduces and eventually eliminates the surplus. When the price of aspirin is $6, the quantity demanded by consumers is 12,000 bottles and the quantity supplied by producers is 12,000 bottles; that is, every consumer who is willing to pay at least $6 for a bottle of aspirin can purchase aspirin, and every supplier who is willing to supply a bottle of aspirin for at most $6 can do so. Since the quantity supplied in the market just equals the quantity demanded in the market, there is neither a shortage nor a surplus of aspirin; consumers are happy, producers are happy, and *ceteris paribus,* there is no reason to expect the quantity or price in the market to change. This is market equilibrium. A price of $6 is a market clearing or equilibrium price, that is, the price at which quantity demanded in the market just equals the quantity supplied in the market.

Figure 8-8 combines our supply and demand schedules and graphically illustrates the process of adjustment to equilibrium. Market equilibrium is indicated by the intersection of the market demand curve DD and the market supply curve SS at point E. The equilibrium price is $6 and the equilibrium quantity is 12,000. At prices above equilibrium price, quantity supplied exceeds quantity demanded and a surplus exists. To sell their output, producers will compete with each other by lowering their prices. As price falls, the surplus is eliminated and equilibrium is achieved. At prices below the equilibrium price, quantity demanded exceeds quantity supplied and a shortage exists. Consumers will compete with each other to get the scarce output that exists, thereby bidding up product price. As price increases, the shortage is eliminated and equilibrium is established. Once the market achieves equilibrium, quantity demanded equals quantity supplied, and there is no tendency for either price or quantity to change.

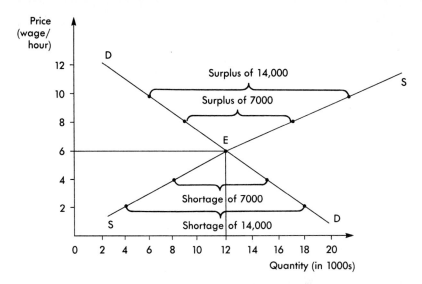

Price (wage/hour) axis with values 12, 10, 8, 6, 4, 2. Labels: D, Surplus of 14,000, S, Surplus of 7000, E, Shortage of 7000, S, Shortage of 14,000, D. Quantity (in 1000s) axis: 0 2 4 6 8 10 12 14 16 18 20.

FIGURE 8-8 Market equilibrium is established at a price wherein quantity demanded just equals quantity supplied. Graphically, this is illustrated at point E, the intersection of the supply and demand curves at the equilibrium price of $6, where quantity supplied equals quantity demanded equals 12,000. At prices greater than $6, a surplus occurs and at prices less than $6 a shortage occurs.

CHANGES IN SUPPLY AND DEMAND

We can use our supply and demand diagram to illustrate the demand and supply concepts we developed earlier. In particular, we will use our market tools to analyze the market for nursing services.

The services of nursing professionals are inputs into the provision of health care. Hospitals, long-term care facilities, and visiting nurse associations are just some of the demanders of nursing services. The demand for nursing services is often referred to as a derived demand, because the demand for nursing services is derived from the demand for health care. The suppliers of nursing services are graduates of nursing schools who decide how many hours in a given week they will devote to their chosen profession. Figure 8-9 illustrates a hypothetical market for nursing services. The vertical axis measures the price of nursing services, the wage, in dollars per hour, while the horizontal axis measures the quantity of nursing services in thousands of hours per month. Market equilibrium is established at a price of $15 per hour and quantity of 60,000 hours per month.

Changes in Demand

Consider first an expected increase in the number of senior citizens. Because senior citizens are major consumers of medical services, an increase in the older population will lead to an increase in the demand for nursing services. This is illustrated in Figure 8-10 as a rightward shift of the demand curve: at every possible price the quantity of nursing services demanded is now larger. In particular, at the initial equilibrium price of $15 per hour, the quantity demanded will increase from 60,000 to 82,000 hours per month. At this price the quantity demanded will now exceed the quantity supplied, and there is a shortage of 22,000 hours. This shortage is the difference between point A on D″D″ and the initial equilibrium, point E, on the supply curve SS. As the result of the shortage, the employers of nursing services, hospitals,

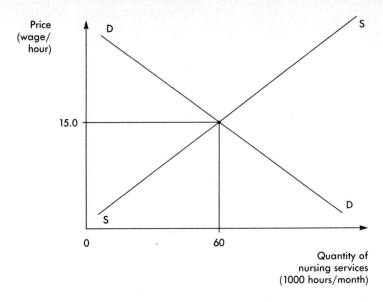

Price (wage/hour)

15.0

0   60

Quantity of
nursing services
(1000 hours/month)

FIGURE 8-9 The graph represents a market equilibrium for nursing services. The quantity of nursing service is measured in thousands of hours per month, and the price of nursing services, the wage, is measured in dollars per hour. Equilibrium is established at a price of $15 per hour; at this wage the quantity of nursing services demanded equals the quantity of nursing supplied equals 60,000 hours.

long-term care facilities, and others will be willing to pay a higher price for nursing services so that they can staff their facilities. When nurses' wages are eventually bid up high enough, equilibrium will once again be established. The new equilibrium is a point E′, the intersection of D″D″, the new demand curve, and SS, the supply curve. The new equilibrium price is $17.50 per hour, and the new equilibrium quantity demanded and supplied is 75,000 hours. An increase in demand, represented by a rightward shift in the demand curve, will increase both price and quantity of nursing services, assuming other things remain the same.

Many other factors could lead to a change in demand for nursing services. For example, a decrease in the wage of other health care workers could lead to a decrease in the demand for nurses, as relatively less expensive health aides and other adjunct health care workers are used to provide services once provided by nurses. A decrease in the income of health care consumers could also lead to a change in the demand for nursing services.

Changes in Supply

We can also use our supply and demand curve diagram to illustrate the impact of a change in supply on a market. Suppose, as a result of the recent nursing shortage, many hospitals begin to subsidize the educational cost of nursing training. For example, hospitals may pay tuition expenses if nursing students agree to work at the hospital after graduation. This subsidization of nursing education will lead to an increase in the supply of nursing services, as prospective students enter nursing to take advantage of the lower education costs. Graphically, the subsidization of nursing education will shift the supply curve SS to the right, to S′S′, in Figure 8-11.

Our initial equilibrium in Figure 8-11 is exactly the same as our initial equilibrium in Figure 8-9: equilibrium price is $15 per hour and equilibrium quantity is 60,000 hours per month, as

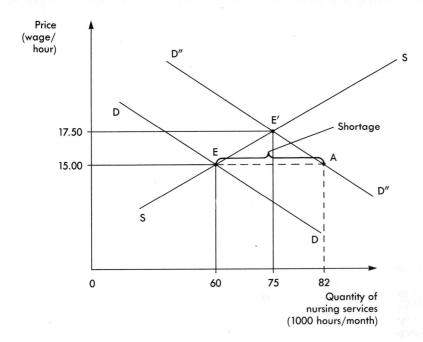

Price
(wage/
hour)

D″

S

D

E′

17.50

Shortage

E

A

15.00

D″

S

D

0

60

75

82

Quantity of
nursing services
(1000 hours/month)

FIGURE 8-10   The market is initially in equilibrium at point E, the intersection of the market demand curve DD and the market supply curve SS; equilibrium price is $15 and equilibrium quantity is 60,000. An increase in demand is indicated by a rightward shift of the demand curve DD to D′D′. At the initial equilibrium price of $15 a shortage of 22,000 hours develops (point E to point A). Employers unable to obtain these needed nursing services bid up the wage. As the wage rises, the quantity of nursing services demanded decreases (point A to point E′), and the quantity of nursing services increase (point E to point E′) just until the new equilibrium is established at a wage of $17.50 and quantity demanded equals quantity supplied equals 75,000 hours.

shown at point E. The subsidization of nursing education and the increase in prospective nursing students will eventually lead to an increase in nursing services and a rightward shift of the supply curve from SS to S′S′. At every possible price, suppliers will now increase the quantity of nursing services they are willing to supply. In particular, at the initial equilibrium price of $15 per hour, they are now willing to supply 85,000 hours of nursing services per month. At this wage, hospitals will only be willing to hire 60,000 hours of nursing services. The quantity supplied therefore exceeds the quantity demanded and a surplus of 25,000 hours, as illustrated by the distance between points B and E, will occur. Unable to find work, some nurses will be willing to work for less than $15 per hour, and the price of nursing services will eventually be bid down to $13.50 per hour. At this price, quantity demanded of nursing services will again equal quantity of nursing services supplied and market equilibrium is restored. The new equilibrium point is now at the intersection of DD and S′S′, indicated by point E′. At the new equilibrium price of $13.50 per hour, the equilibrium quantity bought and sold will be 72,000 hours per month. Hence an increase in supply represented by a rightward shift in the supply curve will decrease price and increase quantity, assuming other things remain the same.

We could easily use our demand-supply diagram to illustrate a decrease in the supply of nursing services. In particular, a decrease in the supply of nursing services will shift the supply curve up and to the left of the original supply curve. The new equilibrium will occur at a higher

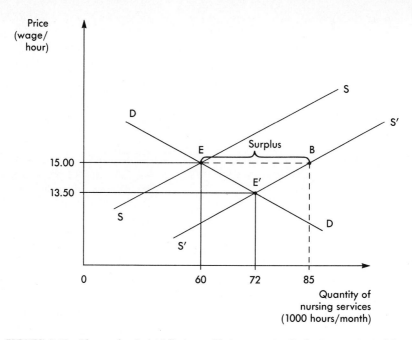

FIGURE 8-11   The market is initially in equilibrium at point E, the intersection of the market demand curve DD and the market supply curve SS; equilibrium price is $15 and equilibrium quantity is 60,000. An increase in supply as indicated by a rightward shift of the supply curve SS to S'S'. At the initial price of $15 a surplus of 25,000 hours develops (point E to point B). Nurses unable to find work at $15 per hour begin to accept lower paying positions. As the wage falls, the quantity of nursing services supplied falls (point B to point E') and the quantity of nursing services demanded increases (point B to point E') just until the new equilibrium is established at a wage of $13.50 and quantity demanded equals quantity supplied equals 72,000 hours.

price and lower quantity than in our initial equilibrium. From your experience in nursing, you might be able to think of a scenario that could explain this decrease in supply.

PRODUCTION THEORY AND COST ANALYSIS

Supply and demand analysis provides some important insight into the interactions of consumers and producers, as well as the determination of equilibrium price and quantity. For purposes of our analysis, we assumed that consumers knew the particular combinations of price and quantity demanded that traced out the demand curve for a particular good. Similarly, we assumed that producers knew the particular combinations of price and quantity supplied that traced out the supply curve. In reality consumers and producers gain this knowledge through a complex series of choices. In this section we discuss some of the important issues and choices producers face when they decide the quantity of a good to supply at a particular price. As a provider of health services, these issues will also be important to you throughout your career.

Production Theory

The providers of health care services, whether an entire hospital, a specific nursing unit within a hospital, or even an individual health care professional, face many decisions when providing health care services. What type of service should we provide and how should we

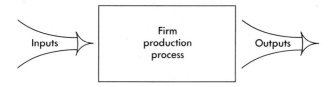

FIGURE 8-12 A representation of the process of choosing services facing health care providers.

provide the chosen service (for example, what combination of medical treatments and services of health care professionals leads to the desired outcome?)? Figure 8-12 provides a simple representation of the process faced by health care providers. There are literally thousands of "inputs" used to produce health care services: medical supplies such as bandages and splints, drugs, the services of health care professionals, and medical equipment such as computed tomography (CT) scanners, laboratory instruments, and so on. There are also as many health service outputs: a "hospital patient day," an "inpatient physician consultation," a physician or clinic "office visit," or a particular test or medical procedure. The job of the health care provider is to select the particular set of inputs that *best* produces a given output. In addition to achieving the best possible clinical outcomes, there are two important economic criteria that will help guide the health care provider in this selection process: technology and economic efficiency.

In our discussion of the supply curve of the firm, we defined technology as the product processes and know-how of the firm. It is the recipe that health care providers use to combine inputs to produce the desired health service outputs. Technology sets the boundaries between the possible and impossible ways to combine inputs to achieve outputs. Therefore our first insight into the determination of the particular quantity supplied of a good involves technology: producers will make the best use of the available technology to combine inputs to provide the feasible set of outputs. Still there are many feasible outputs, and many different combinations of inputs that lead to the same output. For example, a variety of different combinations of RNs, LPNs, and NAs could conceivably be used to provide the nursing services needed on a unit. How do health care providers choose the "best" combination of inputs to provide a particular service? Our second important criterion, economic efficiency, will guide our health care providers in selecting the best combination of inputs.

One of the goals of a health care provider is economic efficiency. What is economic efficiency? *Economic efficiency* is providing the "correct" amount of a good or a service to the "right" consumer at the lowest possible cost. Our definition of economic efficiency has two components, *allocative efficiency*, providing the correct amount of a good or service to the consumers who value the good the most, and *technical efficiency*, producing the good or service at the lowest possible cost. In the face of society's unlimited wants, but scarce and limited resources, it is important to produce the desired level of health services in the most efficient manner.

Now we have another important insight to guide our health care provider in combining inputs to produce health services that can be achieved at the lowest possible cost, given the technically feasible combination of inputs and given input prices. In selecting the least-cost combination of inputs, a health care provider may find it useful to consult other professionals: industrial engineers, who measure technical efficiency in terms of physical units of output, and time and motion analysts, who determine the maximum output achieved for a given combination of inputs. Armed with this technical information, input prices, and legal and standard practices of the health care professional, the health care provider selects the combination of inputs that produces a given service at the lowest possible cost. Thus the economically efficient combination of inputs is the least-cost combination of inputs. To determine the economic efficiency of a particular combination of inputs, it is important to know something about the costs of production. However, the question remains, What is cost?

Cost Analysis

To the economist, the *total cost* of production can be thought of as the market value of the inputs (resources) used in producing the desired output. Costs can be further classified as either fixed or variable. *Fixed costs* are those costs that do not vary with the level of output. Examples might include the lease on a building, debt finances, insurance costs, and the like. *Variable costs* are those costs that vary with the level of output. Examples include labor costs (the wage bill), the cost of supplies and materials, and the operating cost of medical equipment. It is important to be able to define and classify the costs of a firm: understanding a firm's cost structure helps us to describe the economic behavior of the firm and evaluate its use of its scarce resources.

LIMITATIONS OF ECONOMIC THEORY

Before we discuss the solution of our case study in the next section, it is important to discuss some of the limitations of economic theory. In an effort to "describe how things work," economic theory simplifies reality by focusing on the most fundamental and crucial elements of a situation. The complicating "real-world" details are set aside in order to emphasize a few principles that will guide our analysis. Applied economic research involves taking these theoretical principles and applying them in real-world situations together with their complicating details. As you might imagine, this is often a difficult task. The leap from economic theory to applied economic analysis is more difficult in the health industry than in many other U.S. industries. Three factors contribute to this difficulty: lack of clear profit maximization motive in the health industry, physician influence on the demand for health care, and complications surrounding the market price of health services.

Economic theory relies heavily on the profit motive to describe the behavior of firms. Firms evaluate their options on the basis of their impact on profits: a particular option is worthwhile if it increases profits. The health care industry differs for a number of reasons. Price is not market determined, and although health care facilities often seek to have revenue greater than costs, in the strictest sense, profit maximization is not the primary objective. Providing high-quality, comprehensive health care services, regardless of individual profitability, is often more important. Much of the health industry has a nonprofit orientation since a majority of U.S. hospitals are not-for-profit firms. In addition, there are other goals and objectives that provide the focus and direction for health care facilities. These objectives, often established by the hospital board of directors and medical staff, are not necessarily economic in scope, such as increasing the prestige of the hospital by providing costly new procedures or providing high-quality health care to large indigent populations.

The second factor that complicates the use of economic theories in the health industry is physician influence on the demand for health care. Many of the decisions to obtain particular medical care or treatment are orchestrated not by the ultimate consumer, the patient, but by physicians and other health care providers. For example, the method of treatment and hospital admission and discharge decisions are made by physicians, not patients. This complicates the supply and demand analysis of the health field by blurring the distinction between health care demanders and health care suppliers.

Finally, there are many factors that complicate the determination of price in the market for health services. In many cases, market price has only limited impact on the quantity of health services demanded: private and governmental health insurance coverage largely reduces the market price of health care, leaving the insured patient with lower out-of-pocket costs. The role of suppliers in determining the market price of health services is complicated by the limited number of health care providers. Many communities or markets for health care have only one or two hospitals. The smaller the number of health care facilities in a market, the greater the influence of these facilities on market price.

Given these complications—lack of profit motive in the health industry, physician influence on the demand for health care, and complications surrounding the market price for health services—an applied economic analysis of our case study requires careful thought and creativity. Our economic theories will give us basic principles to guide our analysis, but they will not exactly address all the complicating details of a particular situation or environment. Nonetheless the economic theories discussed in this section provide a useful starting point for the analysis of our case study, which follows.

CASE ANALYSIS

In designing the study requested by the administrator, two methodological problems arose: (1) How does one determine or estimate the hospital costs incurred in providing services to obstetrical patients, and (2) How does one control for patient severity or acuity to ensure that patients in the cooperative care unit and the inpatient hospital unit whose costs are being compared are actually medically similar.

Unlike other industries, hospitals have traditionally not been overly concerned with being able to determine the actual or true costs of producing individual units of medical care. There is a clear problem with cost data availability. Therefore, to estimate the cost-effectiveness of the cooperative care unit (problem 1 in methodology), it was necessary to calculate a *proxy measure* (measure to approximate) for the economic costs of production. A major obstacle to this effort in the health care sector is that, unlike other profit-seeking industries, there is no uniform cost-accounting methodology existing that will determine these economic costs. However, there are methods that can be used to estimate hospital costs. In this case, average hospital production costs for obstetrical patients using both the cooperative care unit and the traditional hospital inpatient unit were estimated using the ratio-of-cost-to-charge (RCC) accounting method.* As required in the hospital's annual *Medicare Cost Report,* the costs of labor, supplies, and other direct expenses taken as a whole, are divided among the major cost centers within the institution. Some of these centers, such as the laboratory and the operating rooms, are considered revenue centers because they provide direct medical services that appear as identifiable line items on a patient's bill. Other cost centers, such as housekeeping and general administration, do not bill directly but pass on their expenses in a step-down fashion to the revenue centers. These allocated indirect costs (not directly related to revenue-generating patient services) are added to the direct costs to derive an estimate of total costs for a given center. Within a given center, total cost can be compared with total charges (i.e., the total amount that patients are billed for services rendered by the center). More important, these two figures—costs generated and charges billed—can be used to form a ratio of cost to charge (RCC) for each center. The RCC provides a basis for estimating the cost of the hospital of treating an individual patient. This is accomplished by multiplying the ratios for each center by the

---

*For more details on hospital cost accounting see Neumann, B.R., Suver, J.D. & Zellman, W.N. (1984). *Financial management: Concepts and applications for health care providers.* Owings Mills, MD: National Health Publishing, or Berman, J.H., & Weeks, L.E. (1982). *The financial management of hospitals.* Ann Arbor, MI: Health Administration Press.

corresponding charge for that center as recorded on the patient's bill. For example, using the hospital's hypothetical current fiscal year cost-to-charge ratio of 0.772437 for the labor and delivery center, one would calculate that a patient with a labor and delivery *charge* of $700 would have generated labor and delivery *costs* of 0.772437 × $700 or $540.71. Since each center defines its own units of service for billing purposes, such as days of routine nursing care, minutes of operating room time, or number of laboratory tests, the total cost as derived above for a given patient is directly related to the resources consumed by the patient. In addition to providing an estimate of total cost per patient, the RCC methodology permits a more detailed breakdown of costs into four categories:

1. Direct expenditures of labor and fringe benefits
2. Direct expenditures for supplies
3. Other direct expenditures
4. Allocated indirect expenditures (i.e., overhead costs generated by nonrevenue centers)

These direct and indirect costs should not be confused with the fixed and variable economic costs discussed earlier. The terms *direct costs* and *indirect costs* refer to the accounting costs derived from the RCC methodology. Both direct (patient revenue–related) costs and indirect (nonpatient revenue) costs consist of fixed and variable economic costs. The economic costs relate individual costs to volume of output, while the accounting costs relate individual costs to specific patient revenue–producing and nonrevenue cost centers.

To control for patient severity or acuity (methodological problem 2), obstetrical patients were classified into one of three groups depending on the nature of the delivery: normal, complex, and intraabdominal surgery. As expected, for all obstetrical patients normal deliveries were the least costly, averaging $1309 per case; complex deliveries were more costly at $1489 per case, and those patients requiring intraabdominal surgery were the most costly at $1974 per case. However, for many of the components tested, there were also significant main effects of group. With respect to total cost, patients in the hospital group had an overall average cost of $1508 as compared with an average for the cooperative care group of $1368. Further analysis showed that for both the normal and the complex obstetrical deliveries, there were definite cost savings accruing to the cooperative care patient. These cost savings result from lower costs in the following centers: anesthesiology, blood and intravenous infusions (IV), and routine services. For patients with normal deliveries, nearly two thirds of the savings came from a reduction in routine service costs, and 60% of the savings for the complex cases came from routine services. However, the pattern reverses itself when one considers those patients who required intraabdominal surgery. Here, the cooperative care group had significantly higher total costs than the hospital group and, more specifically, had higher costs in the following centers: blood and IV, medical supplies, drugs, and routine services.

The intraabdominal surgery patients were different from the others with regard to their use of cooperative care, and this may explain their relatively higher costs. Most patients undergoing intraabdominal surgery remained in the hospital for their entire stay. A smaller number of patients used the cooperative care unit as a step-down facility, spending their final day or two in this unit before discharge, and these patients were probably the most severely ill in the category. However, one could hypothesize that the cooperative care for this category of patients actually produced a savings for them as well, compared with what their costs might have been had they stayed in the hospital for their entire stay.

At Metropolitan Hospital, the average cooperative care patient had $140 less in total hospital costs. When multiplied by the 576 obstetrical patients who used the unit, this amounted to a total annual resource savings for the hospital of $80,640. The total savings to the patient in hospital charges amounted to approximately $105,000.

Economic Impact

The exact number of the hospitalized obstetrical patients who were eligible for the cooperative care unit is unknown. However, if we project that 50% of the 1107 hospital patients had instead been in the cooperative care unit (554 patients), the savings would be increased by approximately $77,560. Thus with a projected 50% of the hospital patients using the unit, the combined savings in hospital costs would be approximately $158,200.

The results of this economic analysis confirm that the cooperative care program at Metropolitan Hospital resulted in lower costs to the hospital and the patient when compared with traditional inpatient care. In response to the second question, what was the reason for the decline in use, a survey of the attending physicians who admitted patients to the cooperative care unit indicated that the opening of the new hospital building was the main reason for the decline in occupancy. The new building was farther away from the cooperative care unit, which was located in a nearby hotel. From the physician's perspective, the substitute good, the inpatient unit, was preferred over the cooperative care unit. It took nearly twice as long to walk from the new building to the hotel. If a cooperative care unit is desired, it will need to be located nearer to the offices of the attending physicians. The administrator concurs and believes that more cooperative care unit beds should be made available at Metropolitan. Do you agree? What would you do?

There are a number of economic factors that must be considered before Metropolitan decides to revitalize the cooperative care unit. First, the potential cost savings to the hospital and to society is fully realized only if Metropolitan Hospital is concurrently considering an increase in obstetrical bed capacity or is planning to reduce the number of obstetrical inpatient hospital beds. There must be a relative decline in obstetrical inpatient beds to match the increase in cooperative care unit beds or else the relatively high fixed costs of the empty inpatient obstetrical beds remain. Substituting cooperative care unit beds for inpatient beds does not eliminate the fixed costs of the inpatient beds and they must be covered.

Second, one needs to examine the potential increase in demand that might occur in the future as patients and third-party payers become more aware of the potential savings. The maximum benefit comes when the patient hospitalized in the inpatient unit moves to the cooperative care unit. In addition, as physicians become more aware of the level of quality and the potential savings from using cooperative care units, increased demand may result. As the demand for the cooperative care unit increases (rightward shift of the demand curve), there will be a tendency to increase the price (charge to the patient). With costs remaining constant, this would result in higher net margins to the hospital, but could erode the cost savings and perhaps make the unit less attractive (future demand may be less).

Finally, the administrator should attempt to have the medical staff better informed about the benefits of using the unit, especially for the more complex cases. Efforts should be aimed at having all eligible patients spending a greater proportion of their hospitalization stay in the cooperative care unit. The transfer to the unit needs to take place early in the hospital stay so that the patient can take advantage of the lower costs for routine services (room and board and nursing care). An understanding of the composition of the costs of the cooperative care service and the nature of the demand for cooperative care will lead to a better decision. In health care, demand is not always the sole creation of the patient since the physician makes many of the decisions. In obstetrical care, the hospital needs to better inform both physicians and patients of the service.* The following discussion details further evidence of this need.

*For more details on the cost analysis methodology, see Lingeman, J.E., Saywell, R.M., Woods, J.R. & Newman, D.M. (1986). Cost analysis of extracorporeal shock wave lithotripsy relative to other surgical and nonsurgical treatment alternatives of urolithiasis. *Medical Care, 24*, 1151-1160.

RESEARCH

In a similar study in the same setting evaluating the cost-effectiveness of cooperative care units for gynecology patients (Saywell, Woods, & Benson, 1989), the findings indicated that there were no significant cost savings between clinically similar patients treated in the hospital or in the cooperative care unit. However, further analysis revealed that a cost savings of approximately $450 was generated for those cooperative care patients who were cared for by physicians who were frequent users of the unit. As with the obstetrical patient, most of the savings for this group was achieved through a reduction in the cost of routine services, which included nursing services. It was suggested that the contrasting results in the two studies were primarily due to differences in the features affecting demand. For the obstetrical patient, the patient plays a large role in the decision to use the unit. Many obstetrical patients enter the hospital with some information about the unit; it is a well-publicized option. With the gynecology patient, the physician is the primary decision maker regarding who is eligible to use the unit and when in the stay the patient should be transferred.

To increase use of the unit the hospital needs to:
1. Increase the amount of information available both to patients and physicians.
2. Provide economic incentives to encourage the patient to request cooperative care placement. For patients covered by health insurance, this incentive might include a portion of the "charge saving" being returned to the patient. Unless the hospital and third-party payer cost savings can be passed on to the patient, there will be less demand since there is *no* incentive to choose services that provide few amenities.

Cooperative care units have the potential to reduce the costs of hospitalizations and help alleviate the current problems associated with the nursing shortage but only if they are used to the fullest extent possible. A basic understanding of demand and supply theory *and* production and cost theory is necessary to analyze this case problem. The potential impact on price and quantity of changes in supply and demand and knowledge of the difference in fixed and variable costs is required to offer possible solutions.

REFERENCE

Saywell, R.M., Woods, J.R., & Benson, J.R. (1989). Comparative costs of a cooperative care program versus inpatient care for gynecology patients. *Journal of Nursing Administration, 19,* 29-36.

SUGGESTED READINGS
Selected Economics Texts

Burns, R.T., & Stone, A.W. (1989). *Micro economics* (4th ed.). Glenview, IL: Scott, Foresman.
Dolan, E. (1988). *Micro economics* (5th ed.). Dryden.
Mansfield, E. (1989). *Principles of economics* (6th ed.). Norton.

Other Readings

Bauerschmidt, A.D., & Jacobs, P. (1985). Pricing objectives in non-profit hospitals. *Health Services Research, 20,* 153-162.
Boulding, K. (1971). The concept of need for health services and the concept of shortage. *American Journal of Public Health, 61,* 46-63.
Brown, M.C. (1980). Production and cost relations of Newfoundland's cottage hospitals. *Inquiry, 17,* 268-277.
Daus, K., & Russell, L.B. (1972). The substitution of hospital outpatient care for inpatient care. *Review of Economics and Statistics, 54,* 109-120.
Feldstein, P.J. (1988). *Health care economics* (3rd ed.). New York: John Wiley & Sons.
Goldfarb, M.G., & Coffey, R.M. (1987). Case-mix differences between teaching and non-teaching hospitals. *Inquiry, 24,* 68-84.

Hemenway, D., & Fallon, D. (1985). Testing for physician-induced demand with hypothetical cases. *Medical Care,* *23,* 344-349.

Jones, K.R. (1985). Predicting hospital change and stay variation. *Medical Care, 23,* 220-235.

McGuire, A. (1985). The theory of the hospital: A review of models. *Social Science and Medicine, 20,* 1177-1184.

Wennberg, J.E., Barnes, B.A., & Zubkoff, M. (1982). Professional uncertainty and the problem of supplier-induced demand. *Social Science and Medicine, 16,* 811-824.

Wyszewranski, L., Thomas, J.W., & Friedman, B.A. (1987). Case-based payment and the control of quality and efficiency in hospitals. *Inquiry, 24,* 17-25.

PART II

ORGANIZE

Chapter 9

Theory of Bureaucracy
Max Weber

Pamela C. Levi

▌▌ CASE STUDY

A patient was admitted for an elective surgical procedure at a large urban hospital. Following an uneventful surgery and recovery room period she was admitted to a surgical neurology floor. Three hours later the patient began spiking a temperature. When the floor nurse called the surgeon's office, she was told that he was unavailable but would return the phone call. An hour later the patient's temperature was higher still, and she began to exhibit early signs of confusion. The family was becoming increasingly concerned and wanted the nurses to "do something." The floor nurse again called the physician's office and was told that the surgeon was still unavailable. The floor nurse stressed to the physician's receptionist that it was imperative that she speak with the doctor. When the receptionist refused, the floor nurse insisted she be allowed to speak with the physician's office nurse. The office nurse reaffirmed that the physician was not available. When the hospital floor nurse again explained the urgency of the patient's condition, the office nurse reluctantly admitted that the physician was not in the office and she was unaware of his whereabouts. The physician had not checked out to any other physician that she was aware of. It was now 5 PM, and the patient was becoming increasingly confused and mildly combative. The physician was in practice by himself so no partners could be contacted. The floor nurse contacted her supervisor who in turn tried once again to contact the physician. By this time the office was closed, and the answering service promised to contact the physician. The supervisor called the director of nursing at home and related the situation to her. At 7:30 PM the answering service was recontacted, and it was found that they had been unable to locate the physician. The director of nursing went to the nursing unit, assessed the patient's condition, and immediately called the hospital administrator. The hospital administrator contacted the chief of staff of the medical group. The chief of staff was in surgery and unavailable.

The operating room nurse promised to have him return the phone call as soon as he was available.

At 12 ᴀᴍ the chief of staff called the hospital administrator. The administrator shared the dilemma of what had occurred with the attending surgeon. The chief of staff called the office nurse at home and was able to find out that the patient's surgeon had left town and indeed was out of the country. She denied having knowledge of how to contact him. A very irate chief of staff then went to the nursing unit to assess the patient. The time was 1 ᴀᴍ. Instead of finding a patient very compromised for lack of medical intervention, he found instead a relatively stable, although very ill patient. Although the rules, regulations, and protocols were being followed, a parallel system of events had occurred. An informal but very real system in the hospital had been initiated. The nurses on the floor had recognized how ill the patient was becoming and had begun interventions that departed from standard operating procedures. Fluids, antibiotics, and antipyretics had been started. A surgeon who was trusted and well respected by the nurses had been contacted. Although he had no responsibility to the patient and indeed could suffer for intervening, he did agree to just "stick his head in the door" when he made his own rounds for his patients. The physician wrote orders to cover the medical interventions begun by the nurses and wrote other orders as well. The chief of staff transferred the patient to the intensive care unit at 3 ᴀᴍ, more than 12 hours after the first documentation that there was a problem. The chief of staff brought the incident to the attention of the medical staff organization. Three weeks later the physician who had left his patient unattended when he left the country received a written reprimand but no suspension of privileges.

| | | | | | | | | | | | | | | | | | | | | | | | | | | | | | | | | | | | | | | | | | | | | | | | | | | | | | | | | | | | | | | | | | | | | |

THEORY OF BUREAUCRACY

Bureaucracy has become within the last century the major characteristic of highly complex organizations. The modern world is a bureaucratic world and one in which large hierarchial organizations dominate virtually all spheres of life — from politics and production to education and leisure (Langton, 1984). With only a very few exceptions, large organizations common in today's society did not exist over a hundred years ago. For the student of nursing practice or nursing administration theory, the nature of bureaucracy as a mode of organization is therefore of critical significance.

The person generally credited with providing the classic analysis of bureaucratic structure is Max Weber (1864-1920). Writing in prewar Germany, Max Weber's thinking on bureaucracy can most appropriately be understood as an examination of the characteristics of a system of domination (Weiss, 1983). Weber, a political theorist and sociologist, did not intend to provide advice to managers but rather to address social and political concerns. From his writings, however, has emerged the most significant definition of bureaucracy (Rice & Bishoprick, 1971). Weber considered bureaucracy to be the ideal organizational form to provide a rational and predictable method for organizing the work of human beings. Weber viewed an organization as a particular type of social relationship that either is closed to outsiders or limits their admission and that has regulations enforced by an administrative head. Bureaucracies according to Weber are organizations that have been created, to a very substantial degree, through domination and calculation. Bureaucratization is, in other words, a process of organizational rationalization (Langton, 1984).

Rationalization is a concept that has emerged as a unifying theme in Weber's work. Rationalization is a multifaceted concept that includes (1) the decline of the religious world view and the rise of a rational scientific world view; (2) the decline of peasant agrarian economics and the rise of rational planned economics; (3) the rise of legal-rational authority with a bureaucratic form of administration; and (4) the decline of familial or aristocratic administration (Glassman, 1983).

The practical rational character of bureaucracy occurs because of its dependence on rules, means-end calculations, and "matter-of-factness." Bureaucracy increasingly overtakes structures that are not rational in nature. However, Weber's use of the term *rational* was not synonymous with approval or agreement with the "rightness" of all the ends pursued by bureaucracies. Rather, Weber was convinced that these ends conflicted with ethical and other human values (DeCosmo, 1987). Weber (1958) warned that the process of rationalization tended to lock human beings into an "iron cage" because within a social context, rationalization entails a constriction of options and a decrease in personal freedom and power. Rationalization of an organization in the direction of bureaucratic values makes it more difficult to achieve other competing values (Langton, 1984).

Within the process of rationalization, Weber (1958) describes "peculiar rationalism," which is a historically evolved attitude about the power of the human mind. In essence this view holds that "one can, in principle, master all things by calculation" (Weber, 1967, p. 139). Through calculation better rules, techniques, or principles can always be found for the achievement of any goal or value (Langton, 1984). The characteristics of a bureaucracy as described by Weber (1970) include:

1. A well-defined hierarchy of authority
2. A clear division of work
3. A system of rules covering the rights and duties of position incumbent
4. A system of procedures for dealing with the work situation
5. Impersonality of interpersonal relationships
6. Employment and promotion based on technical knowledge

Weber's theory emphasizes the concepts of authority, domination, command, power, and discipline. These focuses, while not appealing to those within a human relations frame of reference, are nevertheless important concepts for the study of organizational theory (Miner, 1982).

The authority that the organization has over the individual is based on the consent of the individual. According to Weber (1970), there are three bases on which individuals accept the legitimacy of authority. The first is "rational-legal authority" which consists of a body of generalized rules. These rules apply universally and impartially to all persons. Authority of the individual extends only so far as the sphere of office or legitimatized status under the rules. Outside this sphere the individual is treated with no more authority than anyone else. Each member has a specific delineation of powers and a distinct separation of the sphere of office from his or her private affairs. Different offices are organized in terms of a strict hierarchy of authority so that each lower level is subject to control and supervision by the one immediately above it. Rather than being subject to personal authority, administrative officials are subject to an impersonal order. The obligation to obey an individual above them in the hierarchy derives from the office held and not from the person.

The official must, therefore, carry out his duties *sine ira et studio,* without hatred or passion and without affection or enthusiasm (Weber, 1978). Fitness for an office is typically determined by technical competence. This competence is characterized by long periods of formalized training (Sexton, 1970).

Traditional authority, the second type of authority identified by Weber, is based on the sanctity of long-standing rules and powers, on tradition and custom. Traditional authority attaches to the person, not the position. To some extent, tradition may specify the extent of the authority, but there may also be a wide range for individual discretion. Traditional authority tends to be present in family-owned business (Miner, 1982).

Charismatic authority, the third type of authority described by Weber, is also attached to the person and not the position. The great leader, the magnetic personality, will attract people who will follow. Authority is accepted as a result of the person's past record of accomplishments or trust in the person's ability and intention to do the right thing (Rice & Bishoprick, 1971). The powers on which the charisma is based must be frequently demonstrated and serve the needs of the followers if the authority is to continue. Irrationality and emotional ties are more prevalent, while economic considerations are devalued (Miner, 1982).

In practice these different types of authority may exist in the same organization. Rational-legal authority tends to become infused with tradition over time, and bureaucratic organizations tend to be headed at the top level by charismatic leaders (Miner, 1982).

Weber proposed that bureaucratic administration fundamentally attains domination through knowledge (Weiss, 1983). The amount of knowledge and the speed needed to transmit and interpret this knowledge into objective decisions for the organization require a structure supportive of the process. The rapid advancement of the bureaucratic organizational form is due to its suitability for this task, namely, its technical superiority over any other organizational form. The objective discharge of business also requires a structure and process that function according to calculable rules and eliminate from official business all purely personal, irrational, or emotional elements. This is appraised as bureaucracy's special virtue (Sexton, 1970). The result is a climate of formal impersonality. Movement toward such a state is influenced by growth of the organization and as a result of the administrative task to be accomplished (Miner, 1982).

Theoretical elaborations on Weber's theory have been numerous and varied. Many have dealt with the dysfunctional nature of bureaucracy. One of the most significant contributors was Peter Blau. Of particular importance to health care administrators is Blau's attention to the value and role of professionals within an organization. Blau (1974) contends that professional knowledge may enter an organization at relatively low levels on the hierarchical structure. Under such conditions the person in the chain of command may be an expert on the rules/regulations/procedures of the organization but not knowledgeable on the problem in question if the problem is within the professional knowledge realm. Blau recognized this and viewed professional authority as separate from the rational-legal authority described by Weber.

Victor Thompson (1961) also dealt with the concentration of knowledge in specialists and professionals who do not have significant positions of authority. According to Thompson the major problem of modern bureaucracies is the imbalance between ability and authority. This results in continuing confusion and conflict. The rights and responsibilities of the hierarchical superior and the specialized ability and knowledge to solve the problem are vested in different people. Often a supervisor reacts to this situation with an excessive need for control and an exaggerated emphasis on rules, resistance to change, and insistence on the rights of office (Miner, 1982). Thompson describes the resulting behavior as typified by anxiety and insecurity. He suggests establishing two equal salary scales, one for the professionals and one for those in the hierarchy. He also suggests giving persons in supervisory positions some instrumental functions in addition to the exercise of authority. An example of this is the chairperson position in the college setting. The person occupying this position is a member of the hierarchy who also continues to teach and thus remains a part of the professional faculty as well.

Thompson (1961) considered professionalism an alternative to bureaucracy. Professionalizing an organization decreases administration, top-down command, and unquestioning obedience; it improves communication and decreases conflict between units in the organization

(Miner, 1982). Miner (1980) found that the kinds of characteristics that make for managerial effectiveness in bureaucracies are generally distinct from those making for effectiveness in a professional role.

Mahmoudi and Miller (1985) investigated whether hospital organizations have structural characteristics similar to more traditional bureaucratic organizations. When nonprofessional organizations were compared with the hospital structural arrangements, the findings suggest that the theoretical models of organizational structure are relevant to professional organizations. They also indicate that as hospitals grow larger and more specialized, they rely on formalization and automation as impersonal mechanisms of control. Hospitals resemble traditional bureaucratic organizations in this respect. The study goes on to state that the implications for workers may be different, however, since the use of professional standards and rules (an extension of professionalism within the hospital) eliminates somewhat the need for personal supervision and control.

The current knowledge base supports bureaucracy as the structure of choice for large organizations primarily because few alternatives are available. Nonbureaucratic forms of governance seem more suited to small organizations. Critics of bureaucracy state that frequently strict adherence to rules reduces spontaneity, causes rigidity, and discourages innovation. Unless members of the organization have freedom and the initiative to deal with operating problems as they come up, efficiency suffers. Another criticism is that no system's rules and supervision can be so finely written that all situations can be anticipated (Blau & Meyer, 1971). Others contend that employee satisfaction is a component of an effective organization. Winters (1983) found a negative correlation between bureaucratic structure and teacher job satisfaction.

Curry et al. (1986) studied the causal ordering of job satisfaction and organizational commitment in 508 professional hospital employees, 67% of whom were registered nurses. The authors stated that in service organizations such as hospitals, effectiveness and efficiency are related to high employee morale because the services rendered are personal and labor-intensive.

A hierarchy of authority in a bureaucracy is essential for coordination of a complex organization but often produces among the lower level hierarchical workers feelings of apathy and dissatisfaction that impede identification with the organization's objectives. Finally in a democratic society, independence of action as well as equality status are valued. Close supervision is resented and employees tend to become poorly motivated (Blau & Meyer, 1971). Informal relations in work groups can reduce these disruptive tendencies. Once cohesive groups exist in the bureaucracy, they will develop their own standards of conduct and enforce them among its members (Blau & Meyer, 1971). Curry et al. (1986) found a significant association between kinship and satisfaction.

As early as 1954, Gouldner contended that work rules provide cues for employees. Rules establish what unacceptable behavior is and what minimum standards are. Dressler (1980) supports this supposition and gives the example of employees who are told by their manager that they can take only 1 hour for lunch. The manager will find that they rarely take more, but also never less. Katz & Kahn (1966) emphasize:

> For effective organizational functioning, many members must be willing on occasion to do more than their job descriptions specify. If members of the system were to follow the precise letter of job descriptions and organizational protocol, things would soon grind to a halt. Many acts of spontaneous cooperation and many anticipations of organizational objectives are required to make the system viable. (p. 99)

Certainly in the case study described the need to go beyond the minimum expected behavior in order to meet the needs of the hospital organization is evidenced.

CASE ANALYSIS

The case study of the absent physician and the seriously ill patient is an example of how the professional organization, which does not lie entirely within the strictly hierarchical component of the hospital, affects the outcomes of that organization. In the described hospital situation the chain of command is staff nurse, head nurse (or charge nurse), supervisor, director of nursing to hospital administrator; it is a very traditional hierarchy that incorporates individuals who have varying degrees of technical expertise (i.e., knowledge of the standard of care needed). The nursing department within this hospital, like many others, is highly bureaucratized with a variety of relatively independent and clearly defined positions having been established to accomplish the tasks assigned to it. Technical competence frequently establishes an individual's position within the hierarchy. This is congruent with Weber's conceptualization of a bureaucracy as having a well-defined hierarchy of authority and of employment and promotion within the organization being based on technical knowledge. The hospital administrator has final authority within the formal hospital organization. The hospital administrator derives his or her authority from two sources: from legal (positional) authority and from traditional authority. Originally nurses and physicians made up the hospital staff, and nurses carried out the majority of administrative tasks. As hospitals expanded, a separate administrative department was established, but certain aspects of the previous relationship were retained, thus blending traditional authority with legal authority (Malone, 1964). The administrator is dependent, however, on the professional nursing staff to bring to his or her attention a problem with patient care and when a breach of operating procedure with patient care occurs. The professional nurses within the system have an obligation to the organization to protect the interest of that organization. The professional nurse also has an obligation to the client/patient to provide a level of care protective of and beneficial to the patient. The professional nurse has an obligation to the physician as well, which places her or him at the bottom of three lines of authority—that of the hospital administrator, the physician, and the nursing department. This arrangement is not typical of Weber's hierarchical structure. In the case study described these sets of obligations came in conflict.

Procedures within the hospital call for the nurse with primary responsibility for the patient to report any untoward observations to the physician in charge of that patient. If the physician cannot be contacted, then policy dictates that the nurse will report this fact to her or his immediate supervisor, who will attempt to contact the physician. This pattern will continue up the hierarchy until resolution of the problem occurs.

Professional nurses occupy a unique and important position in the modern hospital organization. They are employees of and subject to all rules and regulations of the organization. They are also members of a professional group apart from the hospital structure that is regulated and controlled by a governmental agency, the licensing board of the state. Governmental rules and regulations supersede those of the employing agency. Additionally, many professional nurses identify very strongly with a professional code of ethics that may influence their decision to adhere or not to adhere to any organizational rule or regulation in a specific situation. Although they are rarely cited on organizational charts as appearing within the administrative line, much of their activity is administrative in nature. This is particularly evident at the end of an ordinary work day when members of many other groups leave the hospital and the nursing staff assumes major administrative responsibilities for the hospital (Malone, 1964).

Physicians in the hospital organizations, on the other hand, are often not employees of the hospital but rather are "customers" whose needs and wishes are accommodated whenever possible. No group within the hopsital has power over physicians. Generally physicians spend only a small fraction of their total workday in the institution, yet they are frequently the most powerful group in the organization. Because physicians are not employees, they are not subordinate to the authority of the administrator. Legally their responsibility is to the patient (Malone, 1964). Physicians frequently enjoy a blended authority base. Traditional authority exists because of the historical close alliance between nursing and medicine. Rational-legal authority exists because of the rules governing the responsibilities and rights inherent in the physician role. Charismatic authority may exist because of the physician's demonstrated skill or personality. Because hospitals compete for physicians and thus the patients that the physician admits, a host-guest relationship frequently occurs. The physician in the case study was one who admitted many patients to the hospital and thus generated considerable income for the hospital. The hospital competed with many other hospitals in the same geographical location and was having difficulty in maintaining economic solvency. The loss of the physician's patients to the institution would cause significant financial loss. The professional nurses recognized this and were for the most part very loyal to the institution. The nurses were also aware of this physician's fairly cavalier attitude toward his patients, and they had in the past engaged in "smoothing over" unhappy patients who disliked their treatment by the physician. The physician was frequently difficult to locate, and many of the nurses believed his patients did less well than they should have.

Weber's conception of a bureaucracy as being without emotion is not manifest in this case study. Emotionalism was very high. Detachment and objectivity were not characteristic of the environment in which decision making was occurring.

The professional nurses were angry at the physician's behavior and believed that the hierarchical process they needed to go through to obtain resolution was taking too long. The nurses were frightened that the patient's condition might become critical and that they would be held responsible. The nurses also were genuinely concerned for the patient and were upset over the family's complaints that they "do something." There was an expectation on the family's part and on the nurses' own part that in their role as a professional care giver they should be doing more to alleviate the situation. In response to this pressure the nurses on the hospital unit consciously chose not to adhere strictly to the rules and procedures of the institution. First, based on their professional knowledge of the increasing severity of the patient's illness they instituted treatments, that is, blood work and administration of fluids, antibiotics, and anti-pyretics, that exceeded the sphere of the authority ascribed to them. Second, the nurses went outside the agency to obtain medical help for the patient. Because of the relationship they had developed with other professionals, in this case, the physician who "stuck his head in the door," they were able to obtain help for the patient more rapidly than the formal hierarchy would have provided.

It is significant to note that the nurses' actions were done with a conscious knowledge that they were placing themselves at risk for reprimand and censure. The decision to institute measures aimed at improving the patient's situation even at the risk of losing their jobs should be noted and the motivation for their actions considered, especially in light of what is known about nurses' propensity to take risks (Grier & Schnitzler, 1979).

Certainly, responsive action was needed in this situation. The hierarchy was not ineffective; given time a similar outcome could probably have been attained. However, in a hospital organization, time can become a critical element and employees who adhere strictly to hierarchical structure may endanger human life and adversely affect the effectiveness of the hospital. It is also true that adherence to rules and regulations is generally believed to contribute to a more consistent quality of care for all and to add to the overall effectiveness of the hospital.

If both of these tenets are accepted, that adherence to rules and regulations is beneficial and that at times adherence to rules and regulations is not beneficial and may indeed be detrimental to the effective functioning of an organization, then it appears that the theory of bureaucracy is incomplete. It may be that bureaucracy still is best thought of as a developing theory. Miner (1982) states that Weber's theory of bureaucracy fails to deal with professional systems, knowledge, and authority that exist within bureaucratic organizations. Miner continues that professional components within bureaucratic organizations do not appear to be deviant cases but rather distinct systems having characteristics and sources of authority of their own. Cuff (1978) contends that the search for a distinctive "American type" of bureaucracy continues; a type that is open to control from above and election from below. Lee (1984) suggests that all current theories of bureaucracy are inadequate and require revision if they are to specifically address the burgeoning information technology and the degree to which automation should or can be limited. This is not a futuristic challenge; within today's health care organization technical knowledge related to patient care is being produced at unprecedented levels. The sheer volume of new information becoming available requires that an effective organization be able to respond quickly and to assimilate relevant new technology into its operation.

RESEARCH

Most of the research related to professionals in organizations has been done with nonnurses. A number of descriptive studies have dealt with the nurse as a professional within the tenets of role theory, socialization theory, and professional bureaucratic conflict (Corwin & Taves, 1962; Kramer, 1969, 1970). Dennis (1983) looked at nursing's power in the organization and found a paucity of research. She strongly recommended that nurses identify and examine the basis of their professional power before this base is jeopardized. She also recommended the study of nurses who hold positional power (other than the top executive) within the organization in terms of role use to effect organizational change that deals with professional-bureaucratic conflict.

Dennis (1983) cautioned that decentralization and the concept of shared governance be substantially researched before total endorsement of the concept continues.

Alexander and Bauerschmidt (1987) studied the relationship of technology and structure to the quality of nursing care delivered. Technology was defined as those acts performed by nurses designed to change the status of the individual from hospitalized patient to discharged person. The Overton, Schnesk, and Hazlett (1977) model of technology was used. This model states that technology on nursing units consists of three dimensions: instability, variability, and uncertainty. Instability refers to the unpredictable changes in patients and techniques as indicated by the number of patients susceptible to emergencies, the amount of specialized technical monitoring needed, and the frequency of observations required. Variability represents differences among patients and was measured by the degree to which patients exhibited different problems that required varied and diverse actions from the nurses. Uncertainty expresses the degree to which patients are not well understood and was operationalized as the number of patients who had complex nursing problems and required complex nursing techniques.

Structure consisted of three dimensions: vertical participation, horizontal participation, and formalization. Formalization was defined as the extent to which standardized rules and procedures exist; horizontal participation referred to participation by the individual in decision making, and vertical participation described a hierarchical structure for decision making. The researchers found that the larger the difference between horizontal participation and technical variability, the lower the quality of nursing care. It was suggested that high technological variability should be matched with greater horizontal participation. Integral in this study was the proposal that there is no one most effective structure for all organizations. Organizational structure depends on the degree of technology characteristic of a particular nursing unit.

A bureaucracy structure appears to serve well many of the needs of modern large organizations. However, in large health care organizations it does not seem desirable or possible to have a pure bureaucracy. The answer to the problems of bureaucracy may not be in the adoption of a completely different type of structure, but rather in the need to continue to make modifications specific to the health care setting, and to the roles of professionals within that setting.

REFERENCES

Alexander, J.W. & Bauerschmidt (1987). Implications for nursing administration of the relationship of technology and structures to quality of care. *Nursing Administration Quarterly, 11*(4), 1-10.

Blau, P.M. (1974). *On the nature of organizations.* New York: John Wiley & Sons.

Blau, P.M., & Meyer, M.W. (1971). *Bureaucracy in modern society.* New York: Random House.

Corwin, R.G., & Taves, M.J. (1962). Some concomitants of bureaucratic and profession conceptions of the nurses role. *Journal of Nursing Research, 11,* 223-227.

Cuff, R.D. (1978). Wilson and Weber: Bourgeois critics in an organized age. *Public Administration Review, 38,* 240-244.

Curry, R.G., Wakefield, D.S, Price, J., & Mueller, C.W. (1986). On the causal ordering of job satisfaction and organizational commitment. *Academy of Management Journal, 29,* 847-858.

DeCosmos, J.L. (1987). Alienation and labor in the thought of Karl Marx, Max Weber and Hannah Arendt. (Doctoral dissertation, Florida State University, 1987). *Dissertation Abstracts International.*

Dennis, K.E. (1983). Nursing power in the organization: What research has shown. *Nursing Administration Quarterly, 9*(1), 47-57.

Dressler, G. (1980). *Organization theory: Integrating structured behavior.* Englewood Cliffs, NJ: Prentice-Hall.

Glassman, R. (1983). The Weber renaissance. In S.G. McNall (Ed.), *Current perspectives in social theory* (pp. 239-251). Greenwich, CT: JAI Press.

Gouldner, A.W. (1954). *Patterns of industrial bureaucracy.* Glencoe, IL: Free Press.

Grier, M., & Schnitzler, C.P. (1979). Nurses' propensity to risk. *Nursing Research, 28*(3), 186-191.

Katz, D., & Kahn, R. (1966). *The social psychology of organizations.* New York: John Wiley & Sons.

Kramer, M. (1969). Collegiate graduate nurses in medical center hospital nursing. *Nursing Research, 19,* 428-439.

Kramer, M. (1970). Role conceptions of baccalaureate nurses and success in hospital nursing. *Nursing Research, 19,* 428-439.

Langton, J. (1984). The ecological theory of bureaucracy: The case of Josiah Wedgewood and the British pottery industry. *Administrative Science Quarterly, 29,* 330-354.

Lee, R.M. (1984). Bureaucracies, bureaucrats and information technology. *European Journal of Operations Research, 18,* 293-303.

Mahmoudi, H., & Miller, G.A. (1985). A causal model of hospital structure. *Group & Organization Studies, 10*(2), 209-223.

Malone, M.F. (1964). The dilemma of a professional in a bureaucracy. *Nursing Forum, 3*(4), 36-60.

Miner, J.B. (1980). The role of managerial and professional motivation in the career success of management professors. *Academy of Management Journal, 23,* 487-508.

Miner, J.B. (1982). *Theories of organizational structure and process.* Hinsdale, IL: Dryden.

Overton, P., Schnesk, R., & Hazlett, C.B. (1977). An empirical study of technology of nursing subunits. *Administrative Science Quarterly, 22,* 203-219.

Rice, G.H., & Bishoprick, D.W. (1971). *Conceptual models of organization.* New York: Appleton-Century-Crofts.

Sexton, W.P. (1970). *Organization theories.* Columbus, OH: Charles E. Merrill.

Thompson, V.A. (1961). *A modern organization.* New York: Knopf.

Weber, M. (1958). *The Protestant ethic and the spirit of capitalism.* New York: Scribner's.

Weber, M. (1967). Science as a vocation. In H.H. Gerth & C.W. Mills (Eds.), *From Max Weber* (pp. 129-156). New York: Oxford University Press.

Weber, M. (1970). Bureaucracy. In W. Sexton (Ed.), *Organization theories* (pp. 39-43). Columbus, OH: Charles E. Merrill.

Weber, M. (1978). *Economy and society.* Berkeley, CA: University of California Press.

Weiss, R.M. (1983). Weber on bureaucracy: Management consultant or political theorist? *Academy of Management Review, 8,* 242-248.

Winters, L.L. (1983). A meta-analysis of bureaucratic structure and teacher job satisfaction. (Doctoral dissertation, University of Kansas, 1983). *Dissertation Abstracts International, 44*(11), 240.

Chapter 10

Classical Management Theory
Henri Fayol

Cheryl Pope Long

▮▮ CASE STUDY

Until 1 year ago, the 14 faculty members in the associate degree nursing program of a small private community college had an active voice in decisions affecting curriculum, instruction, and policy. At that time, the program's longtime respected administrator resigned because of failing health and was replaced by a manager whose administrative style has been totally different. Participative management gave way to an autocratic controlling style with top-down communication and strict adherence to the chain of command. Not uncommonly, major decisions have been announced by the administrator to a totally surprised group of faculty, none of whom had been privy to the ideas beforehand. The administrator rarely delegates other than repetitive, noncreative tasks. He is often unduly critical and condemning of faculty. Several have admitted disenchantment in their positions and have begun to prepare resumés for job searches.

Over the course of the last few years, the college, like others nationally, has suffered a decline in enrollment. Recruitment and retention strategies have become priorities. The emphasis on numbers has been pronounced. Consequently the administrator's decision to implement a long-negotiated and well-supported educational mobility option for licensed practical nurses (LPNs) was timely.

The LPN-to-RN curriculum option, popularly known as the "Pathway," has been designed with the nursing course sequence beginning each summer. The program can then be completed in four consecutive academic quarters of study. In preparation for eligibility to this mobility option, LPNs are required to complete general education courses, gain advanced placement in nursing through written examination, and validate their technical proficiency on a clinical performance examination.

Having met the requirements, 10 students enrolled in the initial nursing course. Two experienced nursing faculty were enlisted to teach the course. Both were considered outstanding classroom and clinical educators. Having started as diploma graduates who returned to school for advanced degrees themselves, both valued educational mobility.

Two days before the summer session was due to begin, the program administrator flew cross-country for a week-long professional meeting extended by a week-long vacation. Although it was obvious that there was well-placed confidence in the two faculty teaching the first summer session, the administrator did not delegate authority to either in his absence, nor did he leave a contact number. Shortly thereafter, 11 persons requested entry to the summer course as transfer students. In each case, the student described valid reasons for wishing to transfer. Several were responding to rumors that their own nursing program might be closing.

Privately, the two faculty reviewed the students' records, agreeing that the individuals would be excellent candidates for the program. Despite an earlier suggestion by the administrator that transfer students might ultimately find the "Pathway" appealing, no admission criteria had been proposed for this group. Having witnessed the administrator's wrath on occasions when he was not consulted for major decisions, the faculty were reluctant to admit the students independently. Initially they were unconcerned about the problem, for they believed a resolution would be effected quickly when the administrator called in as their previous superior had always done. Such a call was not forthcoming. Consulting the dean for a decision was briefly considered by the pair but discarded as an alternative because of the college's strong protocol on chain of command and the resolution that matters of admission and progression should be handled autonomously at the department level. There was, as well, some loyalty to the administrator.

Everyone involved in the dilemma recognized a sense of urgency in reaching a decision. This was reinforced not only by inquiries from the director of admissions, hoping to boost sagging admission statistics, but also by the students who insisted on "camping out" in the student lounge. Failure to meet the admission deadline would mean for the students a year-long wait for entry into the special program. Missing the important initial days of class would demand "catching up" in an already challenging course. Despite faculty efforts to the contrary, the 11 students were beginning to feel unwanted. For the student-centered educators, this was perhaps the most frustrating factor in the dilemma as they continued to await a telephone call from the administrator. They were growing quite weary in the discomforture inherent in experiencing responsibility without authority.

What might the program administrator have done to prevent his uncomfortable dilemma?

| | | | | | | | | | | | | | | | | | | | | | | | | | | | | | | | | | | | | | | | | | | | | | | | | | | | | | | | | | | | | | | | |

CLASSICAL MANAGEMENT THEORY

The person who best typifies the theory of classical management is French industrialist Henri Fayol (1841-1925). Born and educated in France, Fayol spent his entire career with the same company, the Commentry-Fourchambault Mining Company, popularly known as Comambault. He began work there in 1860 as a mining engineer and during 12 years in that capacity pioneered work in the fire hazards of coal mining. The following 16 years found Fayol directing a group of mining pits and emerging as an authority on mining geology. Then, in 1888, when the company verged on bankruptcy, Fayol was given the position of Managing Director (Brodie, 1967; Fayol, 1949).

It is interesting that at a time of ultimate crisis for the company, the top administrative post went to a person who had proven expertise in engineering, not in administration. Fayol's son, Henri (cited in Breeze, 1985) explained that his father was asked to conduct a study in anticipation of liquidating the company's assets before closing. On the basis of his findings, Fayol proposed reorganization of the company in accord with sound principles of administration. The board agreed.

Fayol became an outstanding chief executive; the company underwent a rapid turnaround under his leadership. Indeed Fayol believed that his success "in retrieving the firm's fortunes and in guiding it into a period of growth and prosperity, was due to the new style of administration he introduced and to that alone" (Brodie, 1967, p. 3).

Not until he had served as chief executive of Comambault for 12 years did Fayol speak publicly about administration. When he retired in 1918, Fayol popularized his administrative theory, which was reflective of his practical successes in day-to-day administrative experience gleaned over 30 years. This represented the first theory of management.

According to Brodie (1967), Fayol believed that research and practice should continue to guide theory development in administration. Furthermore he was insistent that both theoretical and practical aspects of administration should be taught. Fayol (1949, p. xxi) intended to present his written notions on administration in four parts:

1. The necessity and possibility of teaching management
2. The principles and elements of management
3. Personal observations and experiences
4. Lessons of the war

Only the first two parts, contained in one volume, were completed.

Fayol's theory of management is accessible to an English-reading audience primarily by a translation of his work by Constance Storrs and published as *General and Industrial Management* in 1949. Brodie (1967), who is critical of Storrs's translation, provided updated comprehensive data on Fayol's work through translation of the original manuscript and subsequent writings. Unless otherwise indicated, it will be these two sources that serve as the basis for the following discussion of Fayol's theory of management.

Fayol delineated principles of management that were meant to be flexible, adaptable, and universal. These principles are not only exportable across disciplines but are also well suited to both public and private domains. The principles were offered by Fayol as those factors that he had found effective for management and were not meant to represent an exhaustive list. Yet Fayol (1949, p. 42) contradicted his own notion somewhat when he referred to the principles as "acknowledged truths regarded as proven on which to rely."

Division of Work

Specialization is appropriate to all levels of work, technical and administrative. At the worker level, technical expertise should be unquestionable; however, as workers progress up the chain of command (scalar chain), they need administrative ability to be effective and credible. Specialization decreases the number of matters to which workers or managers must attend or direct their efforts. Consequently the expenditure of effort is the same, but the effectiveness of work increases. The division of work is further enhanced when job routines are well defined.

Authority

Authority refers to the right to give commands and to have them obeyed. One may gain authority from position (statutory authority) or by virtue of such characteristics as intelligence, knowledge, moral worth, and leadership ability (personal authority). For optimal leadership, both types of authority are present.

Responsibility and authority must be commensurate. "Responsibility is a corollary of authority, it is the natural consequence and essential counterpart and wheresoever authority is exercised, responsibility arises" (Fayol, 1949, p. 21).

Further insights into Fayol's ideas on authority may be gained from the content of an address he delivered in 1917. During that address, described by Brodie (1967), Fayol shared an anecdote, which he reported as a basis for the oldest of his notes on administration, dated May 1861. A horse in one of the mines broke a leg and when an attempt was made to get a replacement, the request was denied, for the manager who had to grant such authorization was away. There was a significant loss of output as a result, which prompted Fayol to write, "It seems to me that authority should always be represented" (p. 7). A similar situation later prompted this elaboration, "A substitute should always be appointed in advance, to act in place of a manager who happens to be away or for whatever reason not available" (p. 7).

Discipline

According to Brodie (1967, p. 10), Fayol regarded discipline as a "set of conventions established between an undertaking and its employees." Discipline is essential to an enterprise and includes three components: clear agreements about behavioral expectations, good supervision, and sanctions applied with a sense of fairness and justice. Fayol (1949) suggested the appropriateness of such sanctions as "remonstrances, warnings, fines, suspensions, demotion, [and] dismissals" (p. 23). The individual circumstances in an incident requiring sanctions must receive attention by the manager delivering the sanctions.

Unity of Command

This component of management, which was described as "equal to any other principle" (Fayol, 1949, p. 24), referred to the notion of an employee having only one supervisor giving orders. If this principle is violated, "authority is undermined, discipline is in jeopardy, order disturbed, and stability threatened" (Fayol, 1949, p. 24).

Unity of Direction

"This principle is expressed as: One head and one plan for a group of activities having the same objective. It is the condition essential to unity of action, co-ordination of strength, and focusing of effort" (Fayol, 1949, p. 25). A central authority should take responsibility for preparing an overall plan for the organization. Departmentalization should occur by function, with those individuals working together at the same goal, guided by the same plan, and presenting a united front.

Subordination of Individual Interest to General Interest

In an enterprise, the interest of the employees should not prevail over that of the concern. Pollard (1974, p. 91) summarizes the idea succinctly: "At the individual level the employee or manager must submerge his personal interests or leave them behind at the work place door."

Remuneration of Personnel

A job well done should be rewarded. Staff members should be paid a fair wage, one considered so by both worker and management. Fayol (1949) suggested the appropriateness of bonuses and profit-sharing and seemed to be favoring the idea of fringe benefits with this remark, "The employer should have regards, if merely in the interests of the business, for the health, strength, education, morale, and stability of personnel" (p. 32).

Centralization

The degree of centralization appropriate for an enterprise is likely to vary according to the particular situation and the abilities of the workers and managers. Decentralization increases the role of the worker; centralization reduces it.

Scalar Chain

The scalar chain represents a vertical line of authority and communication from the ultimate superior or decision-making authority to the lowest ranks of the organization. Communication along this chain of command proceeds slowly, especially in larger organizations. Fayol (1949, p. 35) suggests a "gang plank," a means of horizontal interaction between individuals representing two different scalar chains. Although the individuals communicate directly, the scalar chain is not jeopardized because their meeting is preauthorized by their respective superiors. In addition, any decision resulting from such dialogue is reported to the superior, who has ultimate veto power.

Fayol (1949, p. 36) advises, "It is an error to depart needlessly from the line of authority, but it is an even greater one to keep to it when detriment to the business ensues." In the event that a decision must be made and a superior's advice is unavailable, the worker should experience a sense of freedom and comfort to take a risk and adopt a decision in the general interest. For that to occur, however, there must have been a supervisory precedent and example as a guide.

Order

An enterprise must have both material order and social order for effectiveness. Material order refers to "a place for everything and everything in its right place" (Brodie, 1967, p. 11). Resources are carefully chosen and organized; this minimizes loss and promotes the achievement of organizational goals.

Social order refers to personnel appointments—selecting the right person for the task. The presupposition exists that the manager will know the strengths and limitations of personnel and will make use of an organizational chart to ease the processes of selection and assignment.

Equity

That fairness, kindliness, and justice exist within the organization must be evident from the actions taken. Employees wish to be treated fairly and when they are, they are devoted and cooperative. The administrator should strive to assure equity along the entire scalar chain.

Stability of Tenure of Personnel

Orientation of personnel, whether they represent workers or management, is a lengthy and costly process. Without it, however, employees tend to be less secure and less effective in their roles. Once the administrator has ascertained that the employee possesses the prerequisite knowledge and abilities for a position, that person must be given an opportunity to become accustomed to the role before being evaluated. Personnel turnover may cause or be an effect of poor management.

Initiative

Initiative refers to generating a plan and implementing it with success and presupposes the freedom and support to do so. The manager who encourages initiative among subordinates is superior to one who does not. "The manager must be able to sacrifice some personal vanity in order to grant this sort of satisfaction to subordinates" (Fayol, 1949, p. 40). Beyond what such initiative can mean to the individual employee's motivation and sense of satisfaction, it tends to strengthen the organization, especially in times of crisis.

Esprit de Corps

Harmony among personnel must be enhanced and must permeate all of the other management principles. Managers must guard against the pitfall of divide and rule; any dissension should be handled quickly.

Written communications within the organization should not be abused. Face-to-face dialogue facilitates clarity and enhances a sense of cohesion. Fayol (1949, p. 40) further asserts:

> In dealing with a business matter or giving an order which requires explanation to complete it, usually it is simpler and quicker to do so verbally than in writing. Besides, it is well known that differences and misunderstandings which a conversation could clear up, grow more bitter in writing.

ELEMENTS OF THE MANAGEMENT ROLE

Fayol (1949) formulated five elements or functions meant to be representative of the management role: (1) planning, (2) organizing, (3) commanding, (4) coordinating, and (5) controlling. According to Pollard (1974, p. 93), "This constitutes what a manager does when he is actually managing, as distinct from many other non-managerial duties which he will necessarily carry out. The analysis was the first of its kind."

Planning

A sense of futurity is necessary in the foresight associated with administrative planning. Both yearly and 10-yearly forecasts are suggested; the latter are revised every 5 years. Unity, continuity, flexibility, and precision are general features of the planning advised by Fayol. A useful management plan contains anticipated outcomes, interventions, phases for interventions, and methodology. Fayol (1949, p. 50) summarizes the following features of the plan:

> The plan of action facilitates the utilization of the firm's resources and the choices of best methods to use for attaining the objective. It suppresses or reduces hesitancy, false steps, unwarranted changes of course, and helps to improve personnel. It is a precious managerial instrument.

Organizing

The manager's role as organizer implies provision of the material and human resources necessary to the function of the enterprise. Fayol described a line organization and suggested that staff would support the manager by sharing specialized knowledge and by assuming responsibility for some of the daily details of the organization.

Within his examination of the organizing role of administration, Fayol (1949, p. 74) specified requisite qualities for effective managers. These are "health, physical fitness, intelligence, moral fibre, general education, general knowledge of all essential functions, and marked managerial ability."

Commanding

The command function of the administrator involves setting the operation in motion according to its mission and goals and getting the optimal results from each employee in that effort. Command is an art dependent both on personal qualities and familiarity with sound administrative principles.

According to Fayol (1949, pp. 97-98), those in command should be knowledgeable about personnel, ready to eliminate the incompetent, be familiar with personnel contracts, serve as an example, audit the organization periodically, set up conferences among chief assistants to focus effort and provide unity of direction, delegate organizational details, and foster esprit de corps.

The thorough knowledge of personnel so vital to command is made considerably easier by limitations in span of control:

> Whatever his level of authority, one head only has direct command over a small number of subordinates, less than six normally. Only the superior S^1 (foreman or his equivalent) is in direct command of twenty or thirty men, when the work is simple. (Fayol, 1949, p. 98)

Coordinating

Coordination involves harmonizing and balancing the numerous actions and interactions occurring in an organization to assure smooth operation. "It is, in a word, to accord things and actions their rightful proportions, and to adopt means to ends" (Fayol, 1949, p. 103). Weekly conferences wherein departmental heads dialogue are suggested as a means toward coordination. In a well-coordinated enterprise, these features are evident:

1. Individual units work in harmony with each other, enjoying familiarity with necessary tasks and schedules.
2. Units work interdependently, recognizing their shared roles in the total operation.
3. Working schedules of departments and subdivisions are attuned to the circumstances and to organizational goals.

Cues of ineffective coordination are self-contained units working in isolation, departmental interests overriding the general concern, and workers that avoid responsibility by burying themselves in paperwork.

Controlling

Control is the process of verifying whether the operation's actual outcomes are congruent with plans, policy, and administrative directions. Its purpose is to expose errors and take timely corrective action. Such evaluation necessitates impartiality, objectivity, sound judgment, and tact.

CASE ANALYSIS

Classical management theory is sometimes considered outmoded for contemporary practice except for structuring curricula and textbooks for management courses. The theory does indeed lack certain predictive and explanatory components (Miner, 1982). Furthermore a certain degree of ambiguity is associated with Fayol's failure to operationalize many of the theory's variables. The theory has been criticized, too, for the conspicuous inattention to the human relations element. Dessler (1982) and Koontz and O'Donnell (1976) defend against the latter criticism with a suggestion that human relations were not unimportant to Fayol. A strong work ethic that prevailed in that day encouraged instead an emphasis on efficiency, productivity, and fair compensation for a job well done.

Pollard (1974), p. 99) provides a kinder discussion of Fayol's theory than do some other reviewers:

> Inevitably the debt we owe to Fayol diminishes as time and greater complexity make his day and age seem more and more remote. At the time of his attempt, the only one of its kind, to build a basic theory of management was invaluable. It was incomplete . . . it was too narrow, being based solely on his personal experience, but there was a great deal of value in it; . . . there are, for those who can separate the wheat from the chaff, guidelines in Fayol's work which we would do well to remember today.

With such justification, Fayol's theory is applied to analyze the case study. Certain features of the theory seem especially germane to the case: planning, initiative, and authority. To a lesser extent, the principles of esprit de corps, scalar chain, and stability of personnel are applicable.

The kind of sound planning advised by Fayol might have avoided much of the negative aspect of the case situation. First, clearly delineated protocol for student selection, implemented by an admissions committee would have been of incalculable value. This approach would have provided a priori support for decision making by faculty, and strict adherence to protocol would also have guaranteed equity in the selection process. Second, planning with a sense of futurity would seem to imply attention to the sociopolitical milieu in the region surrounding the college. In that case, the administrator should have been aware of rumors concerning closure of a nursing program and the potential impact such an occurrence would have for area schools, including his own.

Positive delegation would also seem an appropriate component in comprehensive planning. Caruth and Pressley (1984, p. 6) define positive delegation as "the art of assigning additional duties, and commensurate authority to employees in a manner so that the assigned work is completed effectively and the employees feel that their time and talents have been used wisely." The operative words here, given the case scenario, refer to authority and the employee's feelings of worth. The program administrator in the case is surrounded by faculty who are obviously capable, talented, and motivated. That they have made a long-term commitment to the organization is evident by their length of tenure. The faculty members, however, are becoming disenchanted with the lack of opportunity for realization of their fullest potential. They aspire to experience authority that matches the responsibility they have been given, miss the participative management they had formerly enjoyed, and hunger for performance reward and recognition of their worth. The initiative, of which Fayol wrote, is sadly missing among these faculty. The administrator would be well advised to work at creating an atmosphere that meets the employees' intrinsic needs to be involved and empowered. He might invite them to try the authority role on a small scale initially as he provides supervision and evaluates their performance. Support would be offered publicly while constructive criticism would be given privately.

Harmony and esprit de corps are conspicuously absent between superior and subordinates in the case scenario. The potential for faculty turnover is very real, caused in large part by poor management. The exit interview will be an unfortunate arena in which to learn of the faculty's disenchantment at not feeling worthwhile to the enterprise. Knowing the harshness of the administrator's criticisms, faculty members do not yet feel comfortable confronting him directly with their concerns and their feelings of professional regression under his controlling leadership approach. They do commiserate privately about their desire to again be more involved in decisions that impact them directly. Until such time that these educators do feel free to express their feelings to the administrator, several practical alternatives exist. For example, they might provide constructively critical input to the administrator using the formal evaluation process, which guarantees anonymity. They may elect to volunteer for specific assignments and clarify which decisions they freely make and what degree of support they can anticipate. Additionally they may solicit feedback on their performance. Faculty might also designate in the format of annual performance objectives how rewarding such opportunities would be.

The case study reinforces the inadequacy of strict adherence to a chain of command, especially when time is critical or there is a potential crisis brewing in the organization. Fayol would have despaired over the lack of freedom and the discomfort experienced by the educators as they considered departing from the scalar chain in an effort to solve the dilemma. They discarded the option on the basis of previous negative experiences, even though this failure conflicted with the general interests of the organization.

The greatest lesson to be gained from Fayol's theory in relation to this case pertains to authority. Fayol maintained that authority should always be represented by the actual administrator or by an appointed substitute. Realizing that no precedent existed for the first summer courses, the case's administrator should have assured that authority was represented in some manner. Either he could have delegated authority during his absence or he could have rescheduled his absence to a less critical time to the nursing program. Otherwise, he might have telephoned at intervals to speak with the faculty involved in the summer session or designated a telephone number where he could be accessible if needed. This is not to suggest that an administrator is not entitled to an uninterrupted vacation; rather that, as Fayol advised, individual interests must at times be subordinated to the general interests of the organization.

Although the actions outlined above would have prevented the specific incident cited in the case study, the uncomfortable working conditions, the larger problem, would continue to exist. The administrator would be well-advised to reexamine his stance with respect to responsibility and its corollary authority. In addition, he would do well to seek faculty participation in decision making for the program and to find ways in which faculty might be rewarded for their effective performance.

RESEARCH

There is a paucity of research bearing specifically on Fayol's work or classical management theory. Fayol's failure to operationalize several of his major variables makes comparison with contemporary research difficult at best. Although the variables may be similarly labeled, one cannot be certain that they are representative of Fayol's conceptualizations.

Stewart (1976) concentrated research on management functions by addressing the differing demands, choices, and constraints, outside specialization, in four management positions: police inspector, bank manager, hospital administrator, and store manager. The assumption preceding Stewart's study was that the problems and needs of all managers would be similar. The behavioral demands in the four managerial positions in Stewart's study were significantly different. "A common feature of the four jobs is the extent to which they are constrained by organizational policies and procedures" (p. 27).

In the design and evaluation of an instrument to measure managerial effectiveness, Morse and Wagner (1978) used several management functions recognizable from Fayol's listing and found that managerial effectiveness was situational. Rather than being held to be designated functions, the more effective managers selected behaviors consistent with their style that tended to yield results in the circumstances.

Dalton, Todor, Spendolini, Fielding, and Porter (1980) surveyed the literature addressing the relationship between the structure of an organization and members' performance, considering variables associated with Fayol's theory. The authors describe this literature "among the most vexing and ambiguous in the field of management and organizational behavior" (p. 60). The quoted conclusions of the review follow:

> An association between levels of formalization and performance has not been convincingly demonstrated. (p. 58)
> An association between specialization and performance has not been clearly demonstrated. (p. 58)
> Limited evidence tends to support a negative relationship between centralization and performance. (p. 59)

Gannon and Paine (1974) studied unity of command in a governmental agency and concluded that when subordinates had two or more superiors, there was a tendency to believe that their employee selections for rewards were not based on ability. Furthermore the authors reported that "as technology becomes more complex, it appears that individuals are more satisfied if more flexibility is provided through violation of the principle of unity of command, since the requirements of the work necessitate such a system (p. 392).

Span of control is likely the variable from Fayol's theory that has been most represented in research studies. Van Fleet and Bedeian (1977), in their historical essay with its 255 references, provide sound evidence that span of control has been widely covered by researchers. Yet results are conflicting (Dalton et al., 1980). Michlitsch and Gipson (1984) are critical that the literature is more philosophic than analytical and that the focus is on numbers of subordinates, not supervisory ability. Their rationale for this stance is that "changing one's span of management is viewed as major organizational surgery because loss of subordinates is tantamount to loss of power" (p. 13).

Udell (1967) used an interview format to study span of control of chief executives in marketing. His conclusions indicate the existence of a "positive relationship between span of control and similarity of functions supervised, geographic dispersion, the use of personal assistants, subordinates' years of experience on the job, and the amount of supervision subordinates receive from others" (p. 438). Span of control and subordinates' formal education were found to be negatively related.

Only one nursing research study is readily accessible that pertains directly to classic management theory. Alidina and Funke-Furber (1988) studied span of control in the nursing division of Juan de Fuca Hospitals in British Columbia. These authors offer two major reasons why the choice of appropriate span of control is valuable (pp. 34, 35):

1. It determines organizational structure.
2. It determines the numbers of managers within a division.

Narrow spans of control are associated with many levels of supervision, while broad spans of control result in organizations with few managers. The former may result in "slow, difficult, and distorted communications" because decisions must traverse several levels before implementation occurs. Too much supervision affects job satisfaction and professional growth negatively. Broad spans of control may be associated with inaccessibility of overtaxed supervisors, who spend time in crisis resolution (p. 35).

Nine key factors were found to be associated with span of control of first-line nursing managers (Alidina & Funke-Furber, 1988, pp. 35-38):

1. Client acuity and the inherent immediacy of necessary decision making
2. Philosophical stance and nursing care delivery system in place within the agency
3. Geographical contiguity of agency (close proximity of clients and subordinates' broadened span of control)
4. Manager style and experience, need for clinical expertise, and human and fiscal resource management abilities
5. Employee profile (professional experts demand more of a manager's time and resources, narrowing the span of control)
6. Job-related factors (task similarity increases span of control; so does task interdependence, number of interactions, and extent of nonsupervisory responsibilities)
7. Maturity of support system (assistants for nonclinical tasks, policies, and procedures broaden effective span of control)
8. Organizational functions (as the program matures and protocols abound, wider span occurs)
9. Environmental functions (social, political, fiscal, and technological)

Fayol's classical management theory may lack predictive validity and may be imprecise for empirical testing. Still, it endures as an organizational framework for management textbooks and courses and offers substantive advice to nursing administrators four decades after it was published.

REFERENCES

Alidina, S., & Funke-Furber, J. (1988). First line nurse managers: Optimizing the span of control. *Journal of Nursing Administration, 18*(5), 34-39.

Breeze, J.D. (1985). Harvest from the archives: The search for Fayol and Carlioz. *Journal of Management, 11,* 43-56.

Brodie, M.B. (1967). *Fayol on administration.* London: Lyon, Grant, & Green.

Caruth, D., & Pressley, T.A. (1984). Key factors in positive delegation. *Supervisory Management, 29, (7),* 6-11.

Dalton, D.R., Todor, W.D., Spendolini, M.J., Fielding, G.J., & Porter, L.W. (1980). Organization structure and performance: A critical review. *Academy of Management Review, 5,* 49-64.

Dessler, G. (1982). *Management fundamentals: Modern principles and practices* (3rd ed.). Reston, VA: Reston.

Fayol, H. (1949). *General and industrial management* (C. Storrs, Trans.). London: Pitman & Sons. (Original work published 1918.)

Gannon, M.J., & Paine, F.T. (1974). Unity of command and job attitudes of managers in a bureaucratic organization. *Journal of Applied Psychology, 59,* 392-394.

Koontz, H., & O'Donnell, C. (1976). *Management — A systems and contingency analysis of managerial functions* (6th ed.). New York: McGraw-Hill.

Michlitsch, J.F., & Gipson, D.L. (1984). Managing the span of control. *Supervisory Management, 29*(6), 12-19.

Miner, J.B. (1982). *Theories of organizational structure and process.* Hinsdale, IL: Dryden.

Morse, D.D., & Wagner, F.R. (1978). Measuring the process of managerial effectiveness. *Academy of Management Journal, 21,* 23-35.

Pollard, H.R. (1974). *Developments in management thought.* London: Heinemann.

Stewart, R. (1976). To understand the manager's job: Consider demands, constraints, choices. *Organizational Dynamics, 4*(4), 22-32.

Udell, J. (1967). An empirical test of hypotheses relating to span of control. *Administrative Science Quarterly, 12,* 420-439.

Van Fleet, D.D., & Bedeian, A.G. (1977). A history of the span of control management. *Academy of Management Review, 2,* 356-372.

Chapter 11

Contingency Theory: Differentiation and Integration Paul R. Lawrence and Jay W. Lorsch

Christine M. Gelb

❙❙ CASE STUDY

Mary Sullivan, Clinical Director of the Maternal Child Nursing Department at St. Luke's Hospital, is in the process of interviewing candidates for the position of Nursing Manager of the Pediatric Intensive Care Unit. St. Luke's is a 500-bed tertiary care hospital in the Midwest. The 15-bed Pediatric Intensive Care Unit cares for a variety of acutely ill children and adolescents with diagnoses ranging from general pediatric medical emergencies to severe multiple trauma.

Mary has narrowed the list of candidates to two persons, each of whom would bring extensive clinical and management experience to the position. Each person has been a successful unit manager in other hospital settings. It has become apparent through interviews as well as references from previous employers that the primary difference between the candidates is related to their use of participative management approaches.

One candidate has made extensive use of a participative management style and is accustomed to functioning in a decentralized setting. The other candidate seems more comfortable with a formalized, centralized approach to management. Mary must decide which of these candidates will be the most effective manager for the Pediatric Intensive Care Unit.

❙❙

CONTINGENCY THEORY

While several earlier researchers examined the relationships among organizational structure, environmental factors such as uncertainty, and organizational performance, Lawrence & Lorsch (1967a, 1967b, 1967c) are credited generally with crystallizing the contingency theory. This theory posits that organizational performance is contingent on an appropriate fit between organizational structure and environmental factors.

Major concepts within the theory were defined by Lawrence and Lorsch as follows:

Organization: "A system of integrated behaviors of people who are performing a task that has been differentiated into several distinct subsystems, each subsystem performing a portion of the task, and the efforts of each being integrated to achieve effective performance of the system" (Lawrence & Lorsch, 1967a, p. 3).

Subenvironment: While no specific definition was provided, this concept was concerned with the "ordering of the environment into three sectors: the market subenvironment, technical-economic subenvironment, and scientific subenvironment" (Lawrence & Lorsch, 1967a, p. 5).

Subsystem: Concerned with differentiation of an organization, with the essential subsystems being sales, production, and research and development (Lawrence & Lorsch, 1967a, pp. 4-5).

Differentiation: "The state of segmentation of the organizational system into subsystems, each of which tends to develop particular attributes in relation to the requirements posed by its relevant external environment" (Lawrence & Lorsch, 1967a, p. 4). Another reference provides an alternative definition: "The difference in cognitive and emotional orientation among managers in different functional departments" (Lawrence & Lorsch, 1967b, p. 11).

Integration: "The process of achieving unity of effort among the various subsystems in the accomplishment of the organization's tasks" (Lawrence & Lorsch, 1967a, p. 3). A second reference provides another definition: "The quality of the state of collaboration that exists among departments that are required to achieve unity of effort by the demands of the environment" (Lawrence & Lorsch, 1967b, p. 11).

Uncertainty: "measured by: (1) the rate of change in environmental conditions, (2) the certainty of information at a given time about environmental conditions, and (3) the time span of definitive feedback from the environment" (Lawrence & Lorsch, 1967a, p. 14).

Degree of formalized structure: "Those aspects of behavior in organizations subject to pre-existing programs and controls" (Lawrence & Lorsch, 1967a, p. 5). This concept was operationalized through the measurement of variables such as span of supervisory control, frequency of review of subsystem performance, and emphasis on rules and procedures.

Orientation of members toward others: "A cognitive and affective orientation toward the objects of work, which is manifested in a person's interpersonal style" (Lawrence & Lorsch, 1967a, p. 7). The researchers identified task accomplishment and social relationships as the primary orientations.

Time orientation: "Related to the modal time span of definitive feedback from the subenvironment on the result of subsystem behavior" (Lawrence & Lorsch, 1967a, p. 8). This concept was concerned with an organization member's short- or long-term time orientation.

Goal orientation: While a specific definition was not provided, this concept was related to differences in objectives among managers in different functional jobs (Lawrence & Lorsch, 1967b). Do production managers and sales managers have different objectives?

Organizational performance: While no specific definition was provided, performance was measured by "change in profits over the five years prior to the study, change in sales volume over the same period, and percentage of current sales volume accounted for by products developed within the last five years" (Lawrence & Lorsch, 1967a, p. 25).

Lawrence and Lorsch proposed the following hypotheses (1967a, pp. 10-12):

Hypothesis 1: The greater the certainty of the relevant subenvironment, the more formalized the structure of the subsystem. . . .

Hypothesis 2: Subsystems dealing with environments of moderate certainty will have members with more social interpersonal orientations, whereas subsystems coping with either very certain environments or very uncertain environments will have members with more task-oriented interpersonal orientations. . . .

Hypothesis 3: The time orientation of subsystem members will vary directly with the modal time required to get definitive feedback from the relevant subenvironment. . . .

Hypothesis 4: The members of a subsystem will develop a primary concern with the goals of coping with their particular subenvironment. . . .

Hypothesis 5: Within any organizational system, given a similar degree of requisite integration, the greater the degree of differentiation in subsystem attributes between pairs of subsystems, the less effective will be the integration achieved between them. . . .

Hypothesis 6: Overall performance in coping with the external environment will be related to there being a degree of differentiation among subsystems consistent with the requirements of their relevant subenvironments and a degree of integration consistent with requirements of the total environment. . . .

Hypothesis 7: When the environment requires both a high degree of subsystem differentiation and a high degree of integration, integrative devices will tend to emerge. . . .

The work of Lawrence and Lorsch as well as that of other researchers has provided a certain amount of support for the major hypotheses of contingency theory. Formal, centralized organizational structures were found to exist in environments of certainty, while uncertain environments were associated with less formalized organizational structures. When this fit between structure and environment occurs, organizational performance has been found to be more effective.

While differentiation is necessary for the successful functioning of modern organizations, it may result in conflict. The Lorsch and Lawrence model emphasizes that such conflict can be resolved through integration methods that include program coordinators, planning directors, and confrontation to resolve conflict (Lawrence & Lorsch, 1967a, 1967c).

Later work by Lorsch and Morse emphasized the importance of the fit among the organization, tasks, and people. Appropriate organizational structure was seen to be contingent on both the nature of the work and the needs of individuals involved. When there is a fit between tasks and the organizational structure, employee competence motivation is enhanced (Morse & Lorsch, 1970).

CASE ANALYSIS

Contingency theory provides an excellent framework that Mary Sullivan can use in making a hiring decision. An initial assessment of the Pediatric Intensive Care Unit environment is required.

Such an evaluation reveals an environment of uncertainty in which conditions change at a rapid rate and information is often uncertain or absent. In applying differentiation and integration to this situation, it is apparent that a decentralized, participative management approach, in combination with this uncertain environment, will yield the most effective performance for the staff and unit. Mary Sullivan's decision to hire the more participative manager should provide the best fit between structure and environment.

RESEARCH

The initial Lawrence and Lorsch studies examined six organizations in the plastics industry, two container companies, and two consumer food businesses (Lorsch & Lawrence, 1965; Lawrence & Lorsch, 1967a). Data were gathered through interview of 30 to 50 managers, examination of organizational documents, and questionnaires such as Fiedler's Least Preferred Coworker instrument.

The research findings supported all hypotheses mentioned previously, with the exception of hypothesis 4. While individuals in sales and production were concerned primarily with the goals of their own subenvironments, research department employees focused on the goals of the production subenvironment (Lawrence & Lorsch, 1967a).

A later study by Morse and Lorsch (1970) examined two container manufacturing companies and two communications technology organizations involved with research and development. The purpose of the study was to "explore more fully how the fit between organization and task was related to successful performance" (p. 62). The researchers were interested in the effects of this fit on worker motivation, as well as individual and organizational performance.

Data were collected through questionnaires and interviews with approximately 40 managers in each of the four organizations. Findings revealed high organizational and individual performance when an appropriate fit existed between organizational structure and environmental uncertainty (high uncertainty with informal structure and low uncertainty with formal structure).

Six other researchers were credited by Lawrence and Lorsch (1967b) with influencing their development of contingency theory. Burns and Stalker (1961) studied 20 industrial organizations using manager interviews to determine (1) the relationship between management approaches and rates of change in scientific techniques and markets, and (2) the effect of this relationship on economic performance. These researchers concluded that "the effective organization of industrial resources, even when considered in its rational aspects alone, does not approximate to one ideal type of management system, but alters in important respects in conformity with changes in extrinsic factors . . . identifiable as different rates of technical or market changes" (p. 96).

Burns and Stalker (1961) identified two management systems. The mechanistic system is characterized by factors such as differentiation, hierarchical structure of control, behavior governed by instructions, vertical communication, and decisions issued by superiors. The organic management system involves a network structure of control, authority, and communication; lateral rather than vertical communication; decision making at lower levels in the organization; and communication characterized by information and advice rather than instructions. The mechanistic system was viewed as appropriate for stable conditions, while the organic structure was effective in changing conditions.

Woodward's study (1958) of 100 diverse production firms in England also influenced the work of Lawrence and Lorsch. Woodward found that technical differences among these organizations were related to patterns of management, especially in the more successful companies. As with other contingency studies, a correlation was noted between task certainty and centralized organizational structure.

Fouraker's research described L and T types of organizations. The L organization is characterized by authoritarian approaches, suppressed conflict, and reliance on discipline. On the other hand, the T organization is represented by independent technical specialists, responsive management, coordination of the outputs of the specialists, limited hierarchy, and reliance on committees.

Fouraker stressed that the L organization is most effective in stable, unfavorable environments, while the T organization is more successful in favorable, changing environments. Like Lawrence and Lorsch, Fouraker was concerned with the need for conflict resolution as organizations attempt to remain differentiated while achieving an adequate level of integration.

Chandler's case histories (1962) of Du Pont, General Motors, Standard Oil, and Sears Roebuck emphasized the development of strategic choices as a result of environmental changes. His writings also stressed the importance of integration for the success of an organization. Centralized organizational structures were viewed as adequate for stable environments, but less appropriate for changing environments.

Udy's study (1964) of 426 organizations in 150 nonindustrial societies was based primarily on data obtained from the Human Relations Area Files. These organizations varied greatly in terms of technological development. Udy's major conclusion was that "certain aspects of authority, division of labor, solidarity, proprietorship, and recruitment structure could be predicted as to general trend from technology alone" (Udy, 1964, p. 126). Udy also concluded from his research that technological complexity limits the number of levels of authority. This finding is certainly consistent with the work of other contingency theorists.

Leavitt's research (1962) involved small-group problem solving under experimentally controlled conditions. The findings were consistent with those of Lawrence and Lorsch. When routine tasks were required, a centralized approach worked well, but when creativity, flexibility, and high morale were needed, a decentralized problem-solving method was more successful. A management-by-task approach was recommended. Leavitt expressed concern that while organizational differentiation was becoming more necessary, communication problems would result from this approach.

One other researcher is cited frequently as a predecessor of Lawrence and Lorsch. Dill's examination (1958) of a Norwegian manufacturing firm and a sales, engineering, and contracting business concluded that "the autonomy of managerial personnel—their decisions for and against independent action—may be influenced by the structure of the environment, the accessibility of information about the environment, and by managerial perceptions of the meaning of environmental information" (p. 409).

At least partial support for the contingency theory is provided by a number of researchers. One study of 30 manufacturing firms in India found that the effectiveness of centralization and decentralization varied with the degree of market competitiveness present (Negandhi & Reimann, 1972). Data were obtained by interviews. The researchers concluded that "dynamic, competitive markets make decentralization more important to organizational effectiveness than do stable noncompetitive conditions" (p. 144). Organizational effectiveness was measured using criteria such as morale, turnover, absenteeism, net profits, and growth in sales.

Yet the data analysis also indicated that, to a lesser degree, in stable environments organizations were also successful when organizational structures were decentralized. The authors attributed this finding to the cultural context of India and still concluded that their study provided support for contingency theory.

In a second study Negandhi and Reimann (1973) again examined interview data from 30 manufacturing firms in India. Although the environment was judged to be stable by the authors, they were especially interested in the effects of the decision makers' perceptions of the environment. Variables studied included degree of centralization/decentralization, organizational effectiveness, and scope of concern. Scope of concern was defined as the amount of organizational concern toward task environmental agents such as consumers, employees, and stockholders.

Results of the study revealed that organizations with a greater scope of concern (maintaining a long-term perspective) had fewer layers of hierarchy, while those taking a short-term perspective were more centralized. This finding supported one of the hypotheses of Lawrence and Lorsch concerning time orientation. Decentralized firms were found to be more effective in both behavioral and economic terms, in contrast to Lawrence and Lorsch's studies, which found centralized structures to be more effective in stable environments.

Khandwalla's examination (1973) of 79 manufacturing firms studied seven organizational variables intended to measure uncertainty reduction, differentiation, and integration, namely, vertical integration, staff support for decision making, delegation of decision-making authority by the chief executive officer (CEO), divisionalization, functional departmentalization, extent of participative management, and use of sophisticated management controls. The criterion for effective performance was profitability. Data were obtained through questionnaires completed by the CEOs of the organizations.

No significant relationship was found between profitability and the other seven variables. There were positive correlations noted between (1) uncertainty reduction and differentiation; (2) differentiation and integration; and (3) uncertainty reduction and integration. The author concluded that environmental uncertainty is an important factor affecting organizational design. Uncertainty and decentralization were found to be related, although these two variables had only a minimal relationship to profitability. Obviously this study provides only mixed support for contingency theory.

Duncan (1972) studied 22 decision groups in three manufacturing and three research and development organizations. Interview and questionnaire data were obtained. The Lawrence and Lorsch definition of uncertainty was expanded to include (1) lack of information about environmental factors associated with a decision-making situation; (2) not knowing the outcome of specific decisions; and (3) inability to assign probabilities.

Duncan (1972) also identified two environmental dimensions. The simple-complex dimension involved the number of factors considered when making a decision, and the static-dynamic dimension represented the degree to which these factors remained the same over time. Study results indicated that perceived uncertainty in decision making was greatest in the dynamic and complex environments.

A further study by Duncan (1974) provided support for the hypothesis that uncertainty and a less structured organizational hierarchy were related.

A study of 40 industrial firms in Italy and Mexico concluded that decentralization was both economically and behaviorally effective in highly competitive environments, while centralization was more economically effective in low competitive environments (Simonetti & Boseman, 1975). Decentralization and behavioral effectiveness (measured by morale, hiring, turnover, and interdepartmental relationships) were related positively in both stable and unstable environments.

Tung's research (1979) added further support for contingency theory. This study examined the relationship between environmental uncertainty and the organizational characteristics of standardization, formalization, and role specialization. These three organizational variables were found to be significant predictors of perceived environmental uncertainty, departmental structure, planning time perspective, and frequency of changes in plans.

While the above studies provide a certain degree of support for the contingency theory, other findings contradict the hypotheses of the theory.

Pennings' study (1975) of 40 brokerage offices found that factors such as competition, uncertainty, and instability did not explain variances in organizational structure. Interestingly complexity and resourcefulness did correlate significantly with organizational power and communication, a finding that lends some support to the general structural-contingency model. With the exception of resourcefulness and complexity in combination with power, environmental variables were not related significantly to organizational effectiveness. Pennings concludes, "From the results obtained, one questions the usefulness of the structural-contingency model" (1975, p. 405).

In Osborn's study (1976) of 26 mechanistic antipoverty agencies no significant relationship was found between organizational effectiveness and most measures of environmental certainty used. Only task environment dependency was found to be correlated significantly.

Schmidt and Cummings (1976) examined the relationships among organizational differentiation, perceived environmental uncertainty, and environmental characteristics such as economic conditions, urbanization, and level of government service. Data were obtained from

23 employment service district offices. One of the researchers' hypotheses was related directly to contingency theory: "the greater the degree of task environment change, the greater the degree of organizational differentiation" (Schmidt & Cummings, 1976, p. 447). This hypothesis was not supported by the data.

Several studies of contingency theory or theoretical concepts such as uncertainty have been conducted by nonnurse researchers using nursing units. Overton, Schneck, and Hazlett (1977) attempted to identify levels of technology among various nursing units. Technology was measured by a 34-item questionnaire and included components such as the number of patients requiring frequent observation, frequency of emergencies, types of nursing skills required, and the degree to which nurses relied on each other to complete their work. The questionnaire was administered to 355 nurses from 71 varying nursing units in hospitals.

Three technological variables were identified using factor analysis: uncertainty, instability, and variability. Uncertainty involved the degree to which patients were not understood because they had complex problems. Instability was related to the number of emergencies that occurred and the amount of observation the patient required. Variability represented the degree to which patients presented different health problems.

Nursing units were then categorized using these variables. Intensive care and psychiatric units were found to be highest in uncertainty, higher than other units in instability, and lowest in variability. Auxiliary units (e.g., long-term care) ranked lowest in instability and variability, but relatively high in uncertainty. Obstetrical units were low in uncertainty and variability, while pediatric rehabilitation units and surgical units were close together on all three factors. The authors suggest these findings as a first step in further examination of the relationship between these technology variables and factors such as organizational success, structural characteristics, and management processes.

In a replication study of the work of Overton et al. 157 nursing units in 24 hospitals were studied using a questionnaire containing 21 items from the original questionnaire (Leatt & Schneck, 1981). One thousand two hundred sixty-five nurses completed the questionnaire. Instability was also measured with a checklist of specialized and technical equipment completed by the head nurse of each unit.

Results indicated a high degree of construct validity for the questionnaire with the three factors of instability, uncertainty, and variability emerging again. The various types of nursing units again were differentiated in terms of these three factors.

Intensive care units were greater than other units in instability, while rehabilitation, auxiliary, and rural units were lowest. Psychiatric, pediatric, obstetrical, surgical, and medical units were intermediate. Psychiatric units were highest in uncertainty, while obstetrical, surgical, and rural were lowest. Units did not differentiate using the factor of variability. The above rankings were generally similar to those found in the original study.

Comstock and Scott (1977) examined 142 nursing units in 16 hospitals. Technological, task, and workflow predictability were examined in relationship to staff qualifications, role differentiation, centralization of decision making, and subunit size. The authors were concerned with examining both individual tasks and subunit workflow because they believed that failure to differentiate various organizational levels had produced confusion in the contingency theory literature. Data were collected through interviews, questionnaires, weekly patient census reports, and independent ratings of nurses regarding predictability of care.

Findings included (1) predictable tasks decreased staff qualifications, increased differentiation, had an insignificant positive relationship to centralization of policy decisions, and had a negative relationship to centralization of routine decisions; and (2) larger size had a positive relationship to differentiation, lower staff qualifications, and centralization of routine administrative decisions. Several of these findings represent a departure from contingency theory. The researchers concluded that "as we move from tasks to workflow, the effects of technology predictability shift from individual job qualifications and specialization to systems of subunit coordination and control. While size continues to have independent effects, it is a less powerful predictor of subunit structure than technology" (Comstock & Scott, p. 177).

An examination of 33 psychiatry departments within general hospitals concluded that "role specialization, centralization, standardization, and mode of conflict resolution were the most important predictors of effectiveness" (Weinman, Grimes, Hsi, Justice, & Schoolar, 1979, p. 32). The uncertainty variable was not included in this study.

Argote's study (1982) of the emergency departments of 30 hospitals examined input uncertainty, means of coordination, and organizational effectiveness. The effectiveness measure included quality of nursing care, quality of medical care, and promptness of care.

Findings indicated that effectiveness in low uncertainty environments was associated with programmed means of coordination that are specified in advance. Nonprogrammed coordination is most effective in high uncertainty environments. Yet the data suggested that many emergency departments were not using the appropriate method of coordination that would contribute to effectiveness.

Only limited nursing research has been conducted using contingency theory as a framework. Alexander and Randolph (1985) studied 27 subunits of varying types in three hospitals with the purpose of examining the fit between technology and structure as a predictor of performance. The authors used the framework of Overton et al. (1977), which includes uncertainty, instability, and variability as measures of technology.

The Leatt and Schneck (1981) tool was used to measure technology. Structure was measured by the adapted Leifer and Huber (1977) questionnaire. Performance was assessed using the Rush-Medicus Nursing Process Monitoring Methodology (Hegyvary, Haussman, Kronman, & Burke, 1979).

Greater variability and horizontal participation were associated with a higher quality of care. Interestingly, greater uncertainty in combination with greater formalization also increased quality of care. A third combination related to quality of care was greater instability with vertical participation.

The authors concluded that "fit between technology and structure is a better predictor of workgroup performance than technology, structure, or technology and structure (Alexander & Randolph, 1985, p. 855). Additionally they suggest, "in nursing subunits where tasks and patient diagnoses vary widely, personnel should be highly involved in decision making and defining tasks. Conversely, in situations with little technological variability among patients, less horizontal participation will enhance the quality of care" (p. 856). Finally, it is suggested that subunits that have high levels of uncertainty in relationship to patient care will benefit from the development of rules and procedures to guide the staff.

Mark (1985) explored the relationships between organizational effectiveness and task and structural variables using 76 private psychiatric hospitals. Task complexity included three dimensions: variability, difficulty, and interdependence. The author noted that these dimensions are often at a high level in the psychiatric setting. Patients and treatment methods are incompletely understood, there are many exceptions, and a high level of interdependence exists among caregivers. Task complexity was measured using the Organizational Assessment Inventory.

Organizational effectiveness (patient care and administrative) was evaluated with Weinman's instrument (Weinman et al., 1979). Patient care effectiveness included measures of treatment response, activities of the treatment program, staff qualifications, quality of treatment planning, and assessment of treatment outcomes. Administrative effectiveness dimensions included assessment of program goals, organizational missions and goals, and use of systematic process to review, evaluate, and modify program goals.

Data were collected through a mailed survey questionnaire. Mark (1985) found that with low task difficulty, centralization and patient care effectiveness were related negatively. With high task difficulty, the relationship between centralization and patient care effectiveness was positive. This is contrary to contingency theory assumptions. Mark suggests that this finding can perhaps be explained by the decision-making structure of the psychiatric multidisciplinary team. While team members may have high levels of input into decision making, the clinical decision making is assumed by the psychiatrist. This phenomenon resulted in a higher centralization score on the survey tool. Yet Mark suggests that "high levels of team input into physician decision making may have mitigated the presumed negative effects of a highly centralized structure" (p. 213).

Findings relative to administrative effectiveness did provide support for the contingency theory. When task difficulty was high, administrative effectiveness was related to low levels of standardization.

Criticism of contingency theory has focused primarily on issues of clarity, assumptions of linearity, definition and measurement of the uncertainty variable, and failure to differentiate the concepts of contingency and congruence. Schoonhoven (1981) faults the theory for lack of clarity in its hypotheses, as well as in its presentation of contingency relationships and interaction effects. Ginsberg and Venkatraman (1985) relates that most researchers have assumed a linear relationship among variables rather than checking for nonlinear relationships.

The research of Tosi, Aldag, and Storey (1973) questioned the internal reliability and construct validity of the Lawrence and Lorsch uncertainty scale. A response from Lawrence and Lorsch refutes the work of Tosi, Aldag, and Storey (Lawrence & Lorsch, 1973).

Other researchers are concerned with the need to include individual perception in defining the uncertainty concept (Duncan, 1972). Lawrence and Lorsch seemed to assume that individual perception and the reality of environmental uncertainty were generally the same.

A variety of measures of uncertainty has appeared in the literature including technological factors, number of product changes, research and development expenditures per net sales dollar, and task uncertainty. Unfortunately, the assumption is made that there is a similar response to each of these different measurements (Downey & Slocum, 1975).

Finally, Drazin and Van de Ven (1985) are concerned that contingency and congruency have not been differentiated in the literature. They view congruence as a simple unconditional association, for example, the greater the task uncertainty, the more complex the structure. A contingent relationship is more complex, involving independent variables such as uncertainty and structure with a dependent variable such as effectiveness. While some of the more recent literature reflects this more complex contingent relationship, other researchers have been content to examine only a congruent relationship without considering performance.

REFERENCES

Alexander, J.W., & Randolph, W.A. (1985). The fit between technology and structure as a predictor of performance in nursing subunits. *Academy of Management Journal, 28,* 844-859.

Argote, L. (1982). Input uncertainty and organizational coordination in hospital emergency units. *Administrative Science Quarterly, 23,* 420-434.

Burns, T., & Stalker, G.M. (1961). *The management of innovation.* London: Tavistock.

Chandler, A. (1962). *Strategy and structure: Chapters in the history of industrial enterprise.* Cambridge, MA: M.I.T. Press.

Comstock, D.E., & Scott, W.R. (1977). Technology and the structure of subunits: Distinguishing individual and workgroup effects. *Administrative Science Quarterly, 22,* 177-202.

Dill, W.R. (1958). Environment as an influence on managerial autonomy. *Administrative Science Quarterly, 2,* 409-443.

Downey, H.K., & Slocum, J.W. (1975). Uncertainty: Measures, research, and sources of variation. *Academy of Management Journal, 18,* 562-578.

Drazin, R., & Van de Ven, A.H. (1985). Alternative forms of fit in contingency theory. *Administrative Science Quarterly, 30,* 514-539.

Duncan, R.B. (1972). Characteristics of organizational environments and perceived environmental uncertainty. *Administrative Science Quarterly, 17,* 313-327.

Fouraker, L.E., unpublished manuscript.

Ginsberg, A., & Venkatraman, N. (1985). Contingency perspective of organizational strategy: A critical review of the empirical research. *Academy of Management Review, 10,* 421-434.

Hegyvary, S.T., Haussman, R.K., Kronman, G., & Burke, M. (1979). User's manual for Rush-Medicus Nursing Process Monitoring Methodology. Appendum to *Monitoring quality of nursing care.* Springfield, VA: National Technical Information Service.

Huber, G.P., O'Connell, M., & Cummings, L.L. (1975). Perceived environmental uncertainty: Effects of information and structure. *Academy of Management Journal, 18,* 725-740.

Khandwalla, P.N. (1973). Viable and effective designs of firms. *Academy of Management Journal, 16,* 481-495.

Lawrence, P.R., & Lorsch, J.W. (1967a). Differentiation and integration in complex organizations. *Administrative Science Quarterly, 12,* 1-47.

Lawrence, P.R., & Lorsch, J.W. (1967b). *Organization and environment.* Boston: Harvard University.

Lawrence, P.R., & Lorsch, J.W. (1967c). New management job: The integrator. *Harvard Business Review, 45,* 142-151.

Lawrence, P.R., & Lorsch, J.W. (1973). A reply to Tosi, Aldag, and Storey. *Administrative Science Quarterly, 18,* 397-398.

Leatt, P., & Schneck, R. (1981). Nursing subunit technology: A replication. *Administrative Science Quarterly, 26,* 225-236.

Leavitt, H.J. (1962). Unhuman organizations. *Harvard Business Review, 40,* 90-98.

Leifer, R., & Huber, G.P. (1977). Relationships among perceived environmental uncertainty, organizational structure, and boundary spanning behavior. *Administrative Science Quarterly, 22,* 235-247.

Lorsch, J.W., & Lawrence, P.R. (1965). Organizing for product innovation. *Harvard Business Review, 43,* 109-122.

Mark, B. (1985). Task and structural correlates of organizational effectiveness in private psychiatric hospitals. *Health Services Research, 20,* 199-224.

Morse, J.J., & Lorsch, J.W. (1970). Beyond theory y. *Harvard Business Review, 48,* 61-68.

Negandhi, A.R., & Reimann, B.C. (1972). A contingency theory of organization re-examined in the context of a developing country. *Academy of Management Journal, 15,* 137-146.

Negandhi, A.R., & Reimann, B.C. (1973). Task environment, decentralization and organizational effectiveness. *Human Relations, 26,* 203-214.

Osborn, R.N. (1976). The search for environmental complexity. *Human Relations, 29,* 179-191.

Overton, P., Schneck, R., & Hazlett, C.B. (1977). An empirical study of the technology of nursing subunits. *Administrative Science Quarterly, 22,* 203-219.

Pennings, J.M. (1975). The relevance of the structural-contingency model for organizational effectiveness. *Administrative Science Quarterly, 20,* 393-407.

Schmidt, S.M., & Cummings, L.L. (1976). Organizational environment, differentiation and perceived environmental uncertainty. *Decision Sciences, 7,* 447-467.

Schoonhoven, C.B. (1981). Problems with contingency theory: Testing assumptions hidden within the language of contingency theory. *Administrative Science Quarterly, 26,* 349-377.

Simonetti, J.L., & Boseman, F.G. (1975). The impact of market competition on organization structure and effectiveness. *Academy of Management Journal, 18,* 631-638.

Tosi, H., Aldag, R., & Storey, R. (1973). On the measurement of the environment: An assessment of the Lawrence and Lorsch environment uncertainty questionnaire. *Administrative Science Quarterly, 18,* 27-36.

Tung, R.L. (1979). Dimensions of organizational environments: An exploratory study of their impact on organization structure. *Academy of Management Journal, 22,* 672-693.

Udy, S. (1964). Administrative rationality, social setting, and organizational development. In W.W. Cooper, H.J. Leavitt, & M.W. Shelley II (Eds.), *New perspectives in organization research.* New York: John Wiley & Sons.

Weinman, M.L., Grimes, R.M., Hsi, B.P., Justice, B., & Schoolar, J.C. (1979). Organizational structure and effectiveness in general hospital psychiatry departments. *Administration in Mental Health, 7,* 32-42.

Woodward, J. (1958). *Management and technology.* London: Her Majesty's Stationery Office.

Chapter 12

Theory of System 4
Rensis Likert

Ann Marriner-Tomey

■| **CASE STUDY**

The shortage of nurses caused the directors of nursing at a large hospital to consider the differences between hospitals that experienced the shortage of nurses and those that were not so troubled by the problem or still had waiting lists of nurses wanting to work there. The major differences they noticed were the use of professional practice and participative management. They decided to plan change toward professional practice and participative management and to study Likert's work to guide them.

||||||||||||||||||||||||||||||||||||||||||||||||||||||||||||||||

THEORY OF SYSTEM 4

Likert's theoretical contributions evolved during his career as Director of the Institute for Social Research at the University of Michigan from 1946 to 1970. His major focus initially was on leadership within a group, but the theory expanded to include vertical and lateral intergroup relationships, organizational climates, and social systems. His theory is presented primarily in three books: *New Patterns of Management* (Likert, 1961), *The Human Organization* (Likert, 1967), and *New Ways of Managing Conflict* (Likert & Likert, 1976). A number of journal articles supplement the books. The program of research conducted at the Institute for Social Research served as both an inductive source and an empirical testing ground for Likert's theoretical statements.

New Patterns of Management (Likert, 1961) was the first comprehensive statement of Likert's views. It contained an extensive discussion of research conducted by the staff of the Institute for Social Research during the late 1940s and the 1950s. Earlier writings dating back to the early 1940s (Likert & Willets, 1940-1941) contain many statements that are similar to those presented more formally in the 1961 book. Key concepts such as the principle of supportive relationships and the value of participative management were clearly presented in external publications in the early 1950s (Likert, 1953; Mann & Likert, 1952) and seem to have guided the research of the staff of the Institute for Social Research from the beginning.

The principle of supportive relationships is the fundamental concept. It assumes an influential role for leadership in organizations. Effective leaders are viewed as employee-centered managers who have ways of creating a perception of supportiveness while transmitting high-performance goals through their own enthusiasm and technical competence. The principle of supportive relationships is stated in various forms throughout Likert's work but the meaning remains similar:

> The leadership and other processes of the organization must be such as to ensure a maximum probability that in all interactions and all relationships with the organization each member will, in the light of his background, values, and expectations, view the experience as supportive and one which builds and maintains his sense of personal worth and importance. (Likert, 1961, p. 103)

The major source of supportive relationships is the work group. Highly effective groups and linking pins are derived from the basic principle, as stated by Likert (1961):

> Management will make full use of the potential capacities of its human resources only when each person in an organization is a member of one or more effectively functioning work groups that have a high degree of group loyalty, effective skills of interaction and high performance goals. . . . Consequently, management should deliberately endeavor to build these effective groups, linking them into an overall organization by means of people who hold overlapping group membership. The superior in one group is subordinate in the next group and so on through the organization. (pp. 104-105)

People who are in positions of dual group membership should exert influence in both groups — upward and downward as members and leaders. This opens up channels of communication throughout the organization through the linking pin function.

Likert identifies three sets of variables: causal, intervening, and end-result. Causal variables include organizational structures, organizational objectives, management practices and behaviors, and such. Intervening variables include personality, perceptions, attitudes, motivational forces, and behavior. End-result variables include production, earnings, absence, turnover, grievances, sales, and so on. Likert particularly emphasizes the intervening variables and how to measure them.

The principle of participation is emphasized by Likert as the best managerial action throughout *New Patterns of Management* (1961). He relates the principle to other management systems, and then compares exploitative authoritative, benevolent authoritative, and consultative types of systems with the participative group system. He places these on a continuum from less to more participation and indicates that "participation should not be thought of as a single process or activity, but rather as a whole range of processes and activities" (p. 242).

Likert's second book, *The Human Organization* (1967) discusses much the same content as the first, elaborates more fully on a number of concepts, and places more emphasis on such facets as establishing high goals, organizational structuring, and accounting for human assets. He labeled exploitative authoritative, benevolent authoritative, consultative, and participative group systems as systems 1, 2, 3, and 4, respectively, and expanded the list of characteristics of these systems. He also expanded the list of causal, intervening, and end-result variables to measure. Likert rejected the classical management view that a person should only have one boss. He suggests horizontally overlapping groups with linking pins for many purposes and comprehensive group decision making for resolving conflicts.

New Ways of Managing Conflict (Likert & Likert, 1976) discusses less organizational theory than the other two books. The central thesis of this book is that system 4 is the best method to deal with conflict. One could hypothesize that as an organization moves toward system 4, productivity and profits would improve and conflict would be reduced. However, system 4T (T refers to total) theory states that there are additional factors beyond position on the system 1 through 4 continuum that determine organizational effectiveness. Likert and Likert state that "if an organization, or a department, scores high on the system 1 to 4 scale and low on one or more of the other dimensions, such as technical competence or level of performance goals, the probabilities are great that it will not be highly effective in conflict management or performance" (p. 50).

System 4T also introduces the concepts of peer leadership and organizational climate. Peer leadership can strengthen or weaken the operating capacity of an organization. It strengthens 4T organizations but can weaken systems 1 or 2 by stimulating behavior oriented to defeating rather than achieving the organizational goals. Peer leadership behaviors tend to reflect the superior's behaviors. Consequently, the leadership behavior of the superior at the top of the organization is mirrored and often magnified by lower levels in the organization. Likert and Likert refer to the effect of the leadership behavior at the top of the organization on all levels of the organization as organizational climate (1976, p. 102; see also Miner, 1982, pp. 18-32).

CASE ANALYSIS

Believing that participative managers need particularly good management skills and to prepare themselves for the planned change, the directors worked with a management consultant to review Likert's theory of system 4, decision-making models, planned change, organization, leadership, motivation, conflict, and stress theories. They decided to implement management by objectives and found their own enthusiasm increased from participating in goal setting. The managers worked with their staffs to set goals for the units, and staff set their own performance goals. The managers were employee centered and used supportiveness toward high-performance goals.

Focus groups were formed for staff to identify strengths and weaknesses of the hospital and to make recommendations for improving working conditions. Shared governance was implemented through the creation of councils and bylaws. The directors functioned as linking pins between the coordinating council and other councils. Managers and staff served as linking pins between councils and unit staff. Peer leadership was used.

Personnel were surveyed with the use of a questionnaire periodically to assess their attitudes and perceptions about the organizational climate, job satisfaction, and quality of care. The organizational climate moved toward system 4 over a period of 2 years and the perception of job satisfaction and quality of care remained high.

RESEARCH

During the 1940s and 1950s, nearly all the research bearing on Likert's theory was conducted by people associated with the Institute for Social Research at the University of Michigan. Likert reported reviews of that research in his books. Almost all of the findings favored the theory. The major approach in the early years was to identify high- and low-producing work groups in organizations and to administer extensive questionnaires to the members for the purpose of identifying leadership practices that differentiated effective from ineffective groups (Likert, 1961).

The best-known research studies were conducted with clerical groups in an insurance company and with railroad section gangs. Kahn and Katz (1960) summarized other research as well. In general, high-producing groups had leaders whose more differentiated role often included planning and interpersonal activities. The leaders did not do the same activities as their subordinates. High production was associated with general rather than close supervision, with a high level of group involvement among members, and with a supportive employee-oriented approach. These conclusions are based on data that vary considerably in the degree to which they differentiate the high and low groups. The correlational nature of the research makes causal interpretations inappropriate.

The Harwood Company, a garment manufacturer, has been the site of considerable behavioral science research since the late 1930s (Marrow, 1972). One study demonstrated the use of participative decision making in overcoming managerial resistance to hiring women over the age of 30 during a labor shortage (Marrow & French, 1945). Another one was a more sophisticated experiment regarding the use of participation in overcoming resistance to introduction of new production processes (Coch & French, 1948). The control group was merely told that certain job changes would be made. A second group was persuaded that a change was needed and was asked to select representatives to receive training. The trainees then taught the other members of the group. All members of the remaining groups received initial training.

Before the change, all groups were producing at about 60 units per hour. All experienced the usual drop in production after the change. The control group never did recover but stabilized at about 50 units. The second group recovered gradually and finally moved up to between 65 and 70 units per hour. The remaining full-participation groups recovered more quickly and stabilized at 70 to 75 units. The differences between the groups seem sizable, but no statistical tests were presented.

Zimmerman (1978) suggests that the Harwood situation was atypical in a number of ways and that generalization of the findings is not advisable. Katzell and Yankelovich (1975) note that no measures of motivation or the effects of participation manipulations on various groups were obtained and question that a causal impact of participation on motivation can be assumed. Gardner (1977) argues that a number of other factors might account for the results. These factors include differences in jobs, group sizes, competition, methods of presenting the need for change, and knowledge of the results.

French, Israel, and As (1960) did a subsequent study in Norway that eliminated a number of the confounding effects and included a measure of the results of the experimental manipulations, but they failed to find significant results. Fleishman (1965) replicated the Harwood study in the United States but failed to support the superiority of participation. French, Ross, Kirby, Nelson, and Smyth (1958) had findings similar to Coch and French (1948) for a more extensive change in the production process at Harwood.

While Likert's linking pin theory extends the role of two-way influence through all levels of an organization, Peltz (1952) dealt only with first-level supervision and satisfaction with the supervisor. Yet his research seems to be the empirical basis for Likert's linking pin hypothesis. Peltz's research findings provide evidence that supervisors with influence on their superiors who also have social closeness with employees and side with employees get greater employee satisfaction than other supervisors.

Morse and Reimer (1956) did a field experiment. In one department decision making was sifted downward to increase employee participation in two divisions and upward to emphasize top-level, hierarchical decisions in two other divisions. Pretests were administered before training supervisors. The divisions operated for a full year before the posttest. In general, there was an increase in satisfaction in the participative divisions and a decrease in satisfaction in the hierarchical divisions. Not all the changes were statistically significant. Productivity increased in both contexts but was greater in the hierarchical groups. Turnover was relatively low in both situations but was greater in the hierarchical divisions. The authors of this research and Likert (1961) hypothesized that the greater productivity increases in the hierarchical groups would not be maintained over time.

Seashore and Bowers (1963) focused in much the same manner as Morse and Reimer (1956) by introducing numerous aspects of the Likert theory. Their findings suggested that the experimental methods did yield results and contributed to greater satisfaction in many areas. However, the experimental and control groups were self-selected, and the data on absenteeism and productivity are hard to interpret.

The Weldon studies (Marrow, 1972; Marrow, Bowers, & Seashore, 1967; Seashore & Bowers, 1970) are an extension of the earlier Harwood studies. They compare changes at Weldon, where participative procedures were first introduced during a period before Weldon's acquisition by Harwood and at the main plant of Harwood, where participation has been practiced for years. The changes were implemented between 1962 and 1964, and a follow-up study was conducted in 1969. The results are perplexing. Weldon appears to have moved from the borderline between systems 1 and 2 to system 4 over the period of the study. A major increase in efficiency and productivity did occur. The overall pattern of motivational and attitudinal change was mixed and varied from measure to measure. A whole battery of changes was introduced almost simultaneously and isolating the precise degree of effect produced by each change was impossible from the methodology used.

The measure of the systems 1 through 4 continuum has changed over the years and is often used in less than its entirety. Even then, it has shown good construct validity. System 4 has correlated with the interpersonal process of informal helping within an organization (Burke & Weir, 1978) and with other measures of similar constructs (Hall, 1972). Golembiewski and Munzenrider (1973) found that Likert profile scores shifted toward system 4 when individuals were exposed to sensitivity training. Likert (1967) reported split-half reliabilities for the profile in the .90s. However, Butterfield and Farris (1974) reported a test-retest value of .52 over a period averaging 1 year. If the instrument is as reliable as the internal consistency suggests, it may be measuring a phenomenon that shows considerable fluctuation over time (Miner 1982, pp. 33-41).

Counte, Barhyte, and Christman (1987) did a field experimental study to determine the effect of increased participation on attendance and job satisfaction of staff nurses. Four units introduced participative management and four served as control units for 1 year. No change was noted in either attendance or job satisfaction. Strasen (1983) addressed how to implement participative management. McClure (1984) even addressed Likert's work specifically.

There is a need for research about participative management in nursing. Does it affect costs, quality of care, productivity, or satisfaction? How does the organizational climate change over time when it is introduced?

REFERENCES

Burke, R., & Weir, T. (1978). Organizational climate and informal helping processes in work settings. *Journal of Management, 4,* 91-105.

Butterfield, D.A., & Farris, G.F. (1974). The Likert organization profile: Methodological analysis and test of system 4 theory in Brazil. *Journal of Applied Psychology, 59,* 15-23.

Coch, L., & French, J.R.P. (1948). Overcoming resistance to change. *Human Relations, 1,* 512-532.

Counte, M.A., Barhyte, D.Y., & Christman, L.P. (1987). Participative management among staff nurses. *Hospital & Health Services Administration, 32,* 97-108.

Dowling, W. (1975). At General Motors: System 4 builds performance and profits. *Organizational Dynamics, 3*(3), 13-38.

Fleishman, E.A. (1965). Attitude versus skill factors in work group productivity. *Personnel Psychology, 18,* 253-266.

French, J.R.P., Israel, J., & As, D. (1960). An experiment on participation in a Norwegian factory: Interpersonal dimensions of decision-making. *Human Relations, 13,* 3-19.

French, J.R.P., Ross, I.C., Kirby, S., Nelson, J.R., & Smyth, P. (1958). Employee participation in a program of industrial change. *Personnel, 35*(6), 16-29.

Gardner, G. (1977). Workers' participation: A critical evaluation of Coch and French. *Human Relations, 30,* 1071-1078.

Golembiewski, R.T., & Munzenrider, R. (1973). Persistence and change: A note on the long-term effects of an organization development program. *Academy of Management Journal, 16,* 149-153.

Hall, J.W. (1972). A comparison of Halpin and Croft's organizational climates and Likert and Likert's organizational systems. *Administrative Science Quarterly, 17,* 586-590.

Kahn, R.L., & Katz, D. (1960). Leadership practices in relation to productivity and morale. In D. Cartwright & A. Zander (Eds.), *Group dynamics research and theory* (pp. 554-570). Evanston, IL: Row, Peterson.

Katzell, R.A., & Yankelovich, D. (1975). *Productivity and job satisfaction: An evaluation of policy-related research.* New York: Psychological Corporation.

Likert, R. (1953). Motivation: The core of management. *American Management Association Personnel Series, 155,* 3-21.

Likert, R. (1961). *New patterns of management.* New York: McGraw-Hill.

Likert, R. (1967). *The human organization: Its management and value.* New York: McGraw-Hill.

Likert, R., & Likert, J.G. (1976). *New ways of managing conflict.* New York: McGraw-Hill.

Likert, R., & Seashore, S.E. (1963). Making cost control work. *Harvard Business Review, 41*(6), 96-108.

Likert, R., & Willets, J.M. (1940-1941). Morale and agency management. Hartford, CT: Life Insurance Agency Management Association.

Mann, F.C., & Likert, R. (1952). The need for research on the communication of research results. *Human Organization, 11*(4), 15-19.

Marrow, A.J. (1972). *The failure of success.* New York: AMACOM.

Marrow, A.J., Bowers, D.G., & Seashore, S.E. (1967). *Management by participation.* New York: Harper & Row.

Marrow, A.J., & French, R.P. (1945). Changing a stereotype in industry. *Journal of Social Issues, 1*(3), 33-37.

McClure, M.L. (1984). Managing the professional nurse: Part 1. The organizational theories. *Journal of Nursing Administration, 14*(2), 15-21.

Miner, J. (1982). *Theories of organizational structure and process* (pp. 18-57). Chicago: Dryden Press.

Morse, N.C., & Reimer, E. (1956). The experimental change of a major organizational variable. *Journal of Abnormal and Social Psychology, 52,* 120-129.

Pelz, D.C. (1952). Influence: A key to effective leadership in the first-line supervisor. *Personnel, 29,* 209-217.

Seashore, S.E., & Bowers, D.G. (1963). *Changing the structure and functioning of an organization: Report of a field experiment.* Ann Arbor, MI: University of Michigan, Institute for Social Research.

Seashore, S.E., & Bowers, D.G. (1970). Durability of organizational change. *American Psychologist, 25,* 227-233.

Stasen, L. (1983). Participative management: A contribution to professionalism. *Critical Care Nurse, 3*(6), 35-40.

Zimmerman, D.K. (1978). Participative management: A reexamination of the classics. *Academy of Management Review, 3,* 896-901.

Chapter 13

Systems Theory
Ludwig von Bertalanffy

Linda Holbrook Freeman
Debra Barker

I| CASE STUDY

Managers at a 500-bed hospital have just completed the budget projection for the new year. Several financial analysts are concerned with revenue losses through insurance companies and other third-party payers. The hospital administrator has observed competitors developing utilization review departments to ensure their hospital's survival and financial viability. Acknowledging the need for this, the administrator has hired Ms. Robins, a registered nurse and financial manager, to develop and implement an additional subsystem, Utilization Management. The mission of the subsystem is to develop effective monitoring systems in patient care utilization to ensure proper reimbursement for services delivered, as well as deliver the most effective health care in the most cost-effective manner. When planning and implementing new subsystems within an organizational structure, the manager needs to consider the possible effects of reorganization.

||||||||||||||||||||||||||||||||||||||||||||||||||||||||||||||

SYSTEMS THEORY

General systems theory was introduced several decades ago by Ludwig von Bertalanffy in an attempt to present concepts that would be applicable across disciplines and would provide a common language; a "doctrine of principles applying to all . . . systems" (1968, p. xix). Such a theory could improve communications among and generally link and facilitate the work of multiple disciplines. The theory was one of wholeness, proposing that "the whole is more than the sum of parts" (p. 55). A system may be defined as "sets of elements standing in interrelation" (p. 38). All systems have elements in common. "The theory of open systems is part of a general system theory" (p. 149). An open system is defined as a "system in exchange of matter with its environment, presenting import and export, building-up and breaking-down of its material components" (p. 141). Open systems theory emphasizes the relationship between a system and its environment and the interrelationships of different levels of systems (Katz & Kahn, 1966, p. 3).

The effects of new subsystems can be analyzed by the open systems theory developed by Daniel Katz and Robert L. Kahn. They contend that "open systems theory emphasizes the close relationship between a structure and its supporting environment" (Katz & Kahn, 1966, p. 3).

One of the basic concepts described is entropy or inputs. Without these energies the system fails or discontinues to thrive. The idea of throughputs is another major concept; throughputs process the inputs to yield an output that is useful to the organization and surrounding environment. The open systems theory includes different levels that work collectively to achieve an outcome. It views the organization as having different hierarchical levels with the higher levels dominating the lower ones.

In Katz and Kahn's theory the system is cyclic. For the system to remain viable it must continually receive and process energy from the external environment. Katz and Kahn describe their theory as "an energic input-output system in which the energic return from the output reactivates the system" (1966, p. 20). The system recognizes boundaries that surround the organization. Boundaries are identified by "following the energic and informational transactions as they relate to the cycle of activities of input, throughput, and output" (1966, p. 21). The open systems theory differs greatly from the earlier system theorists in that this approach deals with temporal and spatial social patterns, uses the concept of an open system, and is dependent on the external environment for a constant flow of energies.

King's theory of goal attainment in nursing is an example of an application of open systems theory to nursing. King has identified "interaction, perception, communication, transaction, role, stress, growth and development, and time and space" as concepts in her theory of goal attainment (1981, p. 144).

The conceptual basis for nursing is a framework of interacting personal, interpersonal, and social systems (King, 1981, p. 11). This framework is illustrated in Figure 13-1. While King's theory of goal attainment is specific for nursing, selected concepts may be redefined to apply to nursing management as a process, rather than to the nursing process.

King defines interaction "as a process of perception and communication between persons and environment and between person and person, represented by verbal and nonverbal behaviors that are goal directed" (1981, p. 145). Figure 13-2 depicts this process. Application to nursing management requires one of the persons in interpersonal systems to be a nurse manager, rather than a client.

Communication is "a process whereby information is given from one person to another either directly . . . or indirectly" (1981, p. 146). This exchange of information between nurse and client or others again may be modified to describe the exchange between the nurse manager and nurse or nurse manager and others in the environment.

Other concepts may be applied to nursing management as originally defined. Perception is "each person's representation of reality" (1981, p. 146). This concept is applicable as presented.

"Transactions are defined as purposeful interactions that lead to goal attainment" (1981, p. 1). Because the subconcept of interaction has been redefined for management, this definition of transaction is appropriate to nursing management as stated.

Stress is "a dynamic state whereby a human being interacts with the environment," and stress "involves an exchange of energy and information between the person and environment for regulation and control of stressors" (1981, p. 147).

King views nursing as "a process of human interactions between nurse and client whereby each perceives the other and the situation; and through communication, they set goals, explore means, and agree on means to achieve goals" (1981, p. 144). Nursing management may be viewed in the same way, again substituting nurse manager for client. The goals may be professional goals of the nurse that contribute to or are congruent with organizational goals.

Health "implies continuous adjustment to stressors in the internal and external environment through optimum use of one's resources to achieve maximum potential for daily

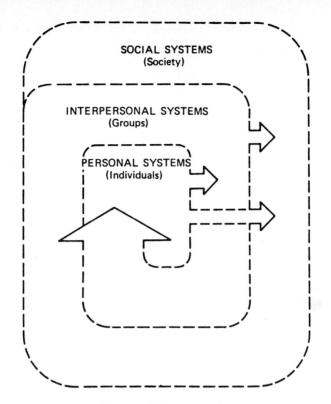

FIGURE 13-1   A conceptual framework for nursing: dynamic interacting systems. *From King, I.M.,* Toward a theory for nursing. © *1981, John Wiley & Sons, Inc.*

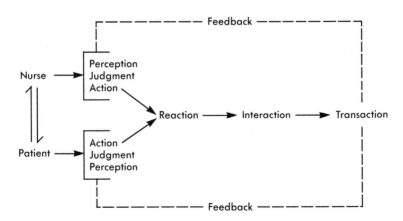

FIGURE 13-2   A process of human interactions. *From King, I.M.,* Toward a theory for nursing. © *1981, John Wiley & Sons, Inc.*

TABLE 13-1   Major Concepts of the Interacting Systems in King's Framework (1989)

Personal systems	Interpersonal systems	Social systems
Self	Communication	Organization
Perception	Interaction	Power
	Transaction	Authority
		Status
		Role
		Control
		Communication
		Decision making

Table developed by Linda Holbrook Freeman from content noted in King, 1989, pp. 39-40.

living" (1981, p. 5). Health may be applied both to the organization and to the individual and may be the function of management-employee interactions to achieve maximum potential.

These concepts, some of which we have redefined, may be used in a theory of goal attainment for nursing management. In 1989 King published a system's framework for nursing administration (King, 1989). This framework, like King's earlier theory, is based on general systems theory.

King uses five characteristics of general systems as a basis for the framework: goals, structure, functions, resources, and decision making (1989, p. 38). The goal in this framework is health, which includes "health promotion, health maintenance, and regaining a functional state of health" (p. 38). "Structure can be viewed as the semipermeable boundaries between" the three systems (p. 38). In open systems, boundaries allow information and energy to move in and out of the system. King states, "Structure provides for the allocation of resources . . . and information flow" (pp. 38-39). Functions are the "action element in the organization . . . carried out by individuals to attain goals" (p. 39). The fourth characteristic, resources, is necessary to perform the work of the system (p. 39). Lastly, decision making "is a process and skill that is required at each level of the three dynamic interacting systems" (p. 39).

While the concept of dynamic interacting systems was retained in the framework for nursing administration, the focus shifts to social systems (King, 1989). The concepts of this new framework for nursing administration include the broad concepts of organization, power, authority, status, role, control, decision making, perception, communication, interaction, and transaction (King, 1989, p. 42). It is necessary to know the major concepts of each of the three interacting systems to facilitate goal attainment (King, 1989). These major concepts are shown in Table 13-1.

The details of the framework, including relevant definitions, are not available in the initial publication by King (1989). King suggests selecting a framework that has relevance for "one's individual and organizational philosophy to implement change" (1989, p. 44).

CASE ANALYSIS

While any open system theory can be used to analyze the case, Katz and Kahn will be used. As Ms. Robins faces her new challenge as Manager of Utilization Management, she recognizes the possible effects of her subsystem on the entire organization. The interrelationships can be best described by the 10 most common characteristics of an open system (Katz & Kahn, 1966). These are input, throughput, output, cycles of events, negative entropy, negative feedback, steady state, differentiation, integration and coordination, and equifinality.

The first characteristic is *input,* or *importation of energy.* This refers to inputs or energy coming from the external environment. According to the theorists, "social organizations must draw renewed supplies of energy from other institutions or people or the material environment. No social structure is self-sufficient or self-contained" (Katz & Kahn, 1966, p. 23). Knowing this, Ms. Robins searches out other organizations that have implemented utilization review and will determine their effectiveness for financial gains for the organization. She will also work closely with the admissions department and the billing department to obtain accurate and current insurance information and will ensure its maintenance on file. Additionally administration will supply all current insurance guidelines for utilization control to ensure prevention of lost funds. To assess the effectiveness and accuracy of the department's monitoring and utilization control, she plans to work closely with Accounts Payable to determine the status of all outstanding accounts.

The second characteristic is *throughput.* This major concept is emphasized, for it is the process of transformation of energy available to the system. Ms. Robins will transform energies from other subsystems in the organization, as well as inputs received from other organizations outside the institution's boundaries. Contact with other subsystems will provide lateral and horizontal communication. Transformation will occur as a result of training of staff for utilization review and monitoring of patient care, computer analysis of outstanding accounts of the previous year in comparison with the present year's financial report as a result of the new program implementation, and continuous implementation and training.

The third characteristic emphasized is *output.* Outputs are the results or outcomes of transformations made. Outputs may reveal themselves as financial reports summarizing yearly progress or changes made in utilization practices. Outputs may also result from changes in knowledge and performance levels of the nurses who perform utilization review. Ms. Robins also must be concerned with the continuation of receiving the desired result. Katz and Kahn believe that this result depends on the receptivity of the members in the organization. Ms. Robins must win the approval for this product from the nursing and physician community. She plans to gain acceptance through education and integration with other subsystems. Nursing opportunities are expected to be found through the development of outpatient surgical suites and home nursing services, which should equally result in meeting established insurance requirements for outpatient treatment. Physicians should also gain incentives to comply with new policy through in-service education to increase knowledge of third-party and insurance regulations, ending in financial growth for the hospital.

The fourth characteristic describes the system as *cycles of events.* By establishing effective utilization controls over patient care, Ms. Robins is aware of its effect on insurance groups, better distribution of governmental tax funds for health care usage by the indigent, and lowering of premiums for insurance holders. As insurance companies are better able to monitor expenditures and usage, these savings are being passed on to the patient for improved health care coverage and more benefits payable to the providers of health care. Ms. Robins's financial report should also show financial gains as a result of improved monitoring and prevention of penalties or lost funds. Financial growth for the organization will furnish the energy to fuel the continued functioning units of the entire system.

The fifth characteristic of an open system is *negative entropy.* "To survive, open systems must reverse the entropic process, they must acquire entropy. The entropic process is the universal law of nature in which all forms of organization move toward disorganization or death" (Katz & Kahn, 1966, p. 25). Ms. Robins is in an organization that is dependent on several organizations outside the boundary of her institution. The outside insurance and governmental agencies supply major financial support to fuel the system's ongoing functions. Virtually every subsystem is dependent on these energies to continue operational processes. Ms. Robins functions at the boundary line with the outside environment to receive inputs selectively to maintain continued existence. This requires continuous updates or changes in hospital requirements to maintain financial homeostasis.

In relation to information input, *negative feedback* is the type of input that allows the system to identify deviations in its functioning processes. Many malfunctions in the present system have been identified as a result of Ms. Robins's assessment, as a new manager, of current procedures. Negative feedback has also been identified to her through access to financial reporting, financial analysis of audit results, and administrative investigation.

Another characteristic of the system is maintenance of the *steady state* or *homeostasis*. The system's homeostasis is maintained through a constant flow of energy exchange. As previously mentioned, this is acquired through avoidance of entropy.

Differentiation occurs as the organization grows. This requires multiplication and changes in established roles. As Ms. Robins continues in her new position as Manager of Utilization Management, she will gain new knowledge and expand her expertise outside the boundaries of the organization to include insurance and other agencies. This activity must create a constant flow of energy exchange as each member also continuously adapts to new functional changes. As a result *integration and coordination* are achieved. This process leads to the establishment of a new organizational structure.

Finally, Katz and Kahn (1966) emphasize the characteristic of *equifinality*. This implies that the goals established can be reached in a variety of ways and not by one method. Ms. Robins will assess the variety of avenues available and select those that meet her own individual management style and still accomplish the desired result.

RESEARCH

Organizational structures and related processes have been investigated by several fields of study. The largest portion of work, however, has been primarily theoretical discussion. Only a few of the studies conducted are actually theory-based research. Most compare structural components but fail to relate results with a theoretical emphasis. Nursing is one field that has just begun presenting an interest in this research in relation to the organizational theories. Most literature reviewed is based on assumptions and not results of research activity. The following is a summarization of the related research.

Mark (1985), from her research of task and structural correlates of organizational effectiveness, explored the relationships between task and structural variables and two dimensions of organizational effectiveness in 76 private psychiatric hospitals. This study showed that high levels of centralization and formulation were associated with patient care effectiveness. The enhancement of organizational structure is suggested to contribute to organizational effectiveness. Data were collected by use of mailed questionnaires to 76 respondents. Mark concluded that the organizational structure may be enhanced instead of constrained by centralization. The use of the centralizing and standardizing tasks resulted in decreasing intraorganizational uncertainty. The researcher contended that as a result of this structure the person may focus on the patient care process and thereby improve the organization's effectiveness.

Rosengren's research (1967) was conducted to explain the relationships that exist between control achieved through structural arrangements and control achieved through supervisory style. Analysis of data was based on comparison between 87 government hospitals and 45 private hospitals. One result showed that structural characteristics most conducive to achieving participant control will occur more frequently in large governmental hospitals rather than smaller ones. Restricted communication was also shown to be the typical pattern of the larger hospitals.

Lawrence and Lorsch (1967) used a theory base and related concepts in the analysis of the relationship of six organizations in the same industrial environment. These researchers looked at three different subsystems: sales, research, and production. Results showed that differentiation and integration had an inverse relationship between the subsystems, implying that only one can be obtained at the expense of the other.

Batchelor (1985) provided a formal discussion of how corporate restructuring is required to meet organizational demands and meet competitive challenges. The researcher concurs that "corporate restructuring allows a hospital to respond to environmental pressures, meet competitive challenges, and expand and diversify into new lines of business" (Batchelor, 1985, p. 202).

The research studies conducted using King's theory of goal attainment have related to nursing, rather than to nursing administration. In the theory of goal attainment "the concepts . . . relate primarily to the interpersonal systems" (King, 1989, p. 40), that of the nurse and client. Research on the interpersonal system of nurse and nurse manager using the theory of goal attainment as adapted has not been done.

King's framework for nursing administration, introduced in 1989, also remains to be tested. King suggests that "knowledge of the concepts of the new theory of administration can be used to analyze one's current organizational structure" (1989, p. 42). King further states, "This theory, when published in detail, will be useful in nursing service administration and in nursing education administration" (1989, p. 42).

REFERENCES

Batchelor, G.J. (1985). Establishing a multicorporate structure. *Nursing Economics, 3,* 201-204.

Katz, D., & Kahn, R.L. (1966). *The social psychology of organizations.* New York: John Wiley & Sons.

King, I.M. (1981). *A theory for nursing: Systems, concepts, process.* New York: John Wiley & Sons.

King, I.M. (1989). King's systems framework for nursing administration. In B. Henry, C. Arndt, M. Vincenti, & A. Marriner-Tomey (Eds.), *Dimensions of nursing administration: Theory, research, education, practice* (pp. 35-45). Boston: Blackwell Scientific Publications.

Lawrence, P.P., & Lorsch, J.W. (1967). Differentiation and integration in complex organizations. *Administration Science Quarterly, 12,* 1-47.

Mark, B. (1985). Task and structural correlates of organizational effectiveness. *Health Services Research, 20,* 199-224.

Rosengren, W.R. (1967). Structure, policy, style: Strategies of organizational control. *Administration Science Quarterly, 12,* 140-164.

von Bertalanffy, L. (1968). *General systems theory: Foundations, development, applications.* New York: Braziller.

Chapter 14

Job Characteristics Theory
Edward E. Lawler III,
J. Richard Hackman, and
Greg Oldham

Phyllis Chafin

I I   CASE STUDY

Ann Winston came to work in the critical care unit on the 3 PM to 11 PM shift shortly after graduation. She worked this shift for several months and then transferred to the 11 PM to 7 AM shift for approximately 8 months. The unit is divided into two sides and each side has the capacity for eight clients and eight telemetry monitors. After orientation to the area and gaining experience she assumed charge duties. Charge duties are usually assigned to the nurse who has the most experience or seniority and the person is responsible for making assignments for the other nurses on the shift. Ann assigned herself the most critical clients because she felt guilty assigning these "difficult" clients to other nurses. During the last 3 months on nights, several of the patients died while Ann was caring for them as a result of numerous medical problems such as terminal cancer, acute myocardial infarction with complications, and multiple problems in elderly patients with poor prognoses. She became unable to cope with death, having charge duties in the unit, or having to help new employees with their nursing care. Ann felt that maybe her ability to deliver quality nursing care was inadequate. She married during this time and later transferred to the 7 AM to 3 PM shift. This did not prove to be any better. Shortly after this Ann considered resigning and moving into the field of home health care.

| | | | | | | | | | | | | | | | | | | | | | | | | | | | | | | | | | | | | | | | | | | | | | | | | | | | | | | | | | | | | | | | | |

JOB CHARACTERISTICS THEORY

The job characteristics theory has gone through numerous revisions since its beginning in the 1950s with Herzberg's work. It is thought that the job characteristics theory is a "different approach to Herzberg's motivation hygiene theory and concerns itself with job enrichment" (Miner, 1981, p. 103). Job enrichment is defined in this chapter as the job providing the worker with a feeling of meaningfulness, responsibility, and feedback (Kraft & Williams, 1975). Job enrichment also enables the worker to have a positive association with the satisfaction derived from the job and the motivation to do the job adequately (Kraft & Williams, 1975).

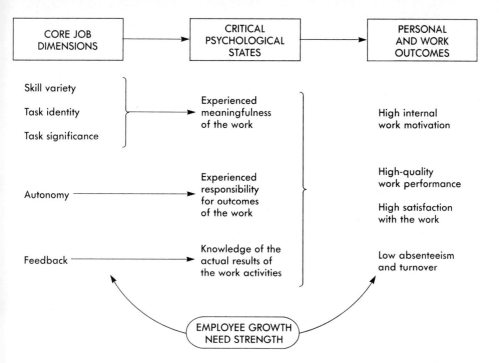

FIGURE 14-1   The job characteristic model of work motivation. *From Hackman, J.R., & Oldham, G.R. (1975). Development of the job diagnostic survey.* Journal of Applied Psychology, 60, 161. *Copyright 1975 by the American Psychological Association. Reprinted by permission.*

There are four characteristics to the first rendition of this particular theory and it is thought by behaviorists that these must be present for a job to be enriched. They are as follows: autonomy, a high degree of task identity, sufficient variety, and feedback (Miner, 1980).

Maslow's hierarchy of needs theory, Alderfer's existence, relatedness, and growth (ERG) theory, and Herzberg's motivation hygiene theory were all part of the human relations movement. Herzberg was also responsible for the beginning development of the job enrichment theory. It was expanded by Lawler's expectancy theory. Following suit with Lawler were Hackman and Oldham. The latter three theorists have published numerous articles and studies regarding the job enrichment theory.

Hackman and Lawler's original theory (1971) was based on five job core characteristics, psychological states, and personal and work outcomes (Figure 14-1). The core job dimensions are defined as follows (Hackman, 1977, pp. 130-131):

Skill variety: the degree to which a job requires a variety of different activities that involve the use of a number of different skills and talents.

Task identity: the degree to which the job requires completion of a whole and identifiable piece of work—that is, doing a job from beginning to end with a visible outcome.

Task significance: the degree to which the job has a substantial impact on the lives or work of other people, whether in the immediate organization or in the external environment.

Autonomy: the degree to which the job provides substantial freedom, independence, and discretion to the individual in scheduling the work and in determining the procedures to be used to carry it out.

$$\text{Motivating potential score (MPS)} = \left[\frac{\text{Skill variety} + \text{Task identity} + \text{Task significance}}{3}\right] \times \text{Autonomy} \times \text{Job feedback}$$

FIGURE 14-2   Motivating Potential Score formula. *From Hackman, J.R. (1977). Work designs. In J.R. Hackman & J.L. Suttle (Eds.),* Improving life at work: Behavioral science approach to organizational change *(p. 131). Santa Monica, CA: Goodyear.*

Feedback: the degree to which carrying out the work activities required by the job results in the individual obtaining direct and clear information about the effectiveness of his or her performance.

The psychological states are responsible for the worker's motivation and satisfaction. They are identified as follows (Hackman, 1977, p. 129):

1. *Experienced meaningfulness:* The person must experience the work as generally important, valuable, and worthwhile.
2. *Experienced responsibility:* The individual must feel personally responsible and accountable for the results of the work he or she performs.
3. *Knowledge of results:* The person must have an understanding, on a fairly regular basis, of how effectively he is performing the job.

These psychological states are present when the worker feels good about himself or herself and has internal rewards. When any of these states are no longer present, the worker no longer regards the internal rewards given for good performance (Hackman, 1977).

Extensive studies have been done regarding job enrichment, and behaviorists agree that job enrichment is most positive for the high-growth-needs individual (Oldham, Hackman, & Pearce, 1976).

The previous five job characteristics have been combined to form the Motivating Potential Score (MPS) to mirror the motivating power of a particular job. This formula is shown in Figure 14-2. To be high in motivating potential, a job must be high on feedback, autonomy, and at least one job dimension that contributes to a job's meaningfulness—skill, variety, task identity, or task significance. A near zero on feedback or autonomy will reduce the overall MPS to near zero, while a near zero on one of the three job dimensions cannot do so.

Hackman and Oldham (1974) also developed a tool to obtain measures of the core characteristics. The Job Diagnostic Survey (JDS) has been revised for different studies conducted by behaviorists (Rousseau, 1977). The question is, does the JDS give reliable measures of variety and autonomy since this tool does differentiate among jobs?

The way a person perceives his or her job and how it is valued varies among persons. The person can, as time goes by, develop a negative perception of his or her job. Job redesign is a chance to enhance the worker's feeling of personal satisfaction or "job enrichment."

Job redesign is a difficult process; therefore, it must include several guidelines to be successful. Hackman (1977) has several ideas for gaining personal and organizational change through job redesign. Job redesign can (1) lessen the negative effect of work that is highly repetitive; (2) supply opportunities for positive and self-sustaining work motivation and productivity; and (3) allow human and industrial attitudes of the workplace to be changed to enrich the content and context of the work simultaneously.

Job redesign can be performed using the job characteristics model but it must be remembered that the

model deals only with aspects of jobs that can be altered to create positive motivational incentives for the job incumbent. It does not directly address the dysfunctional aspects of repetitive work (as

$$\text{Overall group effectiveness} = S_1 \left[\text{Level of effort}\right] + S_2 \left[\begin{array}{c}\text{Amount of}\\\text{knowledge}\\\text{and skill}\end{array}\right] + S_3 \left[\begin{array}{c}\text{Appropriateness of}\\\text{task performance}\\\text{strategies}\end{array}\right]$$

S_1 = 1 — degree of technological constraint on effort
S_2 = 1 — degree of technological constraint on performance strategy
S_3 = 1 — degree of technological constraint on knowledge and skill

FIGURE 14-3   Model of group enrichment. *From Hackman, J.R. (1978). The design of self-managing work groups. In B.T. King, S.S. Streufert, & F.E. Fiedler (Eds.),* Managerial control and organizational democracy *(pp. 78-79). Washington, DC: Winston.*

does activation theory), although presumably a job designed in accord with the dictates of the model would not turn out to be routine or highly repetitive. (Oldham et al., 1976, p. 276)

Job redesign is necessary when there is a weak link in any of the following areas (Kraft & Williams, 1975):

1. *Task combination.* Workers seem to be more satisfied when they are responsible for a whole piece of work rather than fragmented jobs. Job enrichment tries to give whole jobs with clearer outcomes and objectives and greater variety.
2. *Natural units of work.* In some jobs the fragments have no relation to each other; therefore, job enrichment attempts to put the tasks together that belong together.
3. *Client information.* Many workers do not understand the internal operations of the company in which they are employed. Job enrichment tries to help the worker develop an idea of what the services are, who are its potential users, and why they provide these services.
4. *Feedback.* If a worker is not given immediate feedback regarding job performance, he or she does not have internal satisfaction. Job enrichment encourages the use of immediate feedback.
5. *Vertical loading.* When workers have little control of their work, they are deprived of a sense of autonomy. A goal of job enrichment is to increase autonomy and responsibility by giving the worker more control, decision making, and planning.

The job characteristic model has been supported strongly enough in research to be considered a useful tool for job redesign (Nadler, Hackman, & Lawler, 1979). Most of the research on job enrichment has been done on the individual's aspect of what a job means to a person. Many jobs require a team or group effort; therefore behaviorists have moved the research into groups. Research has indicated that it is much more difficult to enrich jobs for groups than for individuals. Hackman (1977) has two criteria for designing work for a group so that the team productivity and satisfaction of each member can be enhanced concurrently. The team or group should be a cohesive group and the environment must allow the group norms that emerge to be of high productivity as well as be able to satisfy interpersonal relationships. The model in Figure 14-3 was developed by Hackman to display how group enrichment is derived (1978, p. 65).

CASE ANALYSIS

Not all jobs are to be enriched and not all jobs need to be enriched. The nursing profession has benefited from the job enrichment theory, in part owing to the fact that nursing is a profession and professionals tend to be high-growth-needs individuals. As stated above, this group of workers respond more positively to job enrichment tactics. However, not all high-growth-needs individuals are enriched.

Job enrichment theory of leadership is introduced into nursing to help lead to employee contentment and motivation. Much of the material written concerning leadership and management is in business journals and other fields of management (Young & Hayne, 1988). Nursing has adopted this information and hopefully will enlarge on it so that the nursing profession can have improved affirmed leadership and management styles. One major misconception of job enrichment for nursing is the idea that if the worker is given more to do, she or he will be motivated. This is the old job enlargement theory (Fuszard, 1984).

Ann came to work motivated and job enriched. In the process of everything that occurred, she became overloaded and lost touch with herself. Job enlargement or simplification is determined by the demands of the job and the workers' capabilities and personal motives (Miner, 1975).

Ann poured herself into her work, wanted to perform well, and wished to see positive results from her clients. Since she assigned herself the terminal clients, there was no one to reinforce the fact that she was giving these people something to make them feel better. She lacked positive feedback.

By looking at the job characteristics model and comparing the core characteristics to the case study, one finds that skill variety was present in Ann's job. Working in the critical care area is closest in proximity to primary nursing; the nurse assigned to the client is primarily responsible for all aspects of care. Task identity was lost with Ann. Task identity is the process of completing a whole job with a positive visible outcome. Most of Ann's clients were terminal; therefore Ann saw very few positive outcomes. Guilt is another feeling Ann had to deal with. She had feelings of guilt if she assigned other nurses to these terminal clients and she felt guilty when they died. She in turn lost confidence in her nursing abilities and became unhappy with herself. Task significance in this case was overwhelming. She felt that her nursing care had a direct impact on the client's well-being. Perhaps by giving herself a break and caring for clients who were less critical, Ann could have felt better about herself. Ann probably never stopped to think that she helped to make these terminal clients' hospital stay easier because of her caring hard work to keep them clean, dry, and as comfortable as possible.

Autonomy was present in Ann's job. She had charge duties when she was the most experienced nurse scheduled. It appears that Ann was not utilizing the other nurses to save her own work stamina. She should have done the assigning differently so that all the staff took turns caring for emotionally draining clients.

Feedback was definitely lacking in this case. Ann's clients could not say, "Thank you, that feels better." Sometimes this is all a nurse needs to push herself forward. Other staff nurses and her supervisors praised her for her work well done, although this did not seem to be enough. What could be done to fix this problem and have Ann's job reenriched? It is more profitable to prevent burnout than to treat it. It is costly in time and money to replace nurses. Satisfaction with supervision and promotion are both highly related to feedback. Overall, satisfaction with work and supervision correlated highest with job characteristics.

RESEARCH

Extensive research and studies have been done in the field of job enrichment theory. Most of the research supports the theory; however, there are some cases in which job enrichment made no difference and some cases in which the situation was worse after job enrichment.

Castellano studied the differences in job response between rural and urban workers. The results provided little support for the hypothesis that worker rural-urban background is related to job attitude and behavior (1976, p. 500). The study indicated that no matter what the worker's background, he or she will adapt and support the organization's value systems, norms, and required behavior patterns.

Umstot, Bell, and Mitchell's research project (1976) examined the effect of job enrichment and goal setting on employee productivity and satisfaction. This study supported the job enrichment satisfaction relationship, but it found little relationship between job enrichment and productivity. People with assigned goals had greater performance and perception of feedback. Goals make work more interesting and therefore jobs are more satisfying.

Sims and Szilagyi (1976) researched the relationship of perceptions of job characteristics and employee expectancies, satisfaction, and performance. The results supported the hypothesis that high-growth-needs individuals are better candidates for job enrichment. These researchers define locus of control as the manner in which an individual perceives contingencies between actions and outcomes (p. 213). Internal locus of control describes a person who thinks he or she has control of himself or herself. External locus of control describes a person who thinks his or her outcomes are controlled by extrinsic factors. It was discovered in this study that low-growth-needs people were found to have stronger relationships between task identity and performance: dealing with others and performance, and friendship and performance. Their locus of control was quite different; those with external locus of control had stronger relationships between autonomy and satisfaction with work, autonomy and satisfaction with supervisor, and also in dealing with others and satisfaction with work. The low-growth-needs individual who is observed to be high on task identity views his or her job as less demanding and performs better.

Sims and Szilagyi (1976) did research to determine the validity and measurement of job characteristics. The results supported the original and revised instruments as a valid and reliable way to research relationships between characteristics and employee attitudes and behavior.

Dunham, Aldag, and Brief (1977) conducted research to measure the dimensionality of task design as measured by the Job Diagnostic Survey (JDS). Results concluded that the JDS was not consistent across samples and conflicting results were produced. The authors feel that there is a most urgent need for further research for the measurement of task design.

Steers and Spencer (1977) examined the effects of job scope and the need for achievement among workers. This study concluded that

> indirectly, enriched jobs may have the effect of contributing to reduced turnover and absenteeism because . . . commitment has been shown to be strongly and inversely related to such behavior. Hence, changes in job design do appear to have very practical consequences for the management of organizations. (p. 117)

This study supports the research found on job enrichment. Behavior modification or reinforcement theory is most successful among low-growth-needs individuals.

Simonds and Orife (1975) focused on work behavior versus the enrichment theory. Their results concluded that pay increases are more important to staff than the differences that job enrichment would introduce.

Salancik and Pfeffer (1978) investigated the social approach to job attitudes and task design. The research found that commitment is important to the worker and this ties him or her to the behavior demonstrated at the workplace.

White (1978) researched the relationship between individual differences and the job quality and worker response relationship. The research reviewed did not prove to be fruitful.

There was a lack of consistency even though extensive studies were reviewed. It was determined by White that further research in these areas are not necessary.

Aldag and Brief (1975) studied the relationship of work values indices to employee affective responses to task characteristics and leader behaviors. Protestant ethic ideals were associated with higher order needs.

Sexton (1967) studied organizational and individual needs. Findings show a significant relationship between the degree of job structure and the satisfaction of high-growth-needs individuals. The findings did not support the popular thesis that the burden of job structure obstructs the worker's satisfaction of his or her higher level needs.

Robey (1974) conducted a study to test Hulin and Blood's hypothesis that job satisfaction and performance are affected by task design and work values. Results support the hypothesis but do not offer "conclusive evidence regarding the effect of job enlargement on work behavior" (p. 272).

Oldham, Hackman, and Pearce (1976) supported the job enrichment theory in their study regarding employee growth need strength and employees' response to enriched work. These behaviorists encourage the study of long-term effects of the theory and how job effects are judged by individual differences and how these differences affect job changes.

Hackman and Lawler (1971) did the renowned AT&T telephone company study to better understand employee reactions to job characteristics. The findings significantly supported the hypothesis of job enrichment; however, not everyone who was employed at the company was enriched.

Locke, Sirota, and Wolfson (1976) researched attitudes and behaviors in the process of job enrichment. They found that job enrichment is not a panacea and that technology limits job enrichment. The results of the study were consistent and showed positive and negative results of job enrichment.

Stone, Mowday, and Porter (1977) focused on the relationship between job characteristics and job satisfactions. The findings of their study also supported the theory. The study revealed that the need for achievement lacked importance as a moderator but had considerable use as an independent forecaster of job satisfaction.

Wanous (1974) was interested in individual differences and reaction to job characteristics. The results support the finding that high-growth-needs individuals respond to enriched jobs. This study used three moderators: (1) job characteristic–job satisfaction relationship showed no difference; (2) job characteristic–job behavior relationship showed no difference; and (3) high- and low-need-strengths group concerned the relationship between task characteristics and specific job facet satisfaction or other attitude variable such as job involvement (p. 620).

Schwab and Cummings (1976) focused on the impact of task scope on employees' performance. They presented a model that linked task scope to employee motivation. This particular study was very involved. It concluded that individual differences have a direct relationship on how a worker perceives his or her task scope. Further research concerning task scope is also encouraged.

Katz (1978) was interested in the overall relationship satisfaction in the workplace and the five task dimensions of job characteristics. The results support the theory and shed light on what new and old employees expect from a job. New employees are interested in being a helpful part of the organization, while older employees want to establish and demonstrate their confidence.

Bishop and Hill (1971) researched low-status workers to determine the effects of job enlargement and job change. They reported that "job enlargement or change may have an overall positive effect on those receiving the manipulation, but it may turn out to be dysfunctional for workers observing but not receiving the treatment" (p. 175). The findings suggested that the changes noted in the workers came about simply because of the Hawthorne effect and not because of any great change. The nonmanipulated workers presented a decrease in status and work satisfaction with an increase in anxiety. The study supports the negative effects of job design on the sample used for this study. Low-status workers were more responsive on the dependent variables to changes in their workplace. The workers' status must be reviewed when the relationship between job design and job satisfaction is examined.

Rousseau (1977) conducted a study to determine the relationship between variety and task significance in relation to job satisfaction. It was determined that skill variety and task significance had the highest association with involvement, alienation, and satisfaction. The results recommend that the completion of a whole job is not a critical factor of positive job response as is the understanding that the task or tasks performed affect the well-being of others.

Job enrichment is not for every job nor for every employee. Occasionally job enrichment fails. Some behaviorists see no need for job enrichment anywhere. Fein (1975) believes that there are two groups of people, the achievers and the nonachievers. Fifteen percent of the workforce are achievers and 85% are nonachievers. The nonachievers work because they have to eat but this does not mean they do not like their work or receive personal satisfaction from a job well done. Fein also reports "deficiencies in the treatment of statistical data and the omission of information by some of the case study reporters which affected their conclusions" (p. 53).

Participation failures stem primarily from the lack of worker interest and is the goal of management. Workers will not respond to participation until they see it as a personal need or feel that it is in their best interest (Fein, 1975).

Job enrichment theory requires time for the whole process to be implemented. Walton remarks that

> the extra effort required for the learning, planning, and persuasion activities probably derive from the desire to create; prove it can be done; collaborate with others; get recognition; and learn and develop new skills. But this investment of energy does not pay off immediately. There is an early period of deferred gratification, while some suffer set-backs and others are taking a wait-and-see stance. (1974, p. 171)

Frank and Hackman (1975) conducted a study using workers in a large bank during the introductory phase of job enrichment. The results showed that some of the workers did not experience job enrichment; some of the workers had jobs deenriched; and most of the workers saw no obvious change at all. This study cannot be noted as a valid test of the job characteristics theory.

Listed below are seven reasons for problems in job enrichment studies: (1) failure to actually change the jobs; (2) job changes intervene with surrounding work systems; (3) inadequate initial diagnosis; (4) management resists change; (5) lack of evaluation; (6) inadequate theoretical knowledge on the part of the behaviorists; and (7) bureaucratic "from the top down" implementation of the changes (Frank & Hackman, 1975; Hackman, 1975).

Little nursing research has been done regarding the job enrichment theory. Other studies have been done in nursing regarding job satisfaction; however, they chose to use other theories.

Sims and Szilagyi's research (1976) states

> that the characteristics of the individual employee, the target of the enrichment movement, has a very strong bearing on the question of whether enriched jobs will lead to improved satisfaction. Current research stresses that both job characteristics and individual employee characteristics should be studied in a thorough examination of the area of job design. (p. 212)

Sims and Szilagyi (1976) conducted two studies at large medical centers to determine the relationship of job enrichment and hospital-employed persons. The results of this study supported its hypothesis that high-growth-needs individuals are more responsive to job enrichment.

Sims and Szilagyi's study (1976) indicated that satisfaction with work was directly related to variety, relationships with co-workers, and performance. Feedback was found to be important in determining the workers' satisfaction with supervision and promotion. Salary was not an important factor in this study sample.

Roedel and Nystrom (1988) focused their study on nursing jobs and satisfaction. The job enrichment core characteristics were measured by the JDS. The findings show that task identity is the key variable and this tends to score lower than the other variables. Task identity is perceived differently by individual nurses.

Nursing is a close personal contact profession and is a high-growth-needs profession. Therefore there are many opportunities for job enrichment studies using all the core dimensions. Research regarding the combination of the job enrichment theory and goal setting theory is needed.

REFERENCES

Aldag, R.J., & Brief, A.P. (1975). Some correlates of work values. *Journal of Applied Psychology, 60,* 757-760.

Bishop, R.C., & Hill, J.W. (1971). Effects of job enlargement and job change on contiguous but nonmanipulated jobs as a function of workers' status. *Journal of Applied Psychology, 55*(3), 175-181.

Castellano, J.J. (1976). Rural and urban differences: One more time. *Academy of Management Journal, 19,* 495-502.

Dunham, R.B., Aldag, R.J., & Brief, A.P. (1977). Dimensionality of task design as measured by the job diagnostic survey. *Academy of Management Journal, 20,* 209-223.

Fein, M. (1975). Job enrichment does not work. *Atlanta Economic Review, 25*(6), 50-54.

Frank, L.L., & Hackman, J.R. (1975). A failure of job enrichment: The case of the change that wasn't. *Journal of Applied Behavioral Science, 11,* 413-436.

Fuszard, B. (Ed.). (1984). *Self-actualization for nurses: Issues, trends, and strategies for job enrichment.* Rockville, MD: Aspen.

Hackman, J.R. (1975). Is job enrichment just a fad? *Harvard Business Review, 53*(5), 129-138.

Hackman, J.R. (1977). Work designs. In J.R. Hackman & J.L. Suttle (Eds.), *Improving life at work: Behavioral science approaches to organizational change.* Santa Monica, CA: Goodyear.

Hackman, J.R. (1978). The design of self-managing work groups. In B.T. King, S.S. Streufert, & F.E. Fiedler (Eds.), *Managerial control and organizational democracy.* Washington, DC: Winston.

Hackman, J.R., & Lawler, E.E. (1971). Employee reactions to job characteristics. *Journal of Applied Psychology, 55,* 259-286.

Hackman, J.R., & Oldham, G.R. (1974). The job diagnostic survey: An instrument for the diagnosis and the evaluation of job redesign projects (Technological Report No. 4). Yale University, Department of Administrative Science.

Herzberg, F. (1987). One more time: How do you motivate employees? *Harvard Business Review, 65,* 109-120.

Katz, R. (1978). Job longevity as a situational factor in job satisfaction. *Administrative Science Quarterly, 23,* 204-223.

Kraft, W.P., & Williams, K.L. (1975). Job redesign improves productivity. *Personnel Journal, 54,* 393-397.

Locke, E.A., Sirota, D., & Wolfson, A.D. (1976). An experimental case study of the successes and failures of job enrichment in a government agency. *Journal of Applied Psychology, 61,* 701-711.

Miner, J.B. (1975). *The challenge of managing* (pp. 205-206). Philadelphia: W.B. Saunders.

Miner, J.B. (1980). *Theories of organizational behavior* (pp. 231-259). Hinsdale, IL: Dryden.

Miner, J.B. (1981). Theories of organizational motivation. In G.W. England, A.R. Negandhi, & B. Wilpert (Eds.), *The functioning of complex organizations.* Cambridge, MA: Oelegeschlarger, Gunn and Harin.

Nadler, D.A., Hackman, J.R., & Lawler, E.E. III. (1979). *Managing organizational behavior* (pp. 81-86). Boston: Little, Brown.

Oldham, G.R., Hackman, J.R., & Pearce, J.L. (1976). Conditions under which employees respond positively to enriched work. *Journal of Applied Psychology, 61,* 395-403.

Robey, D. (1974). Task design, work values, and worker response: An experimental test. *Organizational Behavior and Human Performance, 12,* 264-273.

Roedel, R.R., & Nystrom, P.C. (1988). Nursing jobs and satisfaction. *Nursing Management, 19*(2), 34-38.

Rousseau, D.M. (1977). Technological differences in job characteristics, employee satisfaction, and motivation: A synthesis of job design research and sociotechnical systems theory. *Organizational Behavior and Human Performance, 19,* 18-42.

Salancik, G.R., & Pfeffer, J. (1978). A social information processing approach to job attitudes and task design. *Administrative Science Quarterly, 23,* 224-253.

Schwab, D.P., & Cummings, L.L. (1976). A theoretical analysis of the impact of task scope on employee performance. *Academy of Management Review, 1,* 23-35.

Sexton, W.P. (1967). Organizational and individual needs: A conflict? *Personnel Journal, 46,* 337-343.

Simonds, R.H., & Orife, J.N. (1975). Worker behavior versus enrichment theory. *Administrative Science Quarterly, 20,* 606-612.

Sims, H.P., Szilagyi, A.D., & Keller, R.T. (1976). The measurement of job characteristics. *Academy of Management Journal, 19,* 195-212.

Steers, R.M., & Spencer, D.G. (1977). The role of achievement motivation in job design. *Journal of Applied Psychology, 62,* 472-479.

Stone, E.F., Mowday, R.T., & Porter, L.W. (1977). Higher order need strengths as moderators of the job scope–job satisfaction relationship. *Journal of Applied Psychology, 62,* 466-471.

Umstot, D.D., Bell, C.H., Mitchell, T.R. (1976). Effects of job enrichment and task goals on satisfaction and productivity: Implications for job design. *Journal of Applied Psychology, 61,* 379-394.

Walton, R.E. (1974). Innovative restructuring of work. In J.M. Rosow (Ed.), *The worker and the job: Coping with change* (pp. 612-622). Englewood Cliffs, NJ: Prentice-Hall.

Wanous, J.P. (1974). Individual differences and reactions to job characteristics. *Journal of Applied Psychology, 59,* 616-622.

White, J.K. (1978). Individual differences and the job quality-worker response relationship: Review, integration, and comments. *Academy of Management Review, 3,* 267-280.

Young, L.C., & Hayne, A.N. (1988). *Nursing administration from concepts to practice* (pp. 75-78, 90-96). Philadelphia: W.B. Saunders.

SUGGESTED READINGS

Brief, A.P., & Aldag, R.J. (1975). Employee reactions to job characteristics: A constructive replication. *Journal of Applied Psychology, 60,* 182-186.

Flippo, E.B. (1980). *Personnel management.* New York: McGraw-Hill.

Hackman, J.R. (1969). Nature of the task as a determiner of job behavior. *Personnel Psychology, 22,* 435-444.

Hackman, J.R., Hoffman, L.W., Moos, R.H., Osipow, S.H., & Tornatzky, L.G. (1986). *Psychology and work: Productivity, change, and employment.* Washington, DC: American Psychological Association.

Hackman, J.R., & Oldham, G.R. (1975). Development of the job diagnostic survey. *Journal of Applied Psychology, 60,* 159-170.

Hackman, J.R., & Oldham, G.R. (1976). Motivation through the design of work: Test of a theory. *Organizational Behavior and Human Performance, 16,* 250-279.

Hackman, J.R., Oldham, G.R., Janson, R., & Purdy, K. (1975). A new strategy for job enrichment. *California Management Review, 17*(4), 57-71.

Hulin, C.L. (1971). Individual differences and job enrichment — The case against general treatments. In J.R. Maher (Ed.), *New perspectives in job enrichment.* New York: Van Nostrand Reinhold.

Korman, A.K. (1977). *Organizational behavior* (pp. 296-307). Englewood Cliffs, NJ: Prentice-Hall.

Lawler, E.E. (1969). Job design and employee motivation. *Personnel Psychology, 22,* 426-435.

Lawler, E.E. (1973). *Motivation in work organizations.* Monterey, CA: Brooks/Cole.

McNulty, L.A. (1973, September). Job enrichment: How to make it work. *Supervisory Management,* pp. 7-15.

Pierce, J.L., & Dunham, R.B. (1976). Task design: A literature review. *Academy of Management Review, 1*(4), 83-97.

Porter, L.W., Lawler, E.E., & Hackman, J.R. (1975). *Behavior in organizations.* New York: McGraw-Hill.

Sims, H.P., & Szilagyi, A.D. (1976). Job characteristic relationships: Individual and structural moderators. *Organizational Behavior and Human Performance, 17,* 211-230.

PART III

LEAD

Chapter 15

Theory X and Y
Douglas McGregor

Vicki H. Morgan

CASE STUDY

Jane Roe is a registered nurse with 5 years' experience. She works as a staff nurse in a community health agency. She comes to this position from a previous supervisory position in which she had latitude in implementing changes and new ideas for the better operation of the agency.

The organizational structure of the community health agency is a line and staff type of structure, in which accountability and responsibility are clearly defined. Jane holds a staff nurse position and has a supervisor, who is the lead nurse. She also has a co-worker. Both supervisor and co-worker are within a year or two of retirement. Jane finds it impossible to make changes that she feels are in the best interest for the care of her patients. For example, she would like to develop a teen clinic to provide education to teenagers but permission to do this was denied. Jane feels thwarted at every turn. She feels that she is being used as an assembly-line nurse, without the opportunity to use any of the innovative ideas that would benefit the clients served. Jane has thought of transferring to another job with more autonomy, but enjoys her relationship with the clients and feels that she can make a definite impact on the care in this area, if given the opportunity to do so.

||||||||||||||||||||||||||||||||||||||||||||||||||||||||||||||||||||||

THEORY X AND Y

Most of McGregor's adult life and the important years of his research and teachings were spent at the Massachusetts Institute of Technology where he served as Professor of Industrial Management from 1954-1964. His research years were influenced by colleagues such as Maslow

(1954), Herzberg (1959), Argyris (1957), and Likert (1961), who shared his philosophical views regarding humanism in the workplace.

McGregor created a whole new outlook across the field of management and organizational behavior. In his article "The Human Side of Enterprise" (1957b), he explains his theories of X and Y. He gave us a new theory of man (based on Maslow's hierarchy of needs and the self-actualization theory), a new set of values for the working person, and a new theory of power.

McGregor presented his theories of X and Y in three different publications — an article in 1957, a book in 1960, and supplementary comments in 1964, which were published after his death as a book. According to McGregor, in the original article (1957b), theory X states that most managers believe that people are inherently lazy, stupid, and unambitious. They must be moved to action by either the promise of reward or the threat of punishment. The theory X manager's role, therefore, is to provide security, direction, and control. He or she has the power and can command, reward merit, and punish negligence and inefficiency.

Theory X contained a set of propositions and beliefs about the conventional, accepted role of management in relation to governance of human energy to meet organizational needs and goals. The three propositions are (McGregor, 1957b, p. 23):

1. Management is responsible for organizing the elements of productive enterprise — money, materials, equipment, people — in the interest of economic ends.
2. With respect to people, this is a process of directing their efforts, motivating them, controlling their actions, modifying their behavior to fit the needs of the organizations.
3. Without this active intervention by management, people would be passive — even resistant — to organizational needs. They must, therefore, be persuaded, rewarded, punished, controlled — their activities must be directed. This is management's task.

The five beliefs are (McGregor, 1957b, p. 23):

1. The average man is by nature indolent — he works as little as possible.
2. He lacks ambition, dislikes responsibility, prefers to be led.
3. He is inherently self-centered, indifferent to organizational needs.
4. He is by nature resistant to change.
5. He is gullible, not very bright, the ready dupe of the charlatan and the demagogue.

McGregor believed that the majority of organizational structures reinforced these assumptions. He disagreed with management's view regarding the nature of the working person. After studying the problem extensively, he concludes that "the social scientist does not deny that human behavior in industrial organization today is approximately what management perceives it to be . . . but he is pretty sure that this behavior is not a consequence of man's inherent nature. It is a consequence rather of the nature of industrial organizations, of management philosophy, policy, and practice. The conventional approach of theory X is based on mistaken notions of what is cause and what is effect" (McGregor, 1957b, p. 24).

Instead, McGregor viewed Maslow's hierarchy of needs theory as being more relevant to the nature of man. He believed that what a person wants, he or she works to obtain. When lower level needs are met, the person immediately moves on to satisfying a higher level need. This process is unending from birth to death (McGregor, 1960, p. 36).

According to McGregor, direction and control by management — whether it is hard or soft — are irrelevant and do not motivate the individual. Direction and control are useless in motivating when a person sees his or her needs as social and egoistic (McGregor, 1957b, p. 88).

McGregor (1957a) in his article "An Uneasy Look at Performance Appraisals" gave an alternative approach, in which the responsibility is shifted to the subordinate rather than the superior. The subordinate sets his or her own goals and objectives, while the superior serves as a listener, advising with organizational knowledge and encouraging his employees to develop their own potential.

Therefore McGregor (1957b) proposed a different set of managerial assumptions and practices (theory Y) with an emphasis on releasing potential, encouraging growth, removing obstacles, creating opportunities, and providing guidance. A more humanistic approach to the management process rests on these assumptions (McGregor, 1957b, pp. 88-89):

1. Management is responsible for organizing the elements of productive enterprise—money, materials, equipment, people—in the interest of economic ends.
2. People are not by nature passive or resistant to organizational needs. They have become so as a result of experience in organizations.
3. The motivation, the potential for development, the capacity for assuming responsibility, the readiness to direct behavior toward organizational goals are all present in people. Management does not put them there. It is a responsibility of management to make it possible for people to recognize and develop these human characteristics for themselves.
4. The essential task of management is to arrange organizational conditions and methods of operation so that people can achieve their own goals best by directing their own efforts toward organizational objectives.

Theory Y emphasizes the average person's need to be creative, his or her interest in work, and the desire to be self-directing and to seek responsibility. The shift in management from X to Y does not mean one is relinquishing all managerial control. It means there is more self-control and self-direction exhibited by the employee, who shares to some extent in the managerial role.

McGregor (1960) in his expanded version reviewed his assumptions regarding theory X. The inherent dislike for work, which means most people must be coerced, controlled, directed, threatened with punishment, all continue to be basic assumptions. He also maintained that people prefer being directed, shun responsibility, have little ambition, and continue to want security above all. He felt that management was giving a false impression of moving away from theory X and toward theory Y by using new programs, procedures, and gadgets, when in actuality no changes at all were taking place. In general, he did not believe there has been much progress toward managerial movement away from theory X (McGregor, 1960, p. 42). He did elaborate more on the assumptions relevant to theory Y (McGregor, 1960, pp. 47-48):

1. The expenditure of physical and mental effort in work is as natural as play or rest.
2. External control and the threat of punishment are not the only means for bringing about effort toward organizational objectives. Man will exercise self-direction and self-control in the service of objectives to which he is committed.
3. Commitment to objectives is a function of the rewards associated with their achievement. The most significant of such rewards, e.g., the satisfaction of ego and self-actualization needs, can be direct products of effort directed toward organizational objectives.
4. The average human being learns under proper conditions not only to accept but to seek responsibility.
5. The capacity to exercise a relatively high degree of imagination, ingenuity, and creativity in the solution of organizational problems is widely, not narrowly, distributed in the population.
6. Under the conditions of modern industrial life, the intellectual potentialities of the average human being are only partially utilized.

According to McGregor, such assumptions would lead management to design superior-subordinate relationships in which the subordinate has greater influence over the activities involved in his or her work and greater probability in influencing the superior's actions. He believed that through participatory management, greater creativity and productivity would result, and that the employees would gain a greater sense of personal accomplishment and satisfaction from their work. He came to associate theory Y with a participatory style of management. He believed that people would exercise self-direction and self-control in the achievement of organizational objectives to the degree that they are committed to those objectives (McGregor, 1960).

In his supplementary comments, McGregor (1967) addressed the employee who does not respond to theory Y management. He acknowledged that there is a certain percentage of people who will not respond at all or who will take advantage of a situation, if allowed to do so. He acknowledged that in these cases, firm enforcement of limits and sometimes dismissal are the only solutions to avoid a negative effect on the entire organization. He also reiterated the fact that theory X continued to be much more widely practiced than theory Y.

CASE ANALYSIS

Staff nurse Jane Roe appears to be operating under a theory X type of management, in which the lead nurse operates with an authoritarian type of management, directing the flow of work and employees in the way she feels is best for the organization, with little regard for the ideas of other workers. Indeed as McGregor cited, this style of management is still very widely practiced. It is very understandable that this employee feels thwarted and unable to be creative or use the potential she possesses for the betterment of the organization. Strong feelings of containment are probably particularly felt by this employee since she previously held a position where a theory Y style of management was used and she was allowed to be creative and self-directed and to use her potential for organizational goals.

There are several ways of approaching this problem. Jane can use the chain of command and arrange an appointment with the lead nurse to discuss the reason that her request was denied. There may well be a very good reason for declining her request at this time. If not satisfied, she may continue up the chain of command, but this may not be without consequence. Jane must evaluate how important she feels that the issue is, whether she feels strongly that it should be pursued now, or whether she should bide her time and hope that the lead nurse retires as soon as expected.

RESEARCH

To date, there have been few direct tests of McGregor's theories. This may be due to the fact that many researchers do not consider his theories testable. McGregor did not operationalize concepts to his theories. Being a humanistic theorist, he was not interested in performing research to test his theories.

In a study directed by Morse and Lorsch (1970) at two plants and two research laboratories in Akron, Ohio, and Hartford, Connecticut, the objectives were to explore the goodness of fit between organizations and tasks as related to successful performance and whether or not this goodness of fit increased the motivation of individuals to be more effective performers. They concluded that the employees in Akron, working under a very structured organization with relatively little management participation in decision making were highly motivated. This is inversely related to theory X and theory Y, which states for people to work hard they must be coerced to do so and they should have been involved in decision making to feel so motivated. Conversely, in the low-performing plant in Hartford, the employees were not as highly motivated as the Akron managers even though they were a less structured organization with no participation in decision making. The theory Y assumption would suggest that they should have been more motivated.

As an alternative Morse and Lorsch (1970) proposed the contingency theory, which allowed for the differences inherent in individuals and their different needs. They suggested that the best possibility for managerial action probably is in tailoring the organization to fit the tasks and people.

McGregor's theories were tested in 1972 and again in 1980 for comparison by the management firm of Louis A. Allen Associates, Inc. In both cases a written questionnaire survey of 259 managers from 93 companies was used. The questionnaire was designed to test the congruency of attitudes shared by these managers and McGregor. Topics included "What factors most strongly influence the behavior of people?" "What concerns do most people place first?" "Do most people tend to be lazy or bright? Ambitious or not ambitious? Gullible or hardheaded? Followers or leaders?" (Green, 1981, p. 23).

The results of the two surveys were surprisingly similar (Green, 1981). The majority of those asked disagreed with the standard assumption that people are inherently lazy, gullible, or stupid. Eighty-one percent of the managers believed that the average person is neither highly ambitious nor without ambition at all, but ranges somewhere in the middle. Seventy-four percent polled believed that the average person is neither very bright nor stupid, but falls somewhere in-between in intelligence. A slight majority (54%) of managers polled believed that the average person neither seeks nor shuns responsibility. According to Green's findings, neither theory X nor theory Y in its entirety describes management's attitudes regarding employees.

Bennis (1972) stated two criticisms of McGregor's theory. The first is that theory Y does not appear to be fully human. It allows no room for anger, inconsistency, playfulness, or destructiveness. It does not address loners, weaklings, liars, or villains. People are a mixture of all these feelings. His second criticism is that McGregor's theory of organization operates in an environmental void, depending on a psychologically determined set of manager-employee relationships. He did not address technological factors, norms, groups, legal or political impositions, educational advancement, pollution, conflict, or population growth.

Perhaps one of the most celebrated studies conducted to test McGregor's theories was begun in 1960 at Non-Linear Systems, Inc., of Del Mar, California. The company had been in business for 8 years, was prosperous, and was firmly established in its field before the experiment in participative management was begun. The company's president, Andrew Kay, was a believer in the humanistic approach and was the primary initiator of this change from a traditional hierarchial structure to one of participative management. This experiment drew the attention of management worldwide, including scientists, writers, educators, engineers, consultants, and representatives of governments.

There are many conflicting views regarding the causes of the outcome of this study. McGregor, who spent time at the plant while the study was in progress, noted that productivity increased about 30% and customer complaints decreased by 70%. He noted no quality defects in the first 2 years of the experiment.

Maslow also spent time at the plant 2 years into the study, surveying the results. He agreed with the changes and procedures instituted at Non-Linear Systems, Inc., and agreed that they were consistent with the views of McGregor and himself.

Several years into the study, analysis by various researchers showed different results. The company experienced severe financial problems because of a change in the market. Kay (1973) blamed many of theory Y approaches for the financial problems. He stated, "The experiments caused me to lose touch with what was happening to my company. I assumed that the day-to-day operations of the company would take care of themselves. I found out differently" (Kay, 1973, p. 100).

Malone (1975) concluded that owing to lack of record keeping no reliable conclusions can be drawn from this study. It is his contention that in all probability no actual increase in plant efficiency occurred. In 1965 when the experiment ended, sales volume was down, restlessness was stirring at management levels, there was no increase in productivity, employee layoffs had begun, competition in industry was increasing, and the company had become less profitable. According to Malone, in 1965, Non-Linear Systems, Inc., by abandoning the experiment, retreated to the orthodox methods of management to avoid bankruptcy.

Gray (1978) cited three misconceptions regarding the study. First, it was not a scientific experiment. No dependent or independent variables were identified. All changes were made at once and consequently none could be measured. No records were kept and thus no data were available for analysis. Second, participative management was not tested. Third, it tested theories of leading behavioral writers of the day such as Maslow, McGregor, and Drucker. Gray disagreed with this information, feeling that in all reality nothing could be concluded from the Non-Linear Systems experiment in relation to McGregor's theories.

The largest body of research conducted testing McGregor's theories was from the University of California at Berkeley. This was a worldwide study including 14 countries testing theory X and theory Y assumptions in the managerial world. Information was collected from 3600 managers using a questionnaire to get managers' ideas on the degree to which people are capable of leadership and initiative, as well as on their attitudes toward different managerial practices expected in theory Y orientation toward subordinates. In other words, do different managers from different countries differ from one another?

There was a consistent pattern across all countries that support theory X managerial behavior. Haire, Ghiselli, and Porter (1966) found that managers do not really feel that it is beneficial to use such democratic-type practices as theory Y, but do feel that it is necessary to endorse them lest they be deemed old-fashioned or unorthodox. Although many managers respond in this way on the attitude questionnaire, they seldom put these ideas into practice in actual job situations.

In a study by Caplan (1971), the accounting field was used to test McGregor's theories. According to him, it is impossible to envision any modern industry functioning without communication, planning, and control aides provided by the accounting field. However, this was one of the first changes implemented at Non-Linear Systems. Caplan's findings support the hypothesis that theory X assumptions are widely held.

Research at the Hawthorne Works of the Western Electric Company near Chicago, Illinois, directed by Elton Mayo and reported by Fritz Roethlisberger (1941), began as an attempt to look at the relationship between light illumination in the factory and productivity. These studies have been criticized (Carey, 1971) for using test groups of inadequate size (the most frequent was 5—out of a work force of 29,000); not using true control groups; introducing changes in a cumulative fashion; promanagement bias; and unreliable reporting, in that different members of the research team reported different results when describing the same experiment. They showed that logical, honest analysis of the reported data produced conclusions almost totally in reverse to the human relations theory, which indicates that behavior is influenced more by social than economic factors. They revealed that the Hawthorne researchers (Mayo in particular) ignored or misinterpreted facts that did not support their personal beliefs, and that in fact the Hawthorne studies produced considerable support for the view that money is the prime motivator.

Chris Argyris (1964) supported McGregor and Mayo by saying that managerial domination caused workers to become discouraged and passive and that if employees' self-esteem and independence needs were not met, they would become discouraged and troublesome or they might leave the organization. Argyris stressed the need for employee participation in decision making and flexibility within the organization.

No relevant research could be located in relation to the use of theory X and Y in the nursing field. McGregor's theories are referred to less now than previously in the business literature.

REFERENCES

American Psychological Association. (1983). Ethical principles of psychologist (revised). *American Psychologist.*
Argyris, C. (1957). *Personality and organization.* New York: Harper, 1957.
Argyris, C. (1964). *Integrating the individual and the organization.* New York: John Wiley & Sons.
Bennis, W.G. (1972). Chairman Mac in perspective. *Harvard Business Review, 50,* 140-147.
Caplan, E. (1971). *Management accounting and behavioral science* (pp. 111-112). Reading, MA: Addison-Wesley.
Carey, A. (1971). The Hawthorne studies: A radical criticism. *American Sociological Review, 32,* 403-416.
Gray, E.R. (1978). The Non-Linear Systems experiment: A requiem. *Business Horizons, 21,* 31-36.
Green, J.P. (1981). People management: New directions for the 1980's. *Administrative Management, 42,* 22-26.
Haire, M., Ghiselli, E.E., & Porter, L.W. (1966). *Managerial thinking: An international study* (p. 24). New York: John Wiley & Sons.
Herzberg, F.B. (1959). *The motivation to work.* New York: John Wiley & Sons.
Kay, A. (1973). Where being nice to workers didn't work. *Business Week, 1,* 98-100.
Likert, R. (1961). *New patterns of management.* New York: McGraw-Hill.
McGregor, D. (1957a). An uneasy look at performance appraisals. *Harvard Business Review, 35,* 89-94.
McGregor, D. (1957b). The human side of enterprise. *Management Review, 46,* 22-28, 88-92.
McGregor, D. (1960). *The human side of enterprise* (pp. 33-57, 100). New York: McGraw-Hill.
McGregor, D. (1967). *The professional manager* (pp. 78, 88, 89). New York: McGraw-Hill.
Malone, E. (1975). The Non-Linear Systems experiment in participative management. *Journal of Business, 48,* 52-64.
Maslow, A. (1954). *Eupsychian management.* Homewood, IL: Dorsey Press.
Morse, J., & Lorsch, J. (1970). Beyond theory Y. *Harvard Business Review, 48,* 67-68.
Roethlisberger, F. (1941). *Management and morale.* Cambridge: Harvard University Press.

Chapter 16

Contingency Theory of Leadership Fred Fiedler

Regina K. Bennett
Joanne C. Stratton

I I   CASE STUDY

Ms. Kathryn Adams is the Director of Nursing at Benton Hospital, a large urban hospital. Realizing that the identification and selection of nurse managers constitute a critical task, she is contemplating the two units in the hospital in need of nurse managers. Nursing services represent the largest personnel item in the hospital budget. Management of that resource at this time of the nursing shortage is critical because a highly proficient nurse manager can be a key retention factor. Selection needs to be made with care.

The units involved are 4 West and 4 South. Both units are general medical-surgical settings. The 4-West unit has been without a nurse manager for 2 months. However, problems have existed longer than that. The unit has not had an organized orientation program for new staff. Job descriptions have not been reviewed in over 2 years. Staff evaluations are not on schedule. The policy manual is missing some pages. There has been no consistency to scheduling. Staff are confused about their roles. The daily question is, "Who is in charge today?" Bickering among the staff has begun because of their lack of security. The administrator of nursing services has concerns about the quality of patient care, consumer satisfaction, safety, nurses' satisfaction, and nurses' retention.

The 4-South unit is also in need of a nurse manager. The nurse manager of this unit is scheduled for a maternity leave next month. If she returns to work after her child is born it will be on a part-time basis. As she relinquishes her position the unit is running fairly well. The orientation program and job descriptions are in order. Evaluations are done on a periodic schedule with the staff also doing self-evaluations. The unit has a stable staff who seem to be content. Comments have been heard about a "relaxed" atmosphere. Patient satisfaction seems high judged by the flowers, balloons, and candy gifts to nurses on the unit, as well as by periodic surveys completed by clients after their discharge.

After meeting with the Nurse Recruiter, Ms. Adams decided to fill the vacant positions from external sources. One candidate for these positions, Ms. James, is just moving to the area. Her qualifications meet Benton Hospital's established criteria for nurse managers as far as education and experience. Her last position was a management position. She managed a new unit that opened as a result of hospital expansion. Her references highlight her success at the initial organization and management of the unit for 2 years. A date was set for Ms. Adams to meet with the candidate, Ms. James. It was established that when Ms. James arrived for her appointment the Nurse Recruiter would administer and score testing that would last about 10 minutes. Those results would be given to Ms. Adams before the interview.

Ms. Adams and Ms. James have met as scheduled. Ms. James's references are very positive. Ms. Adams was favorably impressed with Ms. James's precise manner, management experience, and enthusiasm for the job prospect. While Ms. James was on a hospital tour with a unit manager, Ms. Adams reviewed her leadership needs and the test results. An explanation of the perceived unit problems and the designed orientation program for the manager were given to Ms. James. Ms. James had numerous questions. She also offered some quick ideas on restoration of the unit's organization in which staff could be involved.

Ms. Adams has also met with Ms. Barnes, a second candidate for a nurse manager position. Ms. Barnes has had management experience. Her resumé lists experiences in a management position for 2 years on a medical unit. She has also organized and led numerous family support groups on her unit, as well as consulting with other units. Her references highlight her interpersonal skills. She too had some testing before her appointment.

Both candidates have a BSN degree, medical-surgical clinical experience, and management experience. Ms. Adams's task is to match the right manager to the appropriate unit.

||||||||||||||||||||||||||||||||||||||||||||||||||||||||||||

CONTINGENCY THEORY

The Director of Nursing used Fiedler's contingency model of leadership to match leadership style with the needs of the two units. Fiedler, Chemers, and Mahar (1976) state contingency theory:

> This theory holds that the effectiveness of a group or an organization depends on two interacting or "contingent" factors. The first is the personality of the leaders which determine their leadership style. The second factor is the amount of control and influence which the situation provides leaders over the group's behavior, the task, and the outcome. This factor is called "situational control." (p. 3)

A few definitions of Fiedler's major concepts are necessary to understand the contingency model. Fiedler (1967) ascribes to Campbell's 1958 definition of a group as "a set of individuals who are interdependent in the sense that an event which affects one member is likely to affect all" (p. 6). He goes on to say that

> typically the human group shares a common goal, and its members interact in their attempt to achieve this goal. Typically, also, the members are rewarded as a group for achieving their goal; they are punished or they feel that they have failed if their group does not perform as expected. (p. 6)

Fielder (1967) defines the leader as "the individual in the group given the task of directing and coordinating task-relevant group activities or who, in the absence of a designated leader, carries the primary responsibility for performing these functions in the group" (p. 8).

Fiedler (1967) feels that it is important to know the difference between leadership behavior and leadership style in order to understand his theory. Leadership behavior is "the particular acts in which a leader engages in the course of directing and coordinating the work of his group members" (p. 36). Leadership style is "the underlying need-structure of the individual which motivates his behavior in various leadership situations" (p. 36).

There are basically two types of leader managers. The first type tells people what to do and how to do it. Conversely, the second type of manager shares his or her leadership responsibilities with the group members and involves them in the planning and execution of the task. Fiedler et al. (1976) explain that there are all shades of leadership styles in between these two positions.

Experiments (Fiedler, 1967) comparing the performance of both types of leaders have shown that each is successful in some situations and not in others. Researchers have not been able to show that one type of leadership is always superior or effective.

Historically, management has determined what type of leadership style best fits the specific situation, then selected or trained the employee so that his or her leadership style fits the particular job. In contrast, Fiedler (1965) believes that management should "determine the type of leadership style which is most natural for the man in the executive position and then change the job to fit that man" (p. 116). Fiedler found that while a leader's behavior or action changes to meet the situation, his or her basic personality remains constant.

To determine and classify leadership styles, Fiedler et al. (1976) developed the Least Preferred Co-worker (LPC) scale. The LPC scale is an 18-item semantic differential scale (Figure 16-1) that asks the leader to descirbe, favorably or unfavorably, her least preferred co-worker. From the responses, an LPC score is obtained by adding the item scores. Fiedler et al. believe this score reveals the leader's emotional reaction to people with whom he or she cannot work well.

The leader with a high LPC score (score range 64 or above) describes a least preferred co-worker in a favorable manner and tends to be relationship-oriented and considerate of the feelings or his or her workers. He or she obtains major satisfaction from establishing close personal relations with his or her group members. The high LPC leader can tolerate complexity and ambiguity and encourages new ideas from subordinates. Leader and subordinates work together as a team to accomplish the group's objectives.

The leader who describes her least preferred co-worker in negative terms scored low on the LPC scale. The low LPC (score range 57 or below) leader is task oriented and needs to get the job done. Her major satisfaction comes from the successful completion of tasks, even if it comes at the risk of poor interpersonal relationships with the workers.

The group of leaders that fall somewhere between those who are clearly relationship oriented and those who are task oriented are a mix of motivations and goals. Fiedler et al. (1976) wants these leaders to determine for themselves to which group they belong.

SITUATIONAL CONTROL

Each group or team is unique and requires a leader who can effectively guide the group toward the accomplishment of their tasks. To determine which leadership style fits which situation, Fiedler (1967) discovered three major group classifications called situational control. These are leader-member relations, task structure, and position power. It is important for the leader to recognize the particular conditions and situations in which he or she is most effective and how to modify the situation to fit personal style.

Leader-Member Relations

Fiedler (1969) views the leader-member relations as being the most important factor in determining the leader's control and influence over the group. The leader who is liked and has gained the trust and support of the subordinates is able to influence the group's performance. The trusted and well-liked leader does not require special rank or power in order to get things done. Conversely, the leader who is distrusted by subordinates must rely solely on position power to get things done.

	8	7	6	5	4	3	2	1		Scoring
Pleasant									Unpleasant	____
	8	7	6	5	4	3	2	1		
Friendly									Unfriendly	____
	8	7	6	5	4	3	2	1		
Rejecting									Accepting	____
	1	2	3	4	5	6	7	8		
Tense									Relaxed	____
	1	2	3	4	5	6	7	8		
Distant									Close	____
	1	2	3	4	5	6	7	8		
Cold									Warm	____
	1	2	3	4	5	6	7	8		
Supportive									Hostile	____
	8	7	6	5	4	3	2	1		
Boring									Interesting	____
	1	2	3	4	5	6	7	8		
Quarrelsome									Harmonious	____
	1	2	3	4	5	6	7	8		
Gloomy									Cheerful	____
	1	2	3	4	5	6	7	8		
Open									Guarded	____
	8	7	6	5	4	3	2	1		
Backbiting									Loyal	____
	1	2	3	4	5	6	7	8		
Untrustworthy									Trustworthy	____
	1	2	3	4	5	6	7	8		
Considerate									Inconsiderate	____
	8	7	6	5	4	3	2	1		
Nasty									Nice	____
	1	2	3	4	5	6	7	8		
Agreeable									Disagreeable	____
	8	7	6	5	4	3	2	1		
Insincere									Sincere	____
	1	2	3	4	5	6	7	8		
Kind									Unkind	____
	8	7	6	5	4	3	2	1		

TOTAL _____

FIGURE 16-1 Least Preferred Co-Worker (LPC) scale. *From Fiedler, F., Chemers, M., & Mahar, L.* Improving leadership effectiveness: The leader match concept. © *1976, John Wiley & Sons, Inc.*

Circle the number which best represents your response to each item.	Strongly agree	Agree	Neither agree nor disagree	Disagree	Strongly disagree
1. The people I supervise have trouble getting along with each other.	1	2	3	4	5
2. My subordinates are reliable and trustworthy.	5	4	3	2	1
3. There seems to be a friendly atmosphere among the people I supervise.	5	4	3	2	1
4. My subordinates always cooperate with me in getting the job done.	5	4	3	2	1
5. There is friction between my subordinates and myself.	1	2	3	4	5
6. My subordinates give me a good deal of help and support in getting the job done.	5	4	3	2	1
7. The people I supervise work well together in getting the job done.	5	4	3	2	1
8. I have good relations with the people I supervise.	5	4	3	2	1

TOTAL SCORE

FIGURE 16-2 Leader-Member Relations scale. *From Fiedler, F., Chemers, M., & Mahar, L. Improving leadership effectiveness: The leader match concept. © 1976, John Wiley & Sons, Inc.*

The Leader-Member Relations (LMR) scale was designed to measure the degree to which the leader feels accepted and comfortable in the group. The LMR scale is a Likert scale that consists of eight questions with responses that range from "strongly agree" to "strongly disagree" (Figure 16-2). It has been weighted to be worth twice as much as the Task Structure scale and four times as much as the Position Power scale (see in the following sections) because leader-member is considered the most important variable in measuring control. If a leader can rely on his or her subordinates to do their job well and willingly, then he or she will have a considerable amount of control and influence.

Task Structure

The second important factor concerns the structure of the task. Task structure describes the degree to which the task is spelled out for the group to perform. Tasks may be performed step by step according to a detailed standard operating policy or the assignment may be vague, ambiguous, and undefined.

Fiedler (1969) claims that a highly structured task does not need a leader with much position power because the leader's role and that of subordinates are detailed in job descriptions. He states that with a highly structured task, the leader clearly knows what to do and how to do it, and the organization can back him up at each step. Unstructured tasks tend to have more than one right solution that can be reached by any of a variety of methods. (p. 41)

To measure task structure, Fiedler developed a two-part scale. Part 1 of the Task Structure scale consists of 10 questions designed to reflect four aspects of task structure. Marriner-Tomey (1988) describes these variables as followers:

(1) Goal clarity—goal understood by followers; (2) the extent to which a decision can be verified—know who is responsible for what; (3) multiplicity of goal paths—number of solutions; and (4) specificity of solution—number of correct answers. (p. 185)

Responses on the Task Structure scale range in value from 0 to 2 and are subtotaled to complete part 1 (Figure 16-3).

The second portion of the Task Structure scale (Figure 16-4) reflects the training and experience level of the leader. The task structure rating from part 1 is based on the assumption that the leader has had adequate training and education for the managerial position. If the leader lacks one or both of these aspects, points must be subtracted from part 1. The result is the total task structure score.

Position Power

The third variable in determining situational control is position power. According to Fiedler, "Position power is the authority vested in the leader's position" (1969, p. 41) by the organization. This includes the ability to hire and fire, reward and punish, promote and demote. For example, the director of nursing has more position power than the unit managers.

The Position Power scale's rating consists of five questions about the power which the leader has at his or her disposal for directing subordinates. Responses for each question range in value between 0 to 2 (Figure 16-5).

CASE ANALYSIS

Benton Hospital had two vacant units in need of a manager. Ms. Adams as Director of Nursing felt that is was necessary to fill each slot with the individual with the appropriate leadership style to achieve nursing service goals. Ms. James was hired as manager of 4 West. Ms. Barnes accepted the manager position on 4 South. Before making the decision, one of the tools used was Fiedler's tests. Ms. James's score on the LPC scale was low or indicative of a task orientation. Her LMR scale score was interpreted as "good" relations. The Task Structure scale rating had a score revealing high task structure. Position power and situational control were high. According to Fiedler's theory the leadership style assessed for Ms. James is a better fit for the disorganized situation of the 4-West unit. The low LPC leader derives satisfaction from the completion of tasks. This person likes clear guidelines and structure. She is seen as efficient and goal oriented, concerned with achieving success on an assigned task. This low LPC person is concerned with interpersonal relationships in regard to task completion.

The leader-member relations support the leader. The task structure spells out the goal and the position power gives the manager authority to reward and punish.

Fiedler's theory is based on the assumption that one's personality and leadership style do not change. That leadership style should match the situation. The situation control for 4 West favors a high-control person.

Circle the number in the appropriate column.	Usually true	Sometimes true	Seldom true
Is the goal clearly stated or known?			
1. Is there a blueprint, picture, model, or detailed description available of the finished product or service?	2	1	0
2. Is there a person available to advise and give a description of the finished product or service, or how the job should be done?	2	1	0
Is there only one way to accomplish the task?			
3. Is there a step-by-step procedure, or a standard operating procedure which indicates in detail the process which is to be followed?	2	1	0
4. Is there a specific way to subdivide the task into separate parts or steps?	2	1	0
5. Are there some ways which are clearly recognized as better than others for performing this task?	2	1	0
Is there only one correct answer or solution?			
6. Is it obvious when the task is finished and the correct solution has been found?	2	1	0
7. Is there a book, manual, or job description which indicates the best solution or the best outcome for the task?	2	1	0
Is it easy to check whether the job was done right?			
8. Is there a generally agreed understanding about the standards the particular product or service has to meet to be considered acceptable?	2	1	0
9. Is the evaluation of this task generally made on some quantitative basis?	2	1	0
10. Can the leader and the group find out how well the task has been accomplished in enough time to improve future performance?	2	1	0

SUBTOTAL [ ]

FIGURE 16-3 Ratings for Task Structure scale—part 1. *From Fiedler, F., Chemers, M., & Mahar, L.* Improving leadership effectiveness: The leader match concept. © 1976, *John Wiley & Sons, Inc.*

The 4-South unit was assessed to be in need of a "relationship" manager. Ms. Barnes's results from Fiedler's test show her style to be a relationship management style. Fiedler's theory supports that different leaderships are appropriate in different situations.

Ms. James has been the unit manager of 4 West for 6 months. After an orientation period

NOTE: **Do not adjust jobs with task structure scores of 6 or below.**

(a) Compared to others in this or similar positions, how much *training* has the leader had?

3	2	1	0
No training at all	Very little training	A moderate amount of training	A great deal of training

(b) Compared to others in this or similar positions, how much *experience* has the leader had?

6	4	2	0
No experience at all	Very little experience	A moderate amount of experience	A great deal of experience

Add lines (a) and (b) of the training and experience adjustment, then *subtract* this from the subtotal given in Part 1.

Subtotal from Part 1.

Subtract training and experience adjustment

TOTAL TASK STRUCTURE SCORE

FIGURE 16-4 Ratings for Task Structure scale—part 2. *From Fiedler, F., Chemers, M., & Mahar, L.* Improving leadership effectiveness: The leader match concept. © *1976, John Wiley & Sons, Inc.*

she began to understand her superior's standards and expectations. The 4-West unit with group input has set some goals with Ms. James's guidance. Unit morale has improved with the "take charge" attitude of Ms. James. Committees have been formed for job descriptions and the orientation program. The policy manual is being organized. Priorities and timetables are set for task completion. Scheduling is done to allow committees to work. Fielder would say that Ms. James is engineering the job to fit the manager.

Ms. Barnes seems pleased with her management challenge on 4 South. The staff is continuing with self-evaluation. Family support groups are being organized and implemented with staff planning.

Nurse managers have a challenge in their role. There is a need to prioritize the needs of patients while meeting the needs of the staff. The environment needs to be comfortable for their individual leadership styles.

Circle the number which best represents your answer.

1. Can the leader directly or by recommendation administer rewards and punishments to his subordinates?

2	1	0
Can act directly or can recommend with high effectiveness	Can recommend but with mixed results	No

2. Can the leader directly or by recommendation affect the promotion, demotion, hiring or firing of his subordinates?

2	1	0
Can act directly or can recommend with high effectiveness	Can recommend but with mixed results	No

3. Does the leader have the knowledge necessary to assign tasks to subordinates and instruct them in task completion?

2	1	0
Yes	Sometimes or in some aspects	No

4. Is it the leader's job to evaluate the performance of his subordinates?

2	1	0
Yes	Sometimes or in some aspects	No

5. Has the leader been given some official title of authority by the organization (e.g., foreman, department head, platoon leader)?

2	0
Yes	No

TOTAL

FIGURE 16-5 Ratings for position power scale. *From Fiedler, F., Chemers, M., & Mahar, L. Improving leadership effectiveness: The leader match concept. © 1976, John Wiley & Sons, Inc.*

RESEARCH

Fred Fiedler (b. 1922) is a psychologist who began his research in Illinois in the late 1950s and early 1960s. It was applied to the business environment after his theory was presented in 1967.

Fiedler and his collegues have conducted numerous research studies. Minor (1980) has analyzed Fiedler's research and states, "Group performance, leader-member relations, task structure, position power, and even LPC have been measured in many different ways and in different studies" (p. 309). These comprehensive studies support Fiedler's techniques and the

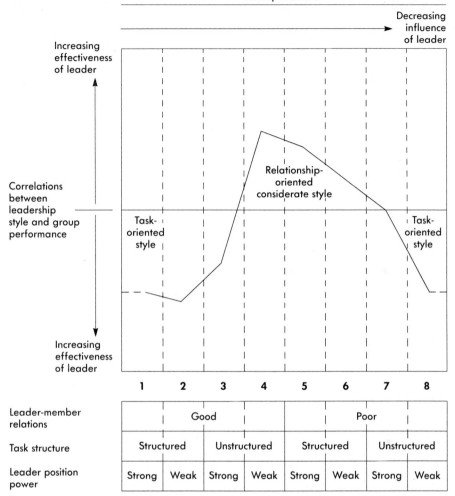

FIGURE 16-6 Fiedler's correlation of leadership style and group situation. *From Fiedler, F. (1969). Style or circumstance: The leadership enigma.* Psychology Today, *2(10), 38-43. Reprinted with permission from* Psychology Today *Magazine, © 1969 American Psychological Association.*

model's validity. Chemers, Harp, Rhodewalt, and Wysocki (1985) report a "meta-analytic review of 125 tests of the contingency model (Strube & Garcia, 1981) provided extremely strong support for the model's validity" (p. 629).

From his studies, Fiedler (1969) was able to determine the groups that had performed their task successfully or unsuccessfully and then correlate the effectiveness of group performance with leadership style (LPC scores).

Fiedler (1965) plotted his correlations of leadership style against a grid of group situations. He was then able to determine what leadership style works best in each situation. Figure 16-6 shows Fiedler's findings. At the bottom of the grid are the eight possible combinations of situational control. Situation 1 represents a group in which the members trust and are loyal to their leader, the job is clearly defined, and the organization has granted the leader strong position power. Moving across the grid, conditions get progressively worse. At the end of the grid, situation 8, the leader is disliked by subordinates, the job is vague and undefined, and the leader has little power.

The upper portion of the grid shows the leadership style that correlates with the eight combinations of situational control. Fiedler (1969) explains his findings:

> The results show that a task oriented leader performs best in situations at both extremes—those in which he has a great deal of influence and power, and also situations where he has no influence and power over the group members.
>
> Relationship oriented leaders tend to perform best in mixed situations where they have only moderate influence over the group. (p. 42)

If the leader works within a situation that fits his or her leadership style, then the leader and the group should successfully perform their duties. However, if there is a mismatch, any one of the situational conditions can be altered to fit the leader's style. Fiedler (1965) advises administrators to "engineer the job to fit the manager" (p. 115). For example, the leader's position power can be reduced by giving subordinates similar power and authority or improved by increasing his or her rank. Task structure can be more detailed and precise or altered to be vague and unstructured. To alter the leader-member relations, the leader can add or subtract subordinates with similar backgrounds and values. Referring to Figure 16-6, one can see that a task-oriented leader assigned to situation 5 would not be very effective and thus would strive to improve leader-member relations in order to be more successful.

Fiedler's contingency model is one of the most thoroughly researched models of leadership, but it has not been without criticisms. Chemers et al. (1985) state that these criticisms concern three primary issues. The first issue concerns Fiedler's extensive use of statistics. The many studies and statistics make it impossible to judge the true validity of the model. The second area of criticism is the flexibility in the choice of variables that have been used to measure task structure. The third issue concerns the use of the LPC scale as an accurate measurement of leadership style. Criticism in this area includes complaints from Kabanoff (1981), Shiplett (1981), Wofford (1985), and Jago and Ragan (1986).

A search of nursing literature reveals no published nursing applications. A doctoral dissertation by Searight (1980) applied Fiedler's theory in the study of leadership styles of selected administrators of accredited and nonaccredited baccalaureate nursing programs. Ross (1985) studied the relationship between leadership style and degree of control over work situations among first-level nurse managers in light of Fiedler's theory for her master's thesis.

REFERENCES

Chemers, M., Harp, R., Rhodewalt, F., & Wysocki, J. (1985). A person-environment analysis of job stress: A contingency model explanation. *Journal of Personality & Social Psychology, 49,* 628-635.

Fiedler, F. (1958). *Leader attitudes and group effectiveness.* Urbana, IL: University of Illinois Press.

Fiedler, F. (1965). Engineer the job to fit the manager. *Harvard Business Review, 43,* 115-122.

Fiedler, F. (1967). *A theory of leadership effectiveness.* New York: McGraw-Hill.

Fiedler, F. (1969). Style or circumstances: The leadership enigma. *Psychology Today, 2*(10), 38-43.

Fiedler, F., & Chemers, M. (1974). *Leadership and effective management.* Glenview, IL: Scott, Foresman.

Fiedler, F., Chemers, M., & Mahar, L. (1976). *Improving leadership effectiveness: The leader match concept.* New York: John Wiley & Sons.

Fiedler, F., & Garcia, J. (1958). Comparing organization development and management training. *Personnel Administrator, 30*(3), 35-47.

Fiedler, F., & Mahar, L. (1979). The effectiveness of contingency model training: A review of the validation of leader match. *Personnel Psycholoyg, 32,* 45-62.

Jago, A., & Ragan, J. (1986). The trouble with leader match is that it doesn't match Fiedler's contingency model. *Journal of Applied Psychology, 71,* 555-559.

Kabanoff, B. (1981). A critique of leader match and its applications for leadership research. *Personnel Psychology, 34,* 749-764.

Marriner-Tomey, A. (1988). *Guide to nursing management.* St. Louis: C.V. Mosby.

Minor, J. (1980). *Theories of organizational behavior.* Hinsdale, IL: Dryden.

Ross, P. (1985). *Relationship between leadership style and degree of control over work situation among first level nurse managers.* Unpublished master's thesis, University of Missouri, Columbia, MO.

Searight, M. (1980). A study of the leadership styles of selected administrators of accredited and nonaccredited baccalaureate nursing programs. *Dissertation Abstracts International, 41B*(3), 896.

Shiplett, S. (1981). Is there a problem with the LPC score in leader match? *Personnel Psychology, 34,* 765-769.

Wofford, J. (1985). Experimental examination of the contingency model and the leader environment-follower interaction theory of leadership. *Psychological Report, 56,* 823-832.

Chapter 17

Path-Goal Theory of Leadership
Robert J. House

Constance F. Buran
Deborah B. Wilson

▌▏   CASE STUDY

Sally Anderson is a manager of a 40-bed medical-surgical unit with an average daily census of 25. The majority of her staff are inexperienced and have less than a year of clinical practice. Upon orientation to the unit, each new employee is precepted for 6 weeks, which includes general hospital orientation. Sally has devised a list of unit-specific expectations that each employee receives during her or his first week of employment. Conferences are scheduled with the employee and manager to determine how the employees are progressing throughout their orientation. As each new policy or procedure is initiated, each employee receives the information through written memos.

For the last month the census has climbed to an average of 37 patients and the nurses are having to take a larger patient assignment. In addition to the increase in patient load, the number of nursing staff is continually changing. Sally found two requests for transfer on her desk from employees who have been on the unit for a year. It seems that the nurses will stay on a medical-surgical unit to obtain experience and then they transfer to specialty areas, such as intensive care, recovery room, or the emergency room. What can Sally do to reverse this trend?

│ │

PATH-GOAL THEORY OF LEADERSHIP

The basis of the path-goal theory as presented by House (1971) is derived from the work of Georgopoulos, Mahoney, and Jones (1957) and from research supporting a broad class of expectancy theories of motivation (Atkinson, 1958; Galbraith & Cummings, 1967; Graen, 1969; Lawler, 1968; Porter & Lawler, 1967; Vroom, 1964). The path-goal theory conceptualizes the relationship between an individual's perception of his or her actions and behaviors (path) and their eventual outcome (goal).

The extent to which the path is seen as helping or hindering the individual in attaining his or her goal is the definition of path-goal instrumentality. A numerical value between $+1$ and -1 is used to represent the degree of help or hindrance perceived. This ranking is then used to make predictions about a person's motivation to engage in a behavior (path). If the person believes a specific path will result in attainment of desired goals, he or she is more likely to engage in that behavior (Evans, 1970). Also factored into an individual's choice of a specific path are the personal gratifications, or valences, associated with the goal (Vroom, 1964). According to House (1971), an individual makes estimates of probability for success of a path-goal and places subjective values on the proposed outcome. The estimated probability of success and gratification will be reflected in the degree of motivation to pursue a goal.

Stated another way, perceived path-goal instrumentality and goal importance determine the level of motivation to follow a path. This motivational level, in combination with environmental variables such as ability, task, and authority, determines the frequency with which a path will be followed. Finally the path frequency, in conjunction with actual path-goal instrumentality, determines the level of goal attainment, a component of job satisfaction (Evans, 1970).

A goal is what a person is consciously trying to achieve. Locke (1968) examined the relationship between the level of difficulty of a chosen goal and the quantitative level of the individual's performance. Each of his studies concluded that the harder it is to achieve a goal, the higher the level of performance. A person's actions are directed by his or her goals. Goals are a result of the person's values, knowledge, anticipation, and priorities. Differences in the goals of individuals are the factors that shape the relationship between past levels of performance and job satisfaction. Locke (1968) proposed that dissatisfaction with one's past performance generates the desire to select another path (set of behaviors) to facilitate goal attainment, while satisfaction with one's past performance encourages replication of previous behaviors.

Locke, Cartledge, and Knerr (1970) examined the hypotheses that satisfaction is predicted from value judgments, goal setting is predicted from satisfaction, and performance is predicted from goals. Generally their premises were supported. However, they did find some cases in which satisfactory past performance did not guide future goal setting. In these cases they found that a person's anticipated satisfaction related to goal attainment and predicted goal-setting behavior.

Participative goal setting was explored by Erez and Arad (1986) using social, motivational, and cognitive perspectives. They examined the relationship between participation in the goal-setting process and subsequent levels of performance, goal commitment, and job satisfaction. This study demonstrated that group discussion, involvement in goal setting, and information sharing all correlate with increases in quantity and quality of work performed and increases in commitment to goals and job satisfaction.

A supervisor may also provide incentives that influence worker performance. Instructions, time constraints, knowledge of performance, competition, pay, evaluation, and participation in decision making can be manipulated directly or indirectly by the supervisor. All these strategies are mechanisms used to convince the worker to set or accept work goals; retain his or her commitment to them; and ensure the persistence of the worker's efforts over time (Earley, Wojnaroski, & Prest, 1987; Locke, 1968).

In a work situation House (1971) demonstrated that the behavior of both the leader and the individual worker has an effect on path choice. House suggested three propositions about the effect of leader behavior on the motivation of an individual. First, motivational functions of a leader are to increase personal rewards to subordinates for path-goal attainment, increase payoffs associated with path choice, and facilitate path instrumentality by increasing opportunities for personal satisfaction en route to goal attainment. Second, the leader facilitates path instrumentality by decreasing role and task ambiguity and by imposing external controls that are perceived positively by subordinates. Finally, a leader's clarification of the obvious is redundant and viewed negatively by subordinates. These propositions provide a framework for understanding the relationship between job performance and job satisfaction.

According to House (1971) there are two important dimensions to supervisory behavior: initiating structure and consideration. The leader initiates structure for subordinates by assigning tasks, specifying procedures to be followed, clarifying expectations, and scheduling the work to be done. Leader consideration occurs when the leader creates an environment of psychological support, warmth, friendliness, and helpfulness, by doing things such as being approachable, looking out for the personal welfare of the group members, and giving advance notice about change (House, 1971).

Leader-initiated structure clarifies path-goal relationships and facilitates goal attainment. Higher occupational jobs are generally more ambiguous in nature. A positive correlation between leader-initiated structure and satisfaction among higher occupational groups has been found because goals are defined by the leader, decreasing job ambiguity. In contrast, lower level jobs are considered more routine and thus path-goal relationships are self-evident and the job itself is not inherently satisfying. When the job is routine and repetitive, leader-initiated structure would be perceived as an imposition of unnecessary external control. While this may increase productivity, it may also result in dissatisfaction among employees (House, 1971).

Consideration leadership is best used to make the path satisfying. That is, it serves as a source of extrinsic social support to employees during the path to the goal attainment process. To contrast, higher level jobs are intrinsically more satisfying and therefore the need for external support is less (House, 1971).

The behavior of the leader affects the worker's degree of motivation. The leader determines the extrinsic rewards (pay raises, promotions, assignment of higher level tasks, or opportunities for personal growth) that are associated with path use and goal attainment. The leader can facilitate path instrumentality by consistently rewarding results of work goal accomplishments and by repeatedly clarifying linkages between path utilized, goal achievements, and rewards. The rewards associated with goal attainment must be perceived to be of value to the person involved in the path-goal process.

In a repetitive or routine situation leader consideration behavior can increase the motivation of the worker. The leader who decreases barriers and increases employee control will increase ego involvement and the willingness of the employee to persevere in his or her efforts to achieve a goal.

Also related to the process of goal attainment is the concept of goal commitment. According to Locke, Shaw, Saari, and Latham (1981), goal commitment is the willingness of a person to expend effort and energy to achieve a goal. This willingness implies perseverant effort over time toward the accomplishment of the goal and a general unwillingness to abandon the goal or the attainment process. It is important to differentiate the concept of commitment from acceptance. Acceptance of a goal does not necessarily include the personal involvement assumed in goal commitment.

Hollenbeck and Klein (1987) used past research in the area of path-goal theory and expectancy theory to develop a model that links antecedents and consequences of commitment to the achievement of difficult goals. Their model followed the work of Locke et al. (1981) and identified variables that affect the expectation and attractiveness of goal attainment. These variables are broken down further into personal or situational factors. The situational factors that tend to increase commitment are "publicness," the degree to which significant others are aware of an individual's goal; volition, the individual's ability to participate in goal setting; explicitness, clearly defined goals; reward structures; and competition (Salancik, 1977).

Personal factors such as needs, beliefs, personality traits, and attitudes also affect a person's commitment to a goal. Hollenbeck and Klein's review of the literature (1987) demonstrated that persons with a high need for achievement, those who demonstrate high levels of endurance, and persons with type A behavior patterns generally set and attain difficult goals. These "high achievers" also demonstrate a link between their personal identification with the goals of the organization and their willingness to commit to organizational goals. Individuals who are highly committed to their job and view goal attainment as a necessary component of this self-esteem will be committed to challenging work goals on both personal and organizational levels.

Locke, Latham, and Erez (1988) looked at the relationship between goal commitment and job performance. Their work supports the idea that goal commitment is affected by external factors, such as authority, rewards, and peer pressure; internal factors, such as expectancy and self-esteem; and interactive factors such as participation and competition.

CASE ANALYSIS

Nursing is considered a higher level job and therefore has some component of ambiguity. A new orientee needs a leader who will initiate structure and thus define the goals and expectations of a new nurse. This is done through written expectations and conferences. The leader must promote attainment of these goals using rewards and positive reinforcement, such as pay raises, increasing responsibility, and praise. However, as the assigned tasks become more familiar, they become more routine and less intrinsically satisfying. The manager then needs to assume the consideration role to provide extrinsic support, making the path of goal attainment easier to travel. In the case study, leader-initiated structure at this time may be viewed as an imposition of external control because more productivity is needed to handle the increased patient census. At the same time this could result in dissatisfaction among employees, causing them to leave after 1 year of employment.

Leader-initiated structure in the case study appears to be related to increased turnover of staff. Because the census is higher, nurses are expected to be more productive, taking responsibility for a greater number of patients. Assuming that the tasks performed by the nurses are less satisfying under conditions of high pressure for output, leader-initiated structure would be viewed as an unnecessary imposition of control. This control was acceptable to the manager because she expected her staff to care for the larger number of patients. The subordinates may have resented this control when it was superimposed by the manager. Leader consideration is more likely to serve as a stress reducer when tasks become more unsatisfying and pressure for output increases. The difference in perception between the manager and employees can be explained in terms of differences in task satisfaction, that is, path valence and pressure for production.

It has been documented that goals influence behavior in both a direct and indirect way. Directly, assigned goals are motivational with a positive correlation between the difficulty of goals and energy expended on the task. Indirectly, goals promote strategic planning. Specific goals foster task mastery by decreasing job ambiguity, and task mastery results in increased commitment to the goals.

There should be no doubt that the staff nurses are committed to the profession of nursing, and it can be assumed that they are concerned with the delivery of quality health care. The question arises whether there is a better way to decrease turnover, maintain staff interest and morale, and still provide quality nursing care.

In analyzing this case it appears that the manager is solely responsible for setting broad goals for the staff and that after a specific formatted orientation, manager-staff communication is minimal. New policies and procedures are sent to the staff, so they are made aware of changes. It does not appear that the staff have input into the creation of policies or procedures.

Information sharing and participative goal setting are two strategies that would be beneficial in this situation. Change, particularly unsolicited change, is difficult for most people. As the workload changes, individual workers need to be involved in the process of planning how to meet the increased need for services without a comparable increase in staff. The manager needs to recognize that an increased inpatient census is a situation that fosters the adoption of functional work habits and is not intrinsically satisfying to the employee. By sharing information about the type of work to be done, staff can set goals for task mastery on an individual basis. It is the responsibility of the leader to use a consideration strategy to recognize and reward persons who are expending energy to become more proficient at their job. As mastery and self-esteem rise, persons will become more committed to the goals of the organization, because the goals will vary with their personal valences. It is only through group process and participative goal setting that a leader can expect his or her staff to demonstrate willingness to commit to the more demanding goals of the institution.

The majority of Sally's nursing staff are new graduates with less than 1 year of clinical experience. To offset the reality shock most new nurses experience as they move from the academic to the work environment, Sally has decided to become more involved in the orientation of new employees. By maintaining a higher profile Sally will convey to the staff that they are not only welcome, but a needed and valued addition to the unit.

Each new employee will receive a precepted orientation of 4 to 8 weeks depending on their need and level of experience. The orientation program will be individually tailored to minimize redundancy while still making each employee feel prepared for her new position on the unit.

As one of her consideration strategies Sally will meet with old as well as new employees at monthly staff meetings. A present agenda item will be the staff's feelings about the orientation process and the role of nursing on the unit. The need for new policies and procedures will also be addressed at the monthly staff meetings. Staff will be asked to participate in writing and implementing new or revised policies. Employees who are encouraged to take an active role in the running of the unit are more likely to support the operation of that unit.

Sally has been informed that the census on her unit is expected to increase to an average of 37 patients per day. This increase is a result of the recent addition of two neurosurgeons to the medical staff and their projected caseloads. Although the hospital administration recognizes that this rise in census will increase the workload of Sally's staff they have not approved the hiring of more nurses.

At the monthly staff meeting Sally candidly informs the staff of the projected changes and asks the staff for suggestions on how they would like to deal with the inevitable change in workload. By informing the staff of an upcoming change Sally is being a considerate leader. Her consideration continues as she asks the staff for their input.

At the meeting staff are able to ventilate their feelings about the rise in census. Through the discussion it becomes obvious to Sally that her staff question their ability to care for the neurosurgical patients. To boost their confidence and make the goal of providing quality patient care attainable Sally has the staff development department provide, on all three shifts, a series of inservices about the special needs of neurosurgical patients. To further increase the personal valences associated with attendance at the inservices, each employee is asked to set personal goals for knowledge attainment and skills acquisition. A reward system is also implemented to support goal attainment.

Through use of the path-goal theory Sally is able to temper her leader initiating style with consideration, the staff nurses are more personally involved in the work of the unit, the staff are supported in their efforts to gain knowledge to deliver quality nursing care, and staff turnover does not become a problem.

RESEARCH

Evans (1970) used nursing as a sample for a study that found empirical evidence suggesting that supervisory behavior relates to path instrumentality, and that the product of path instrumentality and path frequency is related to goal attainment. A finding in the hospital was the lack of a direct relationship between supervisory behavior and path-goal instrumentality. This was attributed to the many other factors that affect path-goal instrumentalities. Evans replicated this study in 1974 and determined that the subordinate's locus of control could moderate the supervisor-subordinate relationship (Evans, 1974).

House and Mitchell (1974) described subordinates in terms of their preference to control or be controlled by factors in the environment. Low authoritarian persons prefer to share in the decision-making process and prefer leaders who will support that participation. High authoritarian subordinates prefer to work in a more externally controlled environment. Participation and authoritarianism is moderated by types of tasks. Highly repetitive tasks are not ego-involving, whereas less repetitive tasks are generally more ambiguous and more ego-involving. Theorizing on the path-goal theory of leadership Schuler (1976) looked at the effect that tasks of differing degrees of repetitiveness had on participation, authoritarianism, and job satisfaction of factory workers of all levels. This research supported House and Mitchell's suggestion (1974) that tasks with a low degree of repetitiveness are conducive to ego involvement, low authoritarianism, and increased job satisfaction.

Sims and Szilagyi (1975) used the path-goal theory of leadership when they examined the relationship between leader-initiating structure and subordinate satisfaction. The two groups involved in the study were hospital-based associate directors of nursing and head nurses. It was hypothesized that at the higher administrative level, roles would be less defined and that strong relationships would exist among leader-initiating behavior, role ambiguity, job expectations, and job satisfaction.

The results of the study supported House's theory (1971) that occupational level does not impact on the relationship between leader behavior and subordinate satisfaction. Sims and Szilagyi (1975) found that leader-initiating behavior was positively correlated with job satisfaction for associate directors of nursing in a high-ambiguity situation and negatively correlated with job satisfaction for head nurses in a low-ambiguity setting. In the high-ambiguity situation clarification of the path resulted in satisfaction for the subordinate and facilitated goal attainment. Leader-initiating structure was not needed to clarify the path to subordinates' goals for the head nurse group; in fact, the clarification was reviewed as an unnecessary imposition of control.

Hedlund (1978) used House's path-goal theory of leadership to explain the work performance and job satisfaction of state legislators. Although legislators have a great deal of autonomy, they do belong to an organization and that organization has leaders. In the legislative environment the role of the leader is to induce cooperation from members, facilitate the decision-making process, and support group members on the path to goal attainment. Hedlund supported House's theory that individuals will select the path that is perceived to produce the goal, as well as provide the greatest degree of personal satisfaction. The research done by Hedlund supports the application of the path-goal theory to legislative settings because the concepts of leader-initiating structure, leader consideration, and role ambiguity are key issues in effective leadership management. Hedlund found a positive correlation between job satisfaction and the previously mentioned leadership variables.

Schriesheim and Schriesheim (1980) tested several of the hypotheses concerning the moderating effects of task structure on goal attainment as presented in the path-goal theory of leadership. The hypotheses tested were (House, 1971):

1. Task structure will have a negative moderating effect on the relationship between initiating leader behavior and subordinate satisfaction.
2. Task structure will have a negative moderating effect on the relationship between initiating leader behavior and subordinate perceptions of clarity.
3. Task structure will have a positive moderating effect on the relationship between considerate leader behavior and subordinate satisfaction.
4. Task structure will have a positive moderating effect on the relationship between considerate leader behavior and subordinate perceptions of role clarity.

The analysis by Schriesheim and Schriesheim (1980) repeatedly showed that task structure did not have a moderating effect on the relationship between leader behavior, subordinate satisfaction, and role clarity. Although initiating leader behavior did not relate well to satisfaction it did impact on role clarity. This work confirmed that consideration leadership does impact on all the dependent variables. Because of the known importance of leadership behavior styles, Schriesheim and Schriesheim recommended further testing of the path-goal theory to explain these results.

In summary, research using the path-goal theory of leadership has determined it to be a viable management theory in a variety of settings. It addresses the relationship between supervisors and subordinates and the factors that affect path choice, goal attainment, and job satisfaction.

REFERENCES

Atkinson, J.W. (1958). Towards experimented analysis of human motivation in terms of motives, expectancies, and incentives. In J.W. Atkinson (Ed.), *Motives in fantasy, action and society.* New York: Van Nostrand.

Early, P.C., Wojnaroski, P., & Prest, W. (1987). Task planning and energy expended: Exploration of how goals influence performance. *Journal of Applied Psychology, 72,* 107-114.

Erez, M., & Arad, R. (1986). Participative goal-setting: Social, motivational, and cognitive factors. *Journal of Applied Psychology, 71,* 591-597.

Evans, M. (1970). The effects of supervisory behavior on the path-goal relationship. *Organizational Behavior and Human Performance, 5,* 277-298.

Evans, M. (1974). Extensions of a path-goal theory of motivation. *Journal of Applied Psychology, 59,* 178-191.

Galbraith, J., & Cummings, L. (1967). An empirical investigation of the motivational determinants of past performance: Interactive effects between instrumentality, valence, motivation and ability. *Organizational Behavior and Human Performance, 2,* 237-257.

Georgopoulos, B., Mahoney, G. & Jones, N. (1957). A path-goal approach to productivity. *Journal of Applied Psychology, 53,* 345-353.

Graen, G. (1969). Instrumental theory of work motivation: Some empirical results and suggested modifications. *Journal of Applied Psychology, 53,* 1-25.

Hedlund, R.D. (1978). A path-goal approach to explaining leadership's impact on legislators' perceptions. *Social Science Quarterly, 59,* 178-191.

Hersey, P., & Blanchard, K. (1982). *Management of organizational behavior: Utilizing human resources.* Englewood Cliffs, NJ: Prentice-Hall.

Hollenbeck, J.R., & Klein, H.J. (1987). Goal commitment and the goal-setting process: Problems and proposals for future research. *Journal of Applied Psychology, 72,* 212-220.

House, R. (1971). A path-goal theory of leader effectiveness. *Administrative Science Quarterly, 16,* 321-338.

House, R., & Mitchell, T. (1974). Path-goal theory of leadership. *Journal of Contemporary Business, 3,* 81-98.

Lawler, E. (1968). A correlation-causal analysis of the relationship between expectancy attitudes and job performance. *Journal of Applied Psychology, 52,* 462-468.

Locke, E.A. (1968). Toward a theory of task motivation and incentives. *Organizational Behavior and Human Performance, 3,* 157-189.

Locke, E.A. (1970). Job satisfaction and job performance: A theoretical analysis. *Organizational Behavior and Human Performance, 5,* 484-500.

Locke, E.A., Cartledge, N., & Knerr, C.S. (1970). Studies of the relationship between satisfaction, goal-setting and performance. *Organizational Behavior and Human Performance, 5,* 135-158.

Locke, E.A., Latham, G.P., & Erez, M. (1988). The determinants of goal commitment. *Academy of Management Review, 13,* 23-39.

Locke, E.A., Shaw, N.K., Saari, L.M., & Latham, G.P. (1981). Goal setting and task performance: 1969-1980. *Psychological Bulletin, 90,* 125-152.

Porter, L., & Lawler, E. (1967). *Managerial attitudes and performance.* Homewood, IL: Irwin Dorsey.

Salancik, G. (1977). Commitment and the control of organizational behavior and belief. In B.M. Straw & G. R. Salancik (Eds.), *New directions in organizational behavior* (pp. 1-54). Chicago: St. Claire Press.

Schriesheim, J.F., & Schriesheim, C.A. (1980). A test for the path-goal theory of leadership and some suggested directions for future research. *Personnel Psychology, 33,* 349-369.

Schuler, R.S. (1976). Participation with supervisor and subordinate authoritarianism: A path-goal theory reconciliation. *Administrative Science Quarterly, 21,* 320-325.

Sims, H.P., Jr., & Szilagyi, A.D. (1975). Leader structure and subordinate satisfaction for two hospital administrative levels: A path analysis approach. *Journal of Applied Psychology, 60,* 194-197.

Vroom, V.H. (1964). *Work and motivation.* New York: John Wiley & Sons.

Chapter 18

Situational Leadership
Paul Hersey and Kenneth Blanchard

Leta M. Holder

▮▮   CASE STUDY

The scenario for this case study is a 30-bed addictive disease treatment unit within a general hospital. The professional nursing staff on this unit consists of a charge nurse, five full-time staff nurses, three part-time staff nurses, one clinical nurse specialist, and one counselor. Staff morale within the unit is low, and communication among staff members is virtually nonexistent. Day-by-day management of the unit is on a needs basis. No long-term planning has been done, and the staff sees no need to do any at this time. A memo from nursing administration has announced that a review team will be auditing the unit within 6 months.

In preparation for this review, the hospital's quality assurance nurse has volunteered to assist the staff in a self-evaluation process. The review of existing policies and protocols indicates that major revisions are necessary. Only limited adaptation of general policies and procedures to meet the needs of this patient population has been accomplished. The charge nurse has previously indicated that she did not see this as her responsibility.

A brief history of the addictive disease unit's staffing pattern and promotion policies may give the reader insight into the situation. The addictive disease unit is viewed by all other units in the hospital as different and with a lighter workload. It is not unusual for the addictive disease unit nursing staff to be detailed to other units in the hospital as needed. Consequently, often the staffing for the unit is less than optimal. The charge nurse had no experience with addictive clients before her assignment to this unit. She has noted on several occasions that she accepted the position as head nurse because she wanted to avoid rotating shifts. It should also be noted that she was the only applicant for the position. The counselor, although counted as nursing staff, actually functions as a primary counselor and carries a full patient caseload. The clinical nurse specialist is a new employee. Her area of expertise is psychiatric nursing, and she too has limited experience with addictive clients. She is highly motivated and willing to assist with the job at hand but readily admits that she needs assistance. One of the part-time staff nurses who currently works on the night shift has past experience as a head nurse on this addictive disease unit. It was reported that she had good managerial skills and communicated well with clients and staff but resigned from the position to spend time with her young children. None of the other staff nurses has had any experience with addictive disease or management.

After deliberation and with the approval of nursing administration, the quality assurance nurse has appointed a task group. The group members selected include the head nurse, clinical nurse specialist, counselor, and nursing service supervisor. It is obvious to both the quality assurance nurse and to adminstration that the task of developing a cohesive working group will not be easy. As leader of this task group, what could the quality assurance nurse do to facilitate this process?

| | | | | | | | | | | | | | | | | | | | | | | | | | | | | | | | | | | | | | | | | | | | | | | | | | | | | | | | | | | | | | | | | | | | |

SITUATIONAL LEADERSHIP THEORY

Situational leadership, a management theory developed by Paul Hersey and Kenneth Blanchard, is based on the interplay of three basic concepts of management: task behavior, relationship behavior, and maturity level. Task behavior, the amount of direction given by the leader to get the task accomplished, and relationship behavior, the amount of emotional support the leader provides to the employee or follower, are directly related to the maturity level exhibited by the employee toward the job at hand (Hersey & Blanchard, 1977).

Hersey and Blanchard postulate that leadership style should be more directive with the immature worker and less directive with the more mature worker. In a similar manner, relationship behavior should increase with the maturity level of the worker until the worker is fully mature. A mature follower is one who has the capacity, willingness, and capability to set individual goals and accomplish the task with minimal direction. The immature follower requires specific step-by-step instructions in order to accomplish a given assignment. A person's maturity level is not constant; rather, it depends on the specific task or objective that must be met. Therefore, a person may be placed on a continuum that ranges from immature to mature. Frequent assessments are required for the appropriate leadership style to be used (Hersey & Blanchard, 1977; Hersey, Blanchard, & Hambleton, 1980).

A major component of situational leadership theory addresses the relationship behavior shared by the leader and follower. This behavior refers to the communication process and the emotional support needed by the follower in a given situation. The immature follower requires a high level of task direction and a low level of social support or relationship behavior from the leader. As the follower's level of task maturity increases, the leader's relationship behavior increases and the task behavior decreases. Essentially within the theory a variance exists in both task behavior and relationship behavior according to the needs of the follower. The more mature follower often needs limited task direction but still requires support or relationship behavior from the leader. As the follower continues to grow and mature, he or she may reach a point at which minimal task direction and emotional support are needed (Hersey & Blanchard, 1977; Hersey et al., 1980). Therefore, as Teasley (1987) noted, an effective leader must have a varied repertoire of leadership styles to meet situational demands.

Situational leadership was initially called life cycle theory. This title alludes to the growth concept that is inherent in the theory. Situational leadership theory acknowledges that leadership style can and should vary not only from individual to individual but also from situation to situation. As the situation changes, the person's level of maturity may change (Hersey & Blanchard, 1977). Furthermore Hersey and Blanchard note that managers are frequently engaged in behaviors focused on producing growth in their followers. Each person should be encouraged to reach a level of task-relevant maturity that surpasses his or her present and/or past level.

Hersey, Blanchard, and Hambleton (1980) have identified the components of maturity. The major factors are psychological maturity and job maturity. They define psychological maturity as the willingness or motivation to complete a task. The person who is psychologically mature has high self-esteem, enjoys the responsibility that comes with an assignment, and likes the satisfaction that results from a job well done. Job maturity refers to a person's ability to do a job adequately. The person with high job maturity has the ability, knowledge, and experience to do a job with minimal task direction from the leader. Using these definitions as descriptions of individuals, these authors have identified four levels by which followers can be classified (Hersey et al, 1980, p. 101):

1. Individuals who are neither willing nor able to take responsibility (low on both psychological and job maturity);
2. Individuals who are willing but not able to take responsibility (high psychological maturity but low job maturity);
3. Individuals who are able but not willing to take responsibility (high job maturity but low psychological maturity); and
4. Individuals who are both willing and able to take responsibility (high on both psychological and job maturity).

Hersey, Blanchard, and Natemeyer (1979) have addressed the leadership styles that are most effective with these levels of maturity. Persons with low maturity need specific directions and guidance. They refer to this style as *telling* because "it requires telling people what, how, when, and where to perform" (p. 422). Persons with moderate maturity respond best to a *selling* style of leadership. These individuals need directions because of their lack of ability but respond best to two-way communication in which the leader offers supportive behavior to complement their willingness. Persons performing at a moderately high level of maturity need a *participating* type of leadership. In these situations the follower may share in decision making, but the leader is the facilitator. Followers functioning at a high level of maturity have both the ability and the motivation to perform well when the task is delegated. They are able to decide "how, when, and where to perform" (Hersey et al., 1979, p. 422).

Hersey and Blanchard (1977) have developed a visual model of situational leadership styles to help the reader conceptualize their theory. This model is illustrated in Figure 18-1. The model illustrates the leadership styles as four quadrants of a graph with relationship behavior and task behavior represented as the horizontal and vertical axes. The maturity level of the follower, shown as a superimposed axis, is illustrated on a continuum from immature to mature. Hersey and Blanchard postulate that effective leadership behavior will move in a curvilinear fashion through the four quadrants as the maturity level of the follower fluctuates from immaturity to maturity.

Based on this model, Hersey and Blanchard (1977) have identified four primary leadership styles that can be conceptualized as the four leadership quadrants:

S1 High task and low relationship
S2 High task and high relationship
S3 High relationship and low task
S4 Low relationship and low task

The bell-shaped curve superimposed over the four quadrants in Figure 18-1 indicates the leadership behaviors needed. Leadership behaviors are viewed on a continuum that reflects the style needed by the follower in relationship to his or her maturity level. The bell-shaped curve illustrates the flexibility needed in leadership. This curve indicates that, as with any bell-shaped curve, quadrants S2 and S3 are the preferred leadership styles because the maturity and readiness levels of most followers fall in R2 and R3 areas and therefore are respectively matched with S2 and S3 correctly.

The basic concept of the individual's level of maturity as is corresponds to the level of leadership behavior is shown below.

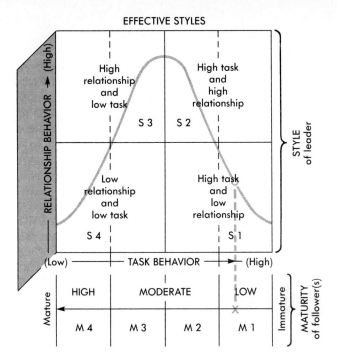

EFFECTIVE STYLES

High relationship and low task **S 3**	High task and high relationship **S 2**
Low relationship and low task **S 4**	High task and low relationship **S 1**

RELATIONSHIP BEHAVIOR ↑ (High)

(Low) ——— TASK BEHAVIOR ——→ (High)

STYLE of leader

HIGH	MODERATE	LOW
M 4	M 3	M 2	M 1

Mature ← → Immature

MATURITY of follower(s)

FIGURE 18-1   Hersey and Blanchard's model of situational leadership styles. *From Hersey, P., & Blanchard, K.H.* Management of organizational behavior: Utilizing human resources *(5th ed.),* © *1988, p. 237. Reprinted by permission of Prentice-Hall, Inc., Englewood Cliffs, NJ.*

Low maturity	→ High task and low relationship
Low moderate maturity	→ High task and high relationship
Moderate maturity	→ High relationship and low task
High maturity	→ Low relationship and low task

In summary, situational leadership takes into account the follower's level of maturity in each situation. Just as followers are categorized on a continuum that indicates their level of maturity, so too does leadership behavior fluctuate according to the needs of the individuals and the organization (Hersey & Blanchard, 1977).

In reviewing nursing theory, situational leadership can be compared to Orem's theory of self-care. Orem (1980) believes that nursing care should be planned and implemented on a level that is congruent with the patient's needs. The patient's needs are directly related to the level of care needed by the client to compensate for any deficiency he or she might have in self-care.

This theory is comparable to Hersey and Blanchard's theory that the amount of supervision needed by the employee is directly related to the employee's level of maturity. The level of maturity is equal to the patient's self-care deficit. The four levels of task direction and relationship behavior identified by Hersey and Blanchard are comparable to Orem's three levels of care (Orem, 1980):

1. *Wholly compensatory.* The patient is unable to participate in his or her self-care, and the nurse provides total care.
2. *Partially compensatory.* The patient is able to cooperate and works with the nurse in his or her care.
3. *Educative/development.* The patient is able to care for self but needs assistance or education.

Orem (1989) states that "the critical difference between the actions of nurses and the actions of nursing administration can be viewed as a difference in their objects or foci" (p. 50). As noted earlier, the major difference in Orem's theory of self-care and Hersey and Blanchard's situational leadership theory is the level and capability of the participants, whether patient or employee.

CASE ANALYSIS

Hersey and Blanchard's situational leadership theory can be used with organizations, families, or groups (Hersey & Blanchard, 1977). In this case analysis, the situational leadership theory will be used to analyze the task group developed to establish policies and protocols for the addictive disease unit.

Initially the quality assurance nurse established a meeting time and place. A review of the Standards of Care required by the Joint Committee on Accreditation of Healthcare Organizations was the first order of business. Committee members listed the noted deficiencies and organized a priority list. The committee agreed that each member should identify a project to develop independently. Each resulting proposal would later be brought before the committee for review and editing.

Priority items for development were identified as the following:
1. Patient handbook
2. Charting protocol
3. Nursing assessment
4. Confidentiality policy
5. Standards of care
6. Safety policies

Several trips had been made by committee members to other hospitals to obtain specific information on the above issues. These resources were made available to committee members.

It became apparent at the first meeting that the quality assurance nurse would have to use varied management tactics appropriate to the individual group members involved. She began by evaluating the environment. As Hersey and Blanchard (1977) stress, in a group situation both the maturity of the group and the maturity level of individual group members must be considered. They further add that the maturity level of a group may be at a different level from that of individuals within the group.

The maturity level of the group was determined as moderate. Even though all members worked together at the hospital, they did not appear comfortable in the small task group setting. The leader therefore took both a task-oriented and a relationship-oriented stance. She gave the group the opportunity to establish their own goals. As Hersey and Blanchard (1972a, 1972b, 1972c) as well as Crowley, Rinker, Neely, and Anderson (1986) have stated, individuals will be more committed to accomplishing a task when they take part in goal setting.

Assessments of group members indicated various levels of maturity. The charge nurse was assessed at a low level of maturity. According to situational leadership theory, she was neither willing nor able to accept a task. The clinical nurse specialist, however, had both the willingness and the ability to accomplish her goal and therefore was rated as having high maturity. The nursing service supervisor was willing to work with the group but lacked knowledge of the addictive disease process and unit. She was assessed as having low-moderate maturity in this particular situation. The nurse counselor was assessed as being somewhat between moderate maturity and high maturity. She was able to perform the task but was hesitant to make a commitment.

In accordance with situational leadership theory, the leader gave group members an opportunity to select task assignments. The clinical nurse specialist readily accepted the responsibility of developing a protocol for charting and developing a nursing assessment tool. The nursing service supervisor volunteered to assist group members with editing and collecting additional background data. The counselor and head nurse made no selection. Consequently the leader assigned the task of developing a confidentiality policy to the counselor and the development of a patient handbook to the charge nurse.

During the interim between task force meetings, the leader frequently offered support and guidance to the members. Analyzing the leader's leadership style according to Hersey and Blanchard's theory, it was obvious that she was varying her tactics according to the maturity level of the members to facilitate growth and change. The clinical nurse specialist needed little assistance and support. She functioned well with low relationship and low task support. She immediately began working on instituting an assessment stamp that could be used by the nurses to do a quick assessment during each shift.

The nursing service supervisor provided the necessary assistance with the protocol required to institute the new policy. The clinical nurse specialist reported on the status of her projects at every task force meeting. Positive reinforcement was always given by the leader and other group members.

Initially the nurse counselor responded best to high relationship and low task support. She had the capability and resources to develop a confidentiality policy but needed reassurance. Blanchard and Lorber (1984) would say that she needed coaching. As she worked on the policy, she frequently asked for feedback from both the leader and the clinical nurse specialist. She attended all task force meetings and was an active participant in all discussions. It soon became apparent that she was the expert concerning the present unit policies and understood the rationale behind existing policies. The leader was careful to give her positive feedback. Blanchard and Johnson (1982) note that followers perform best when they receive specifically focused praise in a timely fashion. They note that as the individual begins to feel valued as a productive and appreciated member of an organization, he or she will be motivated to reach full potential. Blanchard and Lorber (1984) have summarized this theory with their axiom, "People who produce good results feel good about themselves" (p. 18). The counselor's actions support this theory. As her maturity level increased, so did her willingness to accept more responsibility. After completing her first assignment, she volunteered to begin working on additional policies. The leader varied her leadership style to comply with the maturity level of the counselor. A leadership style of low relationship and low task support was effective at this stage of growth.

The leadership style used with the head nurse was high task and low relationship. Specific directions were given on how to develop the patient handbook. A handbook used by a hospital with a similar program was available, and permission had been granted to adapt this handbook for use. The head nurse was asked to edit the book and make the necessary changes. The leader and nursing service supervisor offered their assistance, but the head nurse indicated that she needed no help at this time. The head nurse did not attend the next two meetings. The leader contacted her to determine her progress. The head nurse informed the leader that she had not had an opportunity to work on the project. She cited shortage of staff as a factor. The leader stressed the importance of the project and asked if she had requested additional staff from the nursing service supervisor. The head nurse stated that the addictive disease unit never got any additional help. The leader followed up by contacting the supervisor and asking if staffing was short on the unit. The supervisor reported that the staffing pattern was stable. The supervisor again volunteered to offer her assistance with the project. The head nurse came to subsequent meetings but was usually late. She continued to complain that she did not have adequate time to work on the project. The supervisor confronted the head nurse and told her that she had offered to assist her but to no avail.

The leader noted that the group was fast becoming disgruntled with the lack of progress on the handbook. She determined that her only alternative was to use coercion. The leader announced to the group that a timetable listing responsible parties would be submitted to the director of nurses. Hersey, Blanchard, and Natemeyer (1979) state that a leader must use his or her power base to influence followers. The leader was using both coercive and connection power to influence the lagging worker. It was coercive in that it served as a threat of punishment. The connection power was implied when it was reported that the progress or lack of progress would be noted by the director.

Following the submission of the time plan, progress was noted. The head nurse was able to find time to work on the handbook. However, the quality of work was not always adequate, and the group made numerous editorial changes. As the handbook began to take shape, the head nurse did begin to take pride in her efforts. The leader and group members gave positive reinforcement whenever appropriate. Still, the head nurse was not comfortable in her evolving role. After completing the handbook, she asked for a transfer. Her request was granted.

The head nurse position was filled with a nurse experienced in management and addictive disease. She joined the task force and volunteered to assist other members until she was oriented to the unit and task. An assessment of the group at this time indicated that it was functioning at a high level of maturity. The leader appropriately began to withdraw her support and guidance. Her leadership style became low relationship and low task support.

Tyndall (1979) notes that situational leadership is an appropriate leadership style for nursing. She adds that at any given time a nursing staff is a mix of experienced and inexperienced nurses who need varied leadership styles. This concept was exemplified in the task group described. Only through the expertise of the leader as a facilitator was group cohesion established and the assigned tasks accomplished.

RESEARCH

Situational leadership theory in part was derived from empirical data gathered by researchers studying leadership styles. Studies conducted by the Bureau of Business at Ohio State University in 1945 determined that effective leader behavior was identifiable on two dimensions. These dimensions were structure (task behavior) and consideration (relationship behavior) of the worker. They found that effective leaders did not always score high on both dimensions. These researchers were the first to note that leader behaviors need to be examined in both areas. Hersey and Blanchard (1977) interpreted the data to indicate that no one style of leadership behavior is always the best. They developed the LEAD-Self and LEAD-Other instruments for determining leadership styles.

Hersey and Blanchard's theory adds a third element, the maturity level of the follower. To determine the maturity level of the follower, they developed an instrument, the Manager's Rating Form. Four pilot studies were conducted to test the validity and reliability of this instrument. Using the data gathered from these studies, the tool was revised and additional research was conducted to assess its reliability. They report the test-retest reliability scores as .84 for job maturity and .88 for psychological maturity. The Manager's Rating Form was then revised so that it could be used as a self-rating tool by the follower. Both the Manager's Rating Form and the Self-Rating Form can be used to assist the leader and follower in determining the most effective leadership style. It is suggested that the two tools are very effective in programs utilizing both management by objectives and contracting leadership styles (Hersey et al., 1980).

Guest, Hersey, and Blanchard (1977) report a longitudinal case study of a plant during a period of change. The data were gathered over a 3-year period by Guest and his colleagues when he was working at the Technology Project, Yale Institute of Human Relations. Situational leadership theory was used to analyze the changes that occurred. Data showed that as major changes occurred they were directly influenced by a new manager. The incumbents in the direct line of authority above the plant manager remained constant. Supervisors in the plant and the formal organizational structure remained unchanged. The plant also continued to produce the same product. The scenario began with a plant in serious trouble. Production was low, morale was poor, and turnover was rapid. The resident manager was constantly putting pressure on the supervisors to increase production.

Guest, Hersey, and Blanchard (1977) interpreted the original leadership style as high task and low relationship. The staff resented this leadership style, and consequently an ineffective cycle had developed. A new manager was sent to the plant to reorganize and get the plant functioning on a higher level. The new manager began by assessing the environment. He spent time in the plant getting to know the workers and listening to their complaints and suggestions. He slowly began to develop a high relationship and low task leadership style. As the workers began to respond to his leadership style, they became motivated. At the close of his 3-year tenure, they had moved from low production to high production. In fact, they had moved from sixth to first in production, employee retention, and general efficiency of the six plants within the organization (Guest et al., 1977).

In 1978 Goodin researched the leadership styles of administrators of baccalaureate nursing programs in relationship to selected organizational variables. Using situational leadership as the theoretical framework, she determined that the leadership style of the administrators was independent of the organizational variables studied. The organizational variables identified in this study were group size, group maturity, organizational structure, administrative position, and administrative power.

Two other research studies using situational leadership as a theoretical framework to study academia were conducted by Wakefield-Fisher (1987) and Alexander (1988). Wakefield-Fisher focused her study on the professionalism and scholarly productivity of faculty in relationship to the leadership style of the dean. Her study showed that the dean's leadership style was predominantly low task and high relationship or high task and high relationship. There was no significant relationship between the dean's leadership style and faculty productivity. Alexander focused on the cognitive modes and leadership styles of nursing deans. Her data indicated no significant relationship between cognitive modes and leadership styles.

Duxbury, Armstrong, Drew, and Henly (1984) researched head nurse leadership style in relationship to staff nurse burnout and job satisfaction. These researchers identified four categories of leadership styles: high consideration–high structure, high consideration–low structure, low consideration–high structure, and low consideration–low structure. These classifications are comparable to situational leadership classifications. Results of their research indicated that head nurses in intensive care units who scored high on consideration did positively influence job satisfaction and, to a minimal degree, burnout. Head nurses who scored low on consideration negatively influenced job satisfaction and burnout. Structure, however, had no identifiable effect.

Several studies have been conducted to determine the effectiveness of Orem's theory in guiding practice and research, but few address specifically its use in administration. Dickerson and Lee-Villasnor (1982) used a field study approach to gather data from two private nurse practitioners. They found that analysis of interview sessions yielded data that could be categorized as expression of needs, self-care assets, self-care demands, and self-care measures. They suggested that this data could be used to structure nursing care. Gallant and McLane

(1979) used Orem's theory as a conceptual framework to organize a study focused on validating outcome criteria. Allison (1973) reported on the use of Orem's theory as a framework for organizing a diabetic clinic. Her study focused on answering the question, How can nurses be helped to maintain a nursing focus while assuming new roles and increasing responsibilities for patients in the health care delivery system? (p. 53).

In summary, a review of the pertinent research on situational leadership indicates that this theory is appropriate to nursing management. Limited research is available on Orem's theory, and no studies to date have linked Orem's self-care theory with Hersey and Blanchard's situational leadership theory. Additional research is needed to clarify and refine both situational leadership and Orem's theory of self-care deficit.

REFERENCES

Alexander, J.E. (1988). *The cognitive modes and leadership styles among academic administrators of nursing.* Unpublished Doctoral Dissertation, Indiana University, Bloomington, IN.

Allison, S.E. (1973). A framework for nursing action in a nurse-conducted diabetic management clinic. *Journal of Nursing Administration, 4,* 53-59.

Blanchard, K., & Johnson, S. (1982). *The one minute manager.* New York: Morrow.

Blanchard, K., & Lorber, R. (1984). *Putting the one minute manager to work.* New York: Morrow.

Crowley, J., Rinker, G., Neely, A.E., & Anderson, A.S. (1986). Situational leadership for the laboratory. *Journal of Medical Technology, 3,* 303-306.

Dickson, G.L., Lee-Villasenor (1982, October). Nursing theory and practice: A self-care approach. *Advances in Nursing Science,* pp. 29-40.

Duxbury, M.L., Armstrong, G.D., Drew, D.J., & Henly, S.J. (1984). Head nurse leadership style with staff nurse burnout and job satisfaction in neonatal intensive care units. *Nursing Research, 33*(2), 97-101.

Gallant, B.W., & McLane, A.M. (1979). Outcome criteria: A process for validation at the unit level. *Journal of Nursing Administration, 9*(1), 14–21.

Goodin, M.F. (1978). Relationship among leadership styles of administrative heads of baccalaureate nursing programs and selected variables in the organizational setting. *Dissertation Abstracts International, 39*(11), 6427-A.

Guest, R.H., Hersey, P., & Blanchard, K.H. (1977). *Organizational change through effective leadership.* Englewood Cliffs, NJ: Prentice-Hall.

Hersey, P., & Blanchard, K. (1972a, January). The management of change. *Training Development Journal,* pp. 6-10.

Hersey, P., & Blanchard, K. (1972b, February). The management of change. *Training Development Journal,* pp. 20-24.

Hersey, P., & Blanchard, K. (1972c, March). The management of change. *Training Development Journal,* pp. 28-33.

Hersey, P., & Blanchard, K.H. (1977). *Management of organizational behavior: Utilizing human resources.* Englewood Cliffs, NJ: Prentice-Hall.

Hersey, P., Blanchard, K.H., & Hambleton, R. (1980). Contracting for leadership style: A process and instrumentation for building effective work relationships. In P. Hersey & J. Stinson (Eds.), *Perspectives in leader effectiveness.* Athens, OH: Ohio University, Center for Leadership Studies.

Hersey, P., Blanchard, K.H., & Natemeyer, W.E. (1979). Situational leadership: Perception, and the impact of power. *Group and Organization Studies, 4*(4), 418-428.

Orem, D. (1980). *Nursing concepts of practice.* New York: McGraw-Hill.

Orem, D. (1989). Nursing administration: A theoretical approach. In B. Henry et al. (Eds.), *Dimensions in nursing administration.* Boston: Blackwell.

Teasley, D. (1987). Situational leadership for nurses. *Nursing Management, 8*(1), 112-113.

Tyndall, A. (1979). Situational leadership theory. *Nursing Leadership, 12*(2), 25-29.

Wakefield-Fisher, M. (1987). The relationship between professionalization of nursing faculty, leadership styles of deans, and faculty scholarly productivity. *Journal of Professional Nursing, 3*(30), 155-163.

Chapter 19

Control Theory
Arnold S. Tannenbaum

Katherine S. Russell

❙❙ CASE STUDY

Assistant Director of Nursing Jane Monroe was asked to chair the Nursing Quality Assurance (QA) Committee; the committee was subsequently charged with the task of developing patient care standards that were to be surveyed monthly. Jane appointed nurse managers from each unit as members of the QA Committee and asked that they become involved in planning a quality assurance program for nursing services.

The nurse manager and nursing personnel on each unit were to collaborate in the development of standards from which outcome criteria and process criteria could be established for monitoring and evaluating purposes. In actuality the nurse managers did not get the staff involved in this process, stating that the nurses were "too busy" to participate. At the next meeting of the QA Committee, Jane discovered that little had been accomplished toward writing the standards. Therefore she decided to do the work herself because she was the "best qualified."

Consequently, Jane developed standards, and criteria for monitoring quality and appropriateness of patient care were extracted from the list of standards by the nurse managers. One manager made the suggestion that the staff be involved in auditing the patients' medical records and observing the outcome of care at patients' bedsides. After discussion, however, the decision was made that inspection of the degree of compliance by the staff would instead involve only the nurse manager and Jane functioning as a team. At random intervals, this team would make rounds on the unit, audit the medical records, and observe the patients for evidence of compliance with established criteria. Indicators monitored included admission assessment standards, preoperative teaching protocols, and intravenous (IV) therapy policies.

The new quality assurance program was explained to the nursing staff during a unit meeting. Emphasis was placed on the positive aspects of controlling and improving practice and patient care. The nurses listened quietly and offered neither approving nor disapproving comments.

For 3 months, data were gathered. At the end of this period, Jane correlated and analyzed the results. They revealed that compliance with standards of care was much less than the appropriate threshold that had been established by the committee. For example, compliance with patient teaching criteria was only 30%.

After discussing these results, the committee asked the nurse managers to report the rather dismal findings to the nursing staff at the next unit meeting and to stress the need for compliance. Again, the staff was not asked for input into how to solve the dilemma. Rather, they were told that the situation must be corrected.

A focus survey conducted over the next month did not reveal any change in compliance regarding preoperative teaching standards. The lack of compliance was especially visible on the unit with the most experienced nursing staff.

Could a knowledge of control theory have aided Jane in achieving the overall goals of the quality assurance program?

| | | | | | | | | | | | | | | | | | | | | | | | | | | | | | | | | | | | | | | | | | | | | | | | | | | | | | | | | | | | | | | | | | | | | | | | | | | | |

CONTROL THEORY

In the typical bureaucratic organization, many of the goals of the system and those of the members are viewed as incompatible (Tannenbaum, 1962). Because this situation would lead to limited commitment to and satisfaction with a system, several models for organizations have come into focus in recent years (Likert & Likert, 1976). One such theoretical framework is concerned with organizational control and its relationship to performance and satisfaction (Tannenbaum, 1956, 1962).

Arnold Tannenbaum is credited with the development of control theory as a framework for the study of control in organizations. His initial work with this theory began early in his career at the University of Michigan's Institute for Social Research (Tannenbaum, 1956; Miner, 1982). Early research that he did with Morse and Reimer (1951) led to the notion that understanding the supervisor's role depends on considering events occurring in the organization; he then created the framework of control theory subsequently utilized in the classical investigation of four local unions (Tannenbaum, 1956). The results of the study, which some believe should be viewed as a pilot study, supported the hypotheses for control theory and established Tannenbaum as its authority (Miner, 1982).

In its original usage by the French, the term *control* used in organizations meant "to check" (Tannenbaum, 1956, p. 239). Tannenbaum expanded the classical meaning that focused on control coming from a formal system to a process of interpersonal influence.

Tannenbaum (1966, p. 84) defines control as any process by which a person or group of persons determines (i.e., intentionally affects) what another person or group of persons will do. Essentially it means creating an extended change in the behavior of others — getting them to do something they might not otherwise have done.

A review by Miner offered several postulates that described how control works (1982, p. 61):

1. There must be both a subject and an object; that someone must control something. Controlling is the active aspect; being controlled, the passive.
2. Controlling must be motivated to occur. Thus there must be perception of worthwhile rewards associated with the behavior.
3. Internal control within an organization and external control of the environment are closely related.
4. Control involves several phases of activity; the legislative, in which policies and course of action are decided; the administrative, in which policies and courses of action are interpreted and implemented; the sanctions, in which rewards and punishments are given or withheld.

Therefore control can be accomplished through command, persuasion, policies, technology, or a reward system (Tannenbaum, 1962). It is a pattern of influence in an organization that spans all hierarchical levels of the system. Control may be mutual, whereby persons in a group have control over each other, or unilateral, whereby one member has control for the entire group (Tannenbaum, 1962, 1968).

Power is extended to a member in an organization depending on his or her position. To exercise control in a group, one must have power and responsibility. Tannenbaum (1962) believes that control is viewed by the individual as inversely related to freedom and power. Thus Tannenbaum's control theory deals with the individual's perceptions of and responses to organizational control. A response to the feeling of lack of control can be an emotional issue.

Tannenbaum (1962) offers insight into a person's emotional adjustment to control. Early in a person's life, through the process of socialization, reactions to authority figures are established and modes of behavior in response to control are developed. Here control takes on emotional meanings.

Personality patterns may also suggest how an individual will adjust to a pattern of organizational control. Most persons react favorably when given the freedom to make decisions. Some do not. Workers who receive low scores on measures of authoritarianism adjust well to participative management, but a small number of workers thought to have submissive personalities prefer to depend on rules and the direction of others in decision making (Tannenbaum & Allport, 1958).

Further dimensions of control, personality, and organizational adjustment are described by Tannenbaum (1962). Persons in control are likely to be more enthusiastic about work, ego involved, loyal, and committed on behalf of the organization. Members' reaction to the company can be identified by their favorable attitudes toward the company and work satisfaction. Also, a reduction in dysfunctional reactions such as chronic absenteeism is evident (Rubenowitz, Norrgren, & Tannenbaum, 1983).

Insight into Tannenbaum's beliefs (1962, 1968) on the total amount of organizational control and organizational effectiveness can be seen throughout his work. Generally, organizations that have high total control at all levels (termed by him *polyarchic* organizations) are "best." Voluntary organizations are more effective if control is concentrated at lower hierarchical levels. Therefore, total amount of organizational control and organizational effectiveness have a high reciprocal relationship (Tannenbaum, 1968).

Oganizational effectiveness is the "extent to which an organization as a social system, given certain resources and means, fulfills its objectives without incapacitating its means and resources and without placing undue strain upon its members" (Georgopoulos & Tannenbaum, 1957, p. 535). Georgopoulos and Tannenbaum (1957) formulated three factors that should be present if the organization is to exhibit effectiveness: (1) organizational productivity, (2) organizational flexibility, and (3) absence of intraorganizational strain or tension.

Organizational productivity. As an organization moves progressively toward its goals, it can be viewed as productive. Performance ratings based on established work standards should be the evaluation of productivity. Workers who perceive a manager to be democratic are more productive than those who believe the boss is an authoritarian (Tannenbaum & Allport, 1958).

Organizational flexibility. The "successful adjustment to internal organizational changes" also involves responding appropriately to such change (p. 180). An example would be changes in operating procedures, policies, and equipment introduced successfully by management.

Absence of intraorganizational strain or tension. If problems are handled effectively among the rank and file, conflict is not present. Morale is high among all subsystems of the organization.

The amount and distribution of control in an organization are consistently stressed in Tannenbaum's control theory (Tannenbaum, 1968). Control may vary in total amount and in distribution. Distribution of control is theoretically independent of control (Tannenbaum, 1962, 1968; Levine, 1973). Because the two dimensions may vary independently, distinguishing them from each other is important (Tannenbaum, 1956, p. 55). Distribution is related to control at different organizational levels. High worker and low management control is associated with democracy. In contrast, high management and low worker control indicates an autocratic system. If no one exercises control, a laissez-faire system exists (Tannenbaum, 1956, 1968; Miner, 1982).

When the total amount of control increases, it does so at the expense of neither the rank nor file. Some do not agree with this, as outlined by Wren (1972). Opponents of this theoretical issue proclaim that equalization of power in a system or a polyarchic organization is done so at the expense of management. However, if a system has high mutual influence and trust, management does not relinquish power and authority to workers but rather includes them in decision making (Tannenbaum, 1962, 1968; Tannenbaum & Cooke, 1974). The increase in total amount of control is related positively to the organizational influence over the environment, competition, conflict, work commitment, militancy, member conformity, and rewards (Tannenbaum, 1962, 1968). A factor such as organizational power contributed to the total amount of control. At the same time, high total control correlates with a strong, effective organization that is actively and successfully pursuing its goals (Tannenbaum, 1968).

Patterns of control in an organization can have predictable effects on worker satisfaction (Tannenbaum & Cooke, 1979). Worker satisfaction can be a positive function of control. The total amount of control that an organization exhibits relates positively to measures and feelings of satisfaction among workers. Workers who do not experience control are less satisfied.

In addition, individuals are more satisfied and consider their work to be exhilarating if they have control over only some aspects of their work as opposed to all work activities. In this situation, individuals experience greater satisfaction in those activities in which control is greater (Tannenbaum, 1962).

In contrast, persons who are not allowed to exercise control in the organization are disinvolved, apathetic, and disenchanted with their work and the system in general. However, being given the opportunity to participate in the system increases satisfaction and morale (Tannenbaum, 1962).

Participation by the organization's rank and file is an important concept of control theory (Tannenbaum, 1966). The traditional control concept is usually viewed as a process by which management assures that an organization's activities conform to plan. Tannenbaum's control theory does not correlate increasing total amounts of control with a well-designed, disciplined management process (Miner, 1982). Control theory assumes that increasing control at a lower hierarchical level through the implementation of participative management also increases control at a higher level. Increasing control at the lower level may be the "best" direction for the organization to proceed (Tannenbaum, 1968). However, mutual respect at all hierarchical levels must be present before the total amount of organization control can increase. Management has to believe that increasing control does not mean relinquishing influence. In addition, subordinates need to be willing and able to assume responsibility for increased freedom and decision making. To provide a group with increased freedom and participation when they are not ready generates anxieties that inhibit organizational effectiveness (Tannenbaum, 1962, 1968). Therefore, managers can increase workers' participation in decision making and still maintain necessary authority and control for the overall operation of the organization (Tannenbaum, 1968).

The theory has been criticized because of its lack of guidelines on how to increase the total amount of organizational control and/or the perception of organizational control at lower hierarchical levels (Miner, 1982). Despite this deficiency, the "introduction of participative management seems sufficient" (p. 81).

Organizations do need to be well controlled for the system to be effective, but they do not have to be controlled through centralization and an authoritarian approach (Miner, 1982).

CASE ANALYSIS

Control theory has implications for the case study presented. One of the strongest beliefs of a profession is that its members should have the right and responsibility to control practice. Consequently, evaluation of professional performance requires decision making and other participation from the membership of the group. All levels of hierarchy of the group need to be represented, especially those who are accountable for the final product. If nursing management goals are to increase personal accountability among staff nurses in an organization, participation by the staff enhances the probability of success.

The hospital began the quality assurance program by soliciting participation from all departments. The nursing department was to have control for implementing a plan in nursing. The plan contained the necessary criteria from which to evaluate the nursing staff's compliance to nursing standards. The director of nursing delegated this project to the assistant director, who could have viewed this assignment as an opportunity to involve the entire nursing group in controlling its practice. Instead, she chose to retain this aspect of practice for herself and the nurse managers. She did not believe that participation by all levels of the nursing hierarchy was necessary. Perhaps the assistant director's intent was good. She wanted the program to succeed. However, in conflict with control theory, she perceived that this would be so only if she retained power and authority. Tannenbaum would have suggested that giving subordinates the power to control does not necessarily take power and control from managers. Managers do not exercise less control where there is participation. The success of participative management is increasing the total amount of control, which is more effective toward achieving an organization's goal. In fact, participative schemes enhance management control.

The purpose of a quality assurance program is to coordinate the organization's efforts to reach organizational effectiveness or high-quality, appropriate patient care. In different organizations, nursing quality assurance programs may be coordinated at different levels or by different individuals or groups. Those that are the most effective have participation from all hierarchical groups (Rowland & Rowland, 1988).

An essential step in evaluating patient care is setting standards. Generally, a *standard* is considered to be an agreed-upon level of acceptable nursing practice that constitutes optimum and achievable patient care (Rowland & Rowland, 1988). According to many, standards should come, in part, by observation of the way nursing is actually practiced. Who can describe that reality better than the staff nurse and thereby contribute to standards of practice?

In this case study, standards were carefully developed but were a product of the assistant director of nursing with some input from the nurse managers. According to control theory, some nurses might prefer this approach. Others who are more mature and secure in their practice may resent this scheme. For those, apathy and dissatisfaction will surely follow.

The quality assurance plan was introduced as a "positive step to enhance nursing practice and patient care." However, the staff nurses' practice activities and patient outcomes were to be monitored and evaluated by managers. Most nurses have been socialized to leading and managing their own practice activities, first as students and then as professionals. To take this process from them is to ask that they relinquish control over practice of an autonomous effort that they have been taught and have expected as the rights and responsibilities of their profession. When nursing management decides to make work-related (i.e., patient care–related) decisions for the nursing staff, such actions are viewed as authoritarian and may be resented. The polyarchic system and all it implies are clearly not present in this case study.

The quality assurance program could have been more successful if staff nurses had been included in decision making and determination of standards at the beginning of the project. By increasing control at the lower hierarchical level of a nursing service, the manager can increase control at the upper levels. Nursing managers, when planning for the goals of the organization, should include the nursing staff in the process. Seeking active participation from the staff nurse for any project increases the likelihood of commitment, satisfaction, and overall morale.

RESEARCH

The literature is replete with studies concerning various aspects of control theory, including the control graph method of measurement.

The control graph approach to measuring organizational control structures has been utilized in numerous studies in Europe and the United States in diverse organizational systems. Industrial plants, voluntary organizations, sales industries, churches, brokerage offices, and higher learning centers have been investigated (Tannenbaum & Cooke, 1979; Markham, Bonjean, & Corder, 1984).

The control graph method uses a survey that questions how much control the respondent perceives individuals at various hierarchical levels exert. An average score is obtained from the 5-point rating scale that reflects control at each organizational level (Miner, 1982).

The control graph approach is found to have several beneficial features. The items are brief and easy to understand; the questionnaire is easily administered, and results lend themselves to an attractive graphic format. Questions are stated broadly so that respondents are enabled to consider all aspects of organizational control and reply in terms of what is most agreeable to them (Markham et al., 1984).

Several authorities believe that the control graph approach may successfully integrate a comprehensive theory and link it with organizational variables (Likert, 1961; Likert & Likert, 1976; Tannenbaum & Cooke, 1979; Markham et al., 1984). Others have addressed its beneficial link between human relations theory and structure (Perrow, 1972).

The control graph is not without criticism. One major area of concern is reliance on a single tool for operationalizing variables (Miner, 1982). Other concerns were summarized by the Markham group (1984, p. 265).

1. The global questions about control structure erroneously assume that control is simple and unidimensional.
2. The questions asked do not correspond to Tannenbaum's formal definition of control.
3. Varying forms of the measures have been used by researchers.
4. The questions elicit original responses, but they scored as interval.
5. There may be problems with reliability and validity.

In addition, Miner in his review of control theory reiterated that the problem with the control graph method is that respondents are "free to interpret in their own way" (1982, p. 68); therefore, what is thought to influence at one level may not do so at another level.

The control graph method has also been criticized by its founder. Tannenbaum and Cooke (1979) in their critique of published and unpublished control graph studies acknowledged that the method may be subjective and perceptual rather than structural. At the same time, they continue to argue that the graph is a description of organizational hierarchical levels, not a description of the respondents. Despite the criticism, the control graph method has been used and continues to be used nationally and internationally.

Tannenbaum and Kahn's (1957) study of four labor unions found that the two more effective, active, and influential unions had more total control exerted by the rank and file. The most powerful of the four unions had relatively influential and active members, but the president, executive board, and bargaining group were by no means inactive or uninfluenceable. In later works, Tannenbaum described this polyarchic relationship as one in which the union members and union leaders "attended more meetings, took part in discussions at meetings, communicated informally about union affairs, and heard and considerd the feelings and ideas of others" (1962, p. 250). In contrast, both members and leaders in the least effective group had relatively little influence on union activities. The interaction-influence bond was not present, and apathy seemed to exist in all concerned. Tannenbaum viewed this as a laissez-faire atmosphere as low control was evident among members as well as officers. In the union where high leader influence and low member influence were present, an autocratic system was described. Tannenbaum identified that distribution of control (as reported by members) played an important role, but that the amount of control was more important.

Likert (1961), in his analysis of a study of 31 separate departments of a large industrial service organization, found that this higher degree of control by the workers was not a threat to managerial personnel. In fact, it was part of the process that led to a more effective organization.

The research of Tannenbaum and associates has identified a consistent relationship between the total amount of control exerted by an organizational structure and measures of organizational effectiveness. The major conclusion from these works has been that the more total control an organization exhibits, the higher the overall satisfaction and performance of its members. Satisfaction and performance are related to achievement of the organization's goals. The exercise of control is indicative as a source of satisfaction and is a basis for the psychological integration of its members into the structure (Tannenbaum, 1956; Tannenbaum, 1968; Tannenbaum & Kahn, 1957; Tannenbaum & Cooke, 1974).

Although conflict has not been included as a specific variable in Tannenbaum's research, the conclusions implied that the higher the total control present in the organization, the lower the amount of conflict. Smith and Ari (1968) in their study of service delivery organizations conclude that a consensus of the amount of control in an organization was present. This concept was operationalized as an absence of conflict.

Tannenbaum's (1968) notion of distribution of control and its relationship to organizational effectiveness is supported in a study of voluntary organizations. In this study, members of local Leagues of Women Voters in "effective leagues" had more control than their counterparts in "ineffective leagues." At the same time, leaders of each group did not exercise less control. This was also found to be true by Vroom (1960) in his experiment in a large clerical organization. Increasing control by encouraging participation in decision making was not accompanied by a corresponding decrease in the control attributed to the management.

Despite these studies, interaction between the two control structure variables, amount and distribution, is not well explicated (Levine, 1973). His study of organizational control among 192 undergraduates enrolled in a psychology course found that "balance" of control had to be present for increased effectiveness of a group insofar as freedom for exchange of ideas was concerned.

Distribution of control has been found to affect several areas of work in organizations. Likert & Likert (1976) concluded that high mutual influence forms the basis for an effective integration of the organization. This is demonstrable in highly integrated, tightly knit systems resulting from mutual influence and interaction, as opposed to unilateral influence. Others have agreed with this power equalization approach (Argyris, 1957; Bennis, 1966) and support the exercise of control at lower organizational levels as a correlate of effectiveness. In addition, Lawrence and Lorsch (1969) identified a high total control of influence and a power equalization at all levels of a system.

One study reported by Tannenbaum (1962) compared a newly automated plant with a less automated one. Workers in the more sophisticated plant exercised more control and experienced greater responsibility than did their counterparts in the less automated plant. The group with increased control reported more decision-making responsibilities, which correlated with greater satisfaction with the overall organizational structure.

Other studies reported hierarchical control as a major independent variable affecting organizational effectiveness. All agreed that total amount of control is positively associated with satisfaction, performance, and motivation (Kavcic & Tannenbaum, 1981; McMahon & Perritt, 1973).

Some international studies on aspects of control conducted by Tannenbaum and associates (Bartolke, Eschweiler, Fleshsenberser, & Tannenbaum, 1982; Rubenowitz, Norrgen, & Tannenbaum, 1983). Two forms of participation, direct and indirect, in ten Swedish companies were investigated. In Sweden, all companies have at least one participative body. These bodies are required either by law, through union contract, or through employee-employer agreement. Results demonstrated that direct participation occurs when the employees themselves have decision-making authority and/or are personally involved in the participative process. Workers with direct participation were involved with their supervisors and issues, concentrating on concern of the employee. Participation by the indirect group was through representatives who generally were concerned with company-wide policies, production plans, or personnel policies. Results concluded that direct participative members perceived their companies to be more participative than members of companies with indirect participation. Also, the companies with systems of direct participation had significantly higher worker commitment, company spirit, satisfaction with company policy, and general job satisfaction. Tannenbaum concluded that members are likely to feel committed and satisfied "first and foremost" (p. 254) to the degree that they perceive personal authority to make decisions.

In contrast, the Bartolke group's (1982) study on worker participation and distribution of control in German companies found that workers who perceived less participation did not perceive less control. The researchers concluded that members of German organizations may be more responsive to indirect participation as they are accustomed to and more accepting of a centralized process.

A computer search for evidence of nursing research pertinent to control theory generated no studies on the topic. This area holds promise for future nursing researchers. Until that time, however, control theory appears to serve well as a framework for nursing managers to use in predicting control, organizational effectiveness, and job satisfaction.

REFERENCES

Argyris, C. (1957). *Personality and organizations.* New York: Harper.

Bartolke, K., Eschweiler, W., Flechsenberger, D., & Tannenbaum, A.S. (1982). Worker participation and the distribution of control as perceived by members of ten German companies. *Administrative Science Quarterly, 27,* 380-397.

Bennis, W.G. (1966). *Changing organizations.* New York: McGraw-Hill.

Dachler, P., & Wilpert, B. (1978). Conceptual dimensions and boundaries of participation organizations: A critical evaluation. *Administrative Science Quaterly, 23,* 1-39.

Fulmer, R.M. (1974). *The new management.* New York: Macmillan.

Georgopoulos, B.S., & Tannenbaum, A.S. (1957). A study of organizational effectiveness. *American Sociological Review, 22,* 534-540.

Kavcic, B., & Tannenbaum, A.S. (1981). A longitudinal study of the distribution of control in Yugoslavian organizations. *Human Relations, 34,* 397-417.

Lawrence, P.R., & Lorsch J.W. (1969). *Organization and environment.* Homewood, IL: Dorsey Press.

Levine, E.L. (1973). Problem of organizational control in microcosm: Group performance and group member satisfaction as a function of differences in control structure. *Journal of Applied Psychology, 58,* 188-195.

Likert, R. (1961). *New patterns of management.* New York: McGraw-Hill.

Likert, R., & Likert, J.G. (1976). *New ways of managing conflict. New York: McGraw-Hill.*

Markham, W.T., Bonjean, C.M., & Corder, J. (1984). Measuring organizational control: The reliability and validity of the control graph approach. *Human Relations, 37,* 263-294.

McMahan, J.T., & Perritt, G.W. (1973). Toward a contingency theory of organizational control. *Academy of Management Journal, 16,* 626-637.

Miner, J.B. (1982). *Theories of organizational structure and process,* Hinsdale, IL: Dryden.

Morse, N.C., Reimer, E., & Tannenbaum, A.S. (1951). Regulation and control in hierarchical organizations. *Journal of Social Issues, 7*(3), 41-48.

Perrow, J.L. (1972). *Handbook of organizational measurement.* Lexington, MA: D.C. Heath.

Rowland, H.S., & Rowland, B.L. (1988). *The manual of nursing quality assurance.* Rockville, MD: Aspen.

Rubenowitz, S. Norrgren, F., & Tannenbaum, A.S. (1983). Some social psychological effects on direct and indirect participation in ten Swedish companies. *Organizational Studies, 4,* 243-259.

Smith, C.G., & Ari, O.N. (1968). Organizational control structure and member consensus. In A.S. Tannenbaum (Ed.), *Control in organizations,* New York: McGraw-Hill.

Tannenbaum, A.S. (1956). The concept of organizational control. *Journal of Social Issues, 12*(2), 50-67.

Tannenbaum, A.S. (1962). Control in organizations: Individual adjustment and organizational performance. *Administrative Science Quarterly, 7,* 236-256.

Tannenbaum, A.S. (1966). *The social psychology of the work organization.* Belmont, CA: Wadsworth.

Tannenbaum, A.S. (1968). *Control in organizations.* New York: McGraw-Hill.

Tannenbaum, A.S., & Allport, F.H. (1958). Personality structure and group structure: An interpretative study of the relationship through an event structured hypothesis. *Journal of Abnormal and Social Psychology, 58,* 172-280.

Tannenbaum, A.S., & Cooke, A.A. (1974). Control and participation. *Journal of Contemporary Business, 3*(4), 35-46.

Tannenbaum, A.S., & Cooke, A.A. (1979). Organizational control: A review of studies employing the control graph method. In C.J. Lammers & D.J. Hickson (Eds.), *Organizations: Alike and unlike.* London: Routledge and Kegan Paul.

Tannenbaum, A.S., & Kahn, A.L. (1957). Organizational control structure: A general descriptive technique as applied to four local unions. *Human Relations, 10,* 127-140.

Tannenbaum, R., & Schmidt, W.H. (1973, May-June). How to choose a leadership pattern. *Harvard Business Review,* p. 167.

Vroom, V.H. (1964). *Work and motivation.* New York: Wiley.

Wren, D.A. (1972). *The evoluation of management.* New York: Ronald Press.

Chapter 20

The Bases of Social Power
John R.P. French, Jr.,
and Bertram Raven

Carol Deets
Tamilyn Jones

‖ CASE STUDY

Justine Bates returned for the new fall semester excited about the fact that she was about to apply for promotion and tenure. She had been working toward this action for 5 years and felt that she was in a strong position to make her application. Before the end of the spring semester, she had met with her department chairperson and the chairperson of the school of nursing's promotion and tenure committee. They both indicated that her position was strong. They had also reviewed what needed to be done and gave her suggestions on completing her application.

Once Justine organized her teaching responsibilities for the fall semester, she turned to the task of applying for promotion and tenure. She found that the forms had remained the same, but many of the criteria and expectations for tenure had been changed. A new tenure position statement had been generated over the summer by the university's administration. This position statement included revised criteria and expectations effective immediately.

Justine thought that she could meet the new criteria, but if they had been changed once, what would keep the administration from doing it again? What about academic due process, which she was always hearing about? What should and could she do? After all, she was just an assistant professor and had no real power in the school, much less the university.

‖ ‖

OVERVIEW OF SOCIAL BASES OF POWER THEORY

French and Raven's early efforts were the investigation of the social influence phenomenon (French, 1956; French & Raven, 1959). Expanding on this research, they became involved with the social bases of power. The different effects found in the social influence studies suggested different types of social bases of power. The social bases of power were considered to be reward, coercive, legitimate, referent, and expert.

French and Raven were also interested in understanding the perceptions of the individual on whom the power was being exerted, not the individual exerting the power. French and Raven indicated that their work was influenced by Lewin's (1936), which is based on the belief that behavior is motivated by needs. To understand French and Raven's theory, a grasp of Lewin's theory is necessary.

Lewin

Lewin was concerned with behavior and how an individual's will to act and react was determined by the internal rather than the external environment. Lewin contended that the components of an individual's internal and external environment (life space) would determine that person's behavior. This conceptualization is in contrast to the more popular stimulus-response explanation for behavior.

Lewin was interested in systematizing the information on behavior that had evolved from research. He employed a specific mathematical discipline called *topology* as well as vector psychology in his attempt to systematize the knowledge. In doing so he created new concepts or redefined others with unique meanings.

Life space. Everything that affects a person's current behavior for a specific situation is represented by the life space. Included are those things that are not in an individual's conscious awareness as well as those that are. Components of the life space may stay the same or change, based on the situation.

Regions. Areas in a life space are called "regions." These regions could represent time, reality, physical space, social groups, and almost anything else, depending on the behavior(s) and situation being considered. Regions that have positive or negative valences are called "goals."

Locomotion. One region connects to another by locomotion, which is usually characterized by movement or change within the life space. Locomotion occurs physically (e.g., walking), socially (e.g., upward mobility), and conceptually (e.g., thinking).

Communication. When one region connects with another as if a bridge spanned the two, communication has taken place. It appears to represent the amount of influence one region has on another. The degree of communication is influenced by the kind of communication, properties of the involved regions, and their boundaries.

Boundary. The separation between regions is called a boundary.

Barriers. When a boundary prevents access to a region, a barrier is said to exist. The degree of resistance caused by the barrier depends on the type of locomotion, direction, and point on the boundary.

Paths. Paths are a connection between any two points that do not intersect.

Force. This concept stems from vector psychology and represents a cause of change. It is characterized by strength, direction, and the point of impact on the boundary. When locomotion toward a goal is stopped by a barrier, the usual result is a "force" toward the goal. The strength of the force varies with the amount of influence the exerter of the influence is perceived to have.

Restructuring. When changes in a field do not involve differentiation or integration, restructuring occurs. The number of parts in the region remains the same, and only the region positions change.

Power field. An area of influence is represented by a power field. It is sometimes referred to as a force field.

French and Raven

French and Raven were concerned with dyadic relationship rather than the influence of power among members of a group. One part of the dyadic relation is the individual who experiences the exerted power and the other part of this relation is the exerter of the power. The exerted power could originate from a role or norm (standard), or from a person, group, or part of a group. French and Raven wanted to identify those factors that influenced an individual's response to the experience of responding to exerted power. They employed many of Lewin's concepts such as life space (sometimes they used the term system), locomotion, force, and force field. Only those concepts that are different are defined here (French, 1956; French & Raven, 1959; French, Morrison, & Levinger, 1960; Raven, 1965).

Power. The potential force generated by a social agent (e.g., role, norm, person, or group) upon an individual to create psychological change is power. The potential ability to exert power rather than the amount actually exerted in a situation is conceptualized as strength. In other words, an individual may perceive the person exerting power as having considerable strength and elect to comply to a small amount of exerted power. Conversely, someone perceived of as having little strength may not be complied with even though that person has exerted considerable power. Consequently, the strength of power is a more accurate indicator than the actual power exerted.

Psychological change. This involves an alteration within the life space over time operationalized as the difference in that variable from time one to time two. Psychological change represents changes in behaviors, opinions, attitudes, goals, needs, values, and other aspects composing an individual's life space. The social aspect appears to be related to the reality that someone outside the life space is exerting influence on it that requires some type of response on the part of the individual.

Resultant force. This concept is composed of two components. First, an individual creates a force field by attempting to change someone else's opinion or attitude. Next, the person on whom the force is being exerted responds with a force field to resist the attempts to change his or her attitude or opinion. In other words, resultant force is the amount of force needed to induce change minus that needed to respond to the exerted force. If the resultant force reflects a greater force by component one, then positive control has been exerted and the intended change occurs. In contrast, when the second component prevails, the intended change is in the opposite direction and is labeled *negative control.*

Dependence-independence. This concept is the degree of involvement the perceiver has with the person who is attempting influence. The greater the perceived involvement, the greater the dependence. If no involvement with the exerter of power exists, the situation is an independent one. Information communicated by someone that is acted on without regard for the person providing the information is an instance of independent influence.

Range. This concept indicates the number of different life spaces (systems) where the exerter of power has sufficient power to be influential.

Bases of power. Finally, the authors distinguish among five social bases of power. The bases refer to the relationship between the influenced and the influencer. Although multiple bases are identified, the sum represents the perceived powerful person's amount of power. The five social bases of power usually cited in the literature are: reward, coercive, legitimate, referent, and expert.

Reward. This type of power occurs with a perception that someone has the ability to provide reward(s). The removal of negative valences from the life space is considered a reward. If actual reward is provided and not just promises, the attraction of the recipient to the rewarder is greater. Use of reward power should result in dependence on the rewarder. If a reward system is continued, reward may produce an independence from the rewarder.

Coercive. Obviously, this type of power occurs when someone is perceived as having the ability to punish. If an individual perceives that withholding a reward is a punishment, then that act functions accordingly. If a situation is perceived as a lost opportunity and not punishment, that situation does not function as a punishment. Use of coercive power produces a dependent situation and decreases the attraction for the provider of the punishment.

Legitimate. This type of power occurs when an individual perceives that someone has a right to prescribe for her or him. The behavior is usually the "should" or "ought" behavior arising from socially prescribed behavior. Some individuals have internalized values (a code or set of standards) that dictate that someone else has the right to tell them what to do, while at the same time they become obligated to do it. The use of legitimate power is restricted to life spaces appropriate to the source of the legitimate power; for example, the source is the job description, and the range is all life spaces related to the job.

Referent. This type of power exists when an individual identifies with someone perceived to have power. There must be a strong identification or a "oneness" with the person perceived to have power. The greater the attraction of the perceiver for the person who has power, the wider the range of life spaces that person could influence.

Expert. This type of power is based on the perception that someone has superior knowledge or skills to the perceiver's. This type of power often fosters a dependent relationship and has a limited range based on the areas of superiority. Provision of new information is not an example of expert power. The credibility of the perceived powerful person must be a factor before expert power can become influential.

The relationships of these concepts should explain why an individual responds to attempts to influence him or her. Because of the underdeveloped nature of the theory, most of the suggested relationships are broad, with no specificity to the type of behavior. For instance, the most agreed-upon relationship is that the greater the individual bases of power, the greater the total power. In addition to indicating that the power bases are additive in nature, this relationship indicates that having several bases of moderate power may be better than having one social basis of considerable power.

Two relationships address the interaction of the concepts: (1) the higher the use of reward power over time, the higher the referent power; (2) the higher the use of coercive power over time, the lower the referent power. Obviously, these are opposite relationships having to do with referent power. Interestingly, no specific references were made to relationships of expert and legitimate power to any of the other concepts.

Only one relationship is specified for the concept of range: attempts to use a power basis outside its range reduce the power inherent in that power basis. Concerning the total of the power bases, the range of life space would need to be considered as well. One or two social bases employed outside their ranges would greatly restrict the perceived total power.

Change in behavior is described in three relationships: (1) the higher the overall power, the more likely is psychological change; (2) the higher the use of reward power, the more likely is a cognitive structure change; and (3) the higher the use of expert power, the more likely is a cognitive structure change. These relationships illustrate two things. First, French and Raven tended to conceptualize behavior in terms of internal behavioral changes (such as attitude changes) as much or more than observable behavioral actions. Second, the idea of a cognitive structure may be a concept in the theory that is not usually included in discussions of the theory.

Other possible relationships have not been mentioned specifically by the authors. Each of the above relationships would differ depending upon the independent or dependent relationship of the two persons. There seems to be a logical relationship between having high legitimate and high referent power and the probability of producing the desired behavior.

CASE ANALYSIS

Justine's situation could be conceptualized by employing Lewin's work. Her life space at work included several regions such as teaching, tenure and promotion, university administration, and school of nursing administration. The region of tenure and promotion had become a goal with a positive valence. A path had developed from the region of the school of nursing administration to the tenure and promotion region employing physical (going to committee chairperson) and conceptual (thinking) locomotion. A barrier had been encountered at the university administration region and had created a force.

Justine decided the best way to proceed would be to analyze her position in terms of her power. French and Raven's work is primarily in terms of dyads; Justine was half of the dyad, whereas the committee or administration with which she needed to interact was the other half. The social bases of power were clearly inherent in the university setting in that faculty had specific rights and responsibilities, perhaps even more so than many other settings.

Electing to use French and Raven's ideas about power, Justine had to conclude that she had no reward or coercive power. She decided she had some referent power in that she had been elected to committees and often served as a spokesperson for her colleagues.

The issue of expert power was more difficult to assess. She had been working in the local chapter of the American Association of University Professors (AAUP) but had not been elected to chair any committees or other leadership positions. When she talked to her colleagues at the school of nursing, however, she found that she had a much better understanding of faculty rights and responsibilities than her colleagues. In fact, several friends had already approached her about the change in the criteria for promotion and tenure. She had been able to explain their rights and the appropriate steps to follow, so she did have some expertise in this area.

What about legitimate power? Did she have any by virtue of her role as a faculty member? She had certain rights as well as responsibilities. One such right was participation in decision making with respect to the criteria for promotion and tenure. The established procedure by which criteria for promotion and tenure were to be determined included the right of review and comment.

Three of the five social bases of power were appropriate for Justine to consider employing in her fight to ensure that her application for promotion and tenure was considered fairly. On which type of power should she rely in pursuing her goal? Probably all three were needed because she did not have an abundance in any one type.

How could Justine make use of her power? Because Justine had legitimate power by virtue of her faculty status, that seemed to be the place to start. She reviewed all the faculty council minutes for the last year to determine whether the change in criteria had been discussed. If action had been taken by this group, she would have to admit that their deliberation represented faculty consideration because they had been elected for that role. Her review of the minutes indicated that the criteria for tenure and promotion were never discussed. Because of her involvement with AAUP and her limited expert power as a result of it, she knew that a grievance procedure could be employed to question the appropriateness of the new criteria. She also knew that such a process was time-consuming and tedious.

Several faculty who had planned to apply for tenure and promotion approached Justine. They felt they could not meet the new criteria and that changing them over the summer vacation had not been fair. They wanted to know what they should do and what she was going to do.

They were looking to her for advice and leadership. In other words, Justine had additional evidence of her referent power.

When her three bases of power were considered in total, Justine found that she did indeed have some power. She decided to request a called meeting of the school of nursing's faculty organization to seek the total faculty's support in protesting the creation of the criteria without appropriate faculty input. By virtue of her legitimate power, she was able to seek redress through the faculty organization. Because she had some expert power, she could tell the others what the problem was, explain how it would affect all faculty because this change reduced faculty power if left unchallenged, and suggest reasonable solutions. Because of her referent power, she knew she could influence others to rally support for the cause. By starting with the nursing faculty, she was expanding the social basis of her referent power if they agreed as a group to resist the administration's change in the promotion and tenure position statement. All in all, she had considerable power compared to what she thought she had when she first started to analyze her situation.

RESEARCH

Extensive summaries and critiques of the multiple studies found in the literature focusing on French and Raven's work have been completed by many authors over the years. Podsakoff and Schriesheim (1985) and Bass (1981), two of the more recent ones, are reported rather than the extensive individual studies for the convenience of the reader. Areas of research utilizing French and Raven's power bases are presented in a format organized around major themes rather than the specific social bases.

Podsakoff and Schriesheim (1985) summarized field studies because they utilized explicit and complete operationalizations of French and Raven's power bases. Bass (1981) based his literature review on experimental studies measuring the effects of French and Raven's power bases on influence and leadership. Because Podsakoff and Schriesheim (1985) reviewed field studies and Bass (1981) investigated experimental studies, the two literature reviews have no overlap.

Performance

Studies summarized by Podsakoff and Schriesheim (1985) indicate that reward, coercive, and legitimate power tend to affect performance negatively or not at all. However, expert and referent power tend to produce either positive results or to be unrelated to performance.

Bass (1981) found in his review of literature that, unlike the finding that Podsakoff and Schriesheim (1985) described, reward power had a positive effect on performance. Bass (1981) agreed with Podsakoff and Schriesheim (1985) that coercion had a negative effect or was unrelated to performance.

Satisfaction

Podsakoff and Schriesheim (1985) reported six studies that concluded that coercive power was negatively related or unrelated to satisfaction with supervision and that expert and referent power produced positive effects. Reward and legitimate power results were conflicting and may be distorted; therefore, conclusions were not made about their relationship to satisfaction with supervision. Nonsupervisory satisfaction effects of the five power bases were measured in eight studies indicating that, for the most part, reward and legitimate power were not significantly related. For coercive power, most correlations were nonsignificant; however, two of the eight studies found negative results. Referent power produced mostly nonsignificant correlations as well; however, some positive effects were found in four studies. Expert power results in the eight studies were evenly divided between nonsignificant and positive correlations (Podsakoff and Schriesheim, 1985).

Bass's findings (1981) were similar to those of Podsakoff and Schriesheim (1985) in that expert power tended to have positive effects on satisfaction, and coercion tended to have negative effects. Based on these studies, Bass (1981) contended that referent power often leads to ingratiation, which is defined as "a striving by followers to be valued and rewarded by those they esteem or see as more powerful in other ways as well" (p. 180). If ingratiation is considered to be part of satisfaction, then referent power may also have a positive effect on satisfaction.

Withdrawal

Two studies on withdrawal behavior found that expert and referent power were negatively related to absences, but the other power bases were unrelated. The findings of three studies summarized by Podsakoff and Schriesheim (1985) indicated that reward, coercive, and legitimate power were unrelated to intent to leave an organization, whereas referent and expert power were somewhat negatively related. However, Bass (1981) cited one study that positively related coercion to withdrawal behavior in general.

Influence and Conformity

The findings of two studies summarized by Podsakoff and Schriesheim (1985) were that reward, legitimate, expert, and referent power had positive correlations with influence and that coercive power was unrelated. All of the power bases were positively related to conformity.

Bass (1981) found one study that related expert power to successful leadership if the leader had both perceived and actual expertise. Two more studies concluded that groups often accept an expert's opinion over that of group consensus (Bass, 1981). These studies may indicate that expert power may be positively related to influence. Bass (1981) reviewed one study in which groups with leaders exhibiting referent power tended to be more effective. This result may reflect a positive effect of referent power on conformity. Bass (1981) also cited two studies exploring the effects of reward power on groups. Leadership ability, actual influence, and leader competence were some of the factors favorably affected by reward power. Interdependence effects were also influenced in that rewards motivated members of a group to work harder, even though the reward may have gone to only one member, as indicated by three studies in Bass (1981). Coercive power exerted along with legitimate power tends to have a cumulative effect on increasing conformity, indicating that status is also a significant factor for compliance (Bass, 1981). Two more studies reviewed by Bass (1981) found that threat of punishment tended to induce conformity, although resistance to coercive power tended to be stronger when individuals had the opportunity to observe their peers resist. Influence and conformity may also be affected by legitimate power in that legitimate leaders who were elected by their own members tended to get more accomplished. This finding was inherent in three different studies reviewed by Bass (1981). In summary, the Bass review (1981) provided implications that expert, referent, reward, and legitimate power may positively affect influence and conformity as proposed by Podsakoff and Schriesheim (1985).

Task Clarity

With regard to task-related clarity, Podsakoff and Schriesheim (1985) summarized two studies finding that expert and referent power were associated with task clarity in subordinates, but reward and coercive power tended to be negatively related or unrelated. Legitimate power results were unclear. Bass (1981) did not report any studies addressing this outcome.

Job Tension

One study found that coercive power was directly related to tension and expert power was indirectly related. The other power bases were not significant (Podsakoff and Schriesheim, 1985). No studies in this area were reported by Bass (1981).

Compliance

An investigation of ten studies using a rank-order scale revealed that expert and legitimate power were the strongest reasons for compliance with a supervisor's requests, followed by referent, reward, and coercive power, respectively (Podsakoff and Schriesheim, 1985). This variable was not considered in Bass's review (1981).

Summary

Podsakoff and Schriesheim (1985) summarized the effect of the five power bases on functional subordinate criterion variables (e.g., subordinate performance, satisfaction with supervision, job satisfaction) based upon their analysis of all of the studies. They generally found that expert and referent power were positively related or unrelated to the criterion variables, and reward, coercive, and legitimate power were negatively related or not significant. They contended that making any firm conclusions was a highly questionable activity because of several methodological problems and inconsistencies found in the studies. Bass (1981) reported that expert and referent power, often regarded as personal power, tended to be perceived as being more favorable than the use of reward, coercive, or legitimate power, which was usually exerted as result of position.

Nursing

The remainder of this section is a summary of studies in nursing that were based on French and Raven's work. Much of the literature in nursing that employs French and Raven's work is difficult to identify because it is in the form of unpublished theses. The following is limited to those that were known to us.

Although the following two studies did not test French and Raven's theory directly, their findings in nursing are closely related to the social bases of power. Bennis, Berkowitz, Affinito, and Malone (1958) studied 90 nurses in outpatient departments directly affiliated with hospitals. They found that reward behavior had positive effects on supervisory influence over nurses. Another study conducted by Rosenberg and Pearlin (1962) sampled 1315 nurses employed by a mental hospital. They investigated the power orientations used by nurses on mental inpatients. The results indicated that the orientations used more frequently were persuasion, manipulation, legitimate authority, coercion, and contractual power, respectively. In terms of perceived effectiveness, the orientations of manipulation and persuasion were most effective, followed by contractual power. Legitimate authority and coercion were equally least effective. Nurses in this study indicated that they would like to use persuasion, manipulation, and legitimate authority over contractual power or coercion, despite their perceived effectiveness.

Feistritzter (1980) assessed the power perceptions of directors of nursing. She employed a modification of Dieterly's tool, and her scales demonstrated Cronbach's alphas of .33 to .78. There were no significant differences among director of nurses' perceptions of power on a series of demographic variables except for one. Significantly higher expert power was perceived by those with more previous experience in administration.

Weaver (1981) studied the five types of power to see if a relationship existed among them and Fiedler's situational favorableness variable. Her scale alpha coefficients ranged from .48 to .67. The types of power correlated with favorableness with coefficients ranging from .14 to .24, and four of the five coefficients were significant. The nurse respondents consisting of a sample of head nurses reacted strongly to the implication that they might employ coercion as a power attempt to the extent of writing comments on the tool.

Graham (1982) studied the types of power for a relationship of staff and head nurses' behavior. Her scale alphas ranged from .61 to .75. She was concerned with the relation between perceived power and willingness to stay in a less than optimal job situation. She found that perceptions of legitimate and coercive power were significantly related to tenure in current position. Respondents in the study also indicated that they never employed coercion and wrote specific comments on the tool to that effect.

Arndt (1981) was concerned with school of nursing administrators. She did not assess the reliability of her data. A major concern was if the role descriptors for deans in schools of nursing influenced their perceptions of power. She found no significant differences in perception of power for deans in medical centers and those on other types of campuses. Deans and chairpersons who reported directly to the chief academic officer had significantly higher mean scores for power than those who did not report directly. Lastly, the greater the amount of experience, the higher the perception of power. Instead of legitimate power being the primary power basis, referent power was consistently the primary source of power.

George and Deets (1986) modified the Dieterly and Arndt work to create a scale specific to top nurse executives in hospitals. They conducted a content and construct validity study. In the content validity study, they found obtaining consensus difficult on items, especially for the coercive and reward items when reversed and the expert and legitimate items. In the construct study (Deets & George, 1987), expert and legitimate items factored into one factor. Their scales demonstrated Cronbach alphas of .76 for referent, .76 for legitimate, .76 for expert, and .78 for reward. When the expert and legitimate items were combined as indicated in the factor analysis, the alpha was .83.

Miller and Deets (1989) employed the George and Deets tool to measure the power of 52 faculty members in a school of nursing. They were interested in testing for construct validity of the tool in another setting and in determining if combining legitimate and expert power would recur as in the Deets and George study (1987). They hypothesized that faculty who were dissatisfied and willing to take action to resolve the problem perceived themselves to have legitimate, expert, reward, and referent power. The possibility that rank and tenure status influenced faculty perceptions of power was also considered. Only the scales that measured legitimate, referent, and expert power demonstrated construct validity via factor analysis. Reliability employing Cronbach's alpha ranged from .77 for referent to .81 for legitimate and .83 for expert, which were the highest reliabilities reported to date. Willingness to take action was unrelated to the social bases of power. No significant differences occurred because of faculty rank, but tenure status resulted in significant differences for referent power.

Although the first two nursing studies did not attend to measurement issues much like research in other areas, the remaining studies did. Even though the evidence for validity and reliability improved slightly, there was no support for the hypothesis based on the theory. The fact that all of these studies were conducted on nurses who regard themselves as professionals may explain why results were not replicated from earlier studies that were done mostly on different populations such as factory workers.

EVALUATION OF THEORY

Lewin's concern for theory development was reflected in his use of mathematical symbols to designate his variables and the relationships among them. French and Raven were as interested in theory development and employed similar techniques. Unfortunately, the use of these symbols may have resulted in confusion for many readers because of unfamiliarity with the mathematical conventions. In addition, the use of mathematical symbols does not ensure that a theory was developed.

Although the bases of power are defined separately, in reality they are often intertwined. For example, one exercising reward and coercive power may acquire legitimate power through internalization. In organizations, increasing legitimate power in one or several levels tends to result in more control. The effectiveness of expert power must be interpreted with caution because studies may be interpreted incorrectly. This problem was compounded by the fact that usually only two or three of the social bases of power, rather than all five, are assessed in any one study. For instance, Raven and French (1958a) studied the role of social influence as it impacted legitimate and coercive power. Raven and French (1958b) also addressed the role of group support on legitimate power. None of the data from these studies supported their hypothesis that coercive power would reduce perceptions of legitimate power. When only some of the social bases are assessed, the total power is not determined nor the relationships among the social bases of power.

Degree of dependence upon the individual exerting power is a variable that is seldom addressed in current literature. The amount of dependence changes with reference to the perceptions of the person attempting to influence and the life space of the person being influenced. French and Raven focused upon the dependence of the individual on the person with power and attempted to operationalize this concept by observing what happened once the influence was withdrawn from the life space. If the behavior returned to pre-influence levels, then it was dependent; however, if the behavior continued, it was independent.

Instead of addressing the relationships within the theory, most researchers have employed the theory as a way of thinking about power. Most design a study with its component concerning power to test some other theory or model or to answer a question that is usually situation specific and not theoretical. Use of the theory in this manner does not add to the body of knowledge about it. Less sophisticated consumers of the literature see these articles and assume that the reported study findings add support for the theory. Soon the perception is that the theory has been tested and holds true, but in actuality the only part of the theory that has been used is the idea of the five social bases of power.

Although French and Raven consistently discussed change in terms of attitudes and opinions, most of the studies that have tested or used the theory have done so with explicit behavioral outcomes. The direct connection between attitude and behavior is tentative at best. No matter what the intention (which is based on the opinion or attitudes), the real world intervenes, and the behavior may or may not be attempted. Assessing the social bases of power as they relate to behavior may be questionable in terms of the original theory, which addressed psychological change, not behavioral change.

Poor measurement has plagued this work from the beginning. Almost 20 years elapsed before attempts at consistent measurement were made. Dieterly (1975) developed scales to measure each of the social bases of power and tested them for reliability and validity. Many of the later nursing studies built on his work and revised and improved the scales. Podsakoff and Schriesheim (1985) stressed the problem of measurement and emphasized the importance of employing the right type of scale (Likert rather than a rank-order technique).

Another factor became clear in the nursing studies. To measure the subjects' perceptions of power effectively, the items in the tool needed to measure the perceptions in a specific life space situation. Slight rewording of items would be needed for each study to ensure that the specific life space situation was adequately measured.

In summary, evaluating the research support for this theory is difficult because most of the studies employed inconsistent and inappropriate measurement. Results from flawed measurement are by definition flawed. The other reason that the support is difficult to evaluate is that very little real support is evident. Most researchers employ the five bases of power because they need to assess power for their study, not because they are testing the theory.

Conceptually, the theory has much to offer. Specific relationships could be tested; however, researchers would have to address the fact that French and Raven were interested in psychological change rather than behavioral change. The later work in nursing appears to support fewer power bases than suggested. French and Raven tended to name both ends of continuums, such as independence and dependence. This continuum phenomenon seems to exist for reward and coercive power as well. Apparently the continuum of reward has a positive end (reward) and a negative end (coercive). Efforts such as these to clarify the theoretical concepts should lead to a better evaluation of the theory.

CONCLUSION

Although the perception is that many studies have been conducted that support French and Raven's work, in truth there are few. Most of these have major problems with measurement, and few have attempted to employ the same measurement approach, which would allow comparability. The major criticism Podsakoff and Schriesheim (1985) had was that even when measured with an instrument, incorrect measurement techniques were employed. They reanalyzed several studies and found that expert and referent power were positively related or unrelated to certain outcomes (e.g., performance or satisfaction). Reward, coercive, and legitimate power, conversely, were negatively related or unrelated to the same outcomes. Although these findings may have lent some support for the theory, Podsakoff and Schriesheim (1985) caution against making any firm conclusions because of inconsistent and problematic measurement.

The most common finding is that a relationship exists among the five types of power. In fact, reward and coercive power may be at opposite ends of a reward continuum. Because this interrelationship of the powers was a basic assumption of the theory, that finding is not surprising.

Continued use of the theory without further testing is ill advised. Perpetuating the belief that the theory has been tested decreases the possibility of studies being developed to test it. Emphases in the future should be on assessing psychological changes and the types of power or total power needed to create them.

REFERENCES

Arndt, M.J. (1981). *Sources of social power for administrators of baccalaureate and higher degree programs in nursing.* Unpublished doctoral dissertation, Ball State University, Muncie, IN.

Bass, B. (1981). *Stogdill's handbook of leadership: A survey of theory and research.* New York: Macmillan.

Bennis, W.G., Berkowitz, N., Affinito, M., & Malone, M. (1985). Authority, power, and the ability to influence. *Human Relations, 11,* 143-155.

Deets, C., & George, S. (1987). Power—Can it be measured? Paper presented at Midwest Research Society, St. Louis.

Dieterly, D. (1975). *Research on power in organizations: A measurement technique and pilot study.* Detroit, MI: University Microfilms International.

Feistritzer, K. (1980). *The perception of power by directors of nursing.* Unpublished master's thesis, Indiana University, Indianapolis.

French, J.R.P. (1956). A formal theory of social power. *Psychological Review, 63,* 181-193.

French, J.R.P., Morrison, H.W., & Levinger, G. (1960). Coercive power and forces affecting conformity. *Journal of Abnormal & Social Psychology, 61,* 93-101.

French, J.R.P., & Raven, B. (1959). The bases of social power. In D. Cartwright (Ed.), *Studies in social power.* Ann Arbor, MI: Institute for Social Research.

George, S., & Deets, C. (1986). Personal communication.

Graham, J.V. (1982). *Exit and voice: The prediction behavior by nurses engaged in hospital practice.* Unpublished dissertation, Indiana University, Indianapolis.

Lewin, K. (1936). *Principles of topological psychology.* New York: McGraw-Hill.

Miller, C.L., & Deets, C. (1989). *Faculty perceptions of power: A construct validity study.* Unpublished manuscript, Indiana University School of Nursing, Indianapolis.

Podsakoff, P.M., & Schriesheim, C.A. (1985). Field studies of French and Raven's bases of power: Critique, reanalysis, and suggestions for future research. *Psychological Bulletin, 97,* 387-411.

Raven, B. (1965). Power and leadership. In I.D. Steiner & M. Fishbein (Eds.), *Current studies in social psychology.* New York: Holt, Rinehart, & Winston.

Raven, B., & French, J.R.P. (1958a). Legitimate power, coercive power, and observability in social influence. *Sociometry, 21,* 83-97.

Raven, B., & French, J.R.P. (1958b). Group support, legitimate power and social influence. *Journal of Personality, 26,* 400-409.

Rosenberg, M., & Pearlin, L.I. (1962). Power-orientation in the mental hospital. *Human Relations, 15,* 335-350.

Weaver, D.J. (1981). *The relationship of situational favorableness and the bases of social power in first-level nurse managers.* Unpublished dissertation, Indiana University, Indianapolis.

Chapter 21

Structural Theory: Women in Management Roasabeth Moss Kanter

Genevieve E. Chandler

❙❙ CASE STUDY

Ms. Russo was the only female vice president at Forest Hospital. She was the new VP for nursing who was regarded highly by those in the nursing department. Ms. Russo had come up through the ranks at Forest and was the nurses' first choice for their new leader. The day Ms. Russo stepped into the VP position was a victory for nursing. The nurses felt administration had finally listened to them.

A year into the job things were quite different at Forest Hospital. Now, when the nurses were being kind they referred to Ms. Russo as the little dictator. When they were not so kind, they used more colorful terms to describe the VP's behavior. While a group of nurse managers were waiting for their weekly meeting with Ms. Russo to begin, the following conversation could be overheard:

JENKINS: She was such a great supervisor. Now that she's making good money and is one of the boys, she has sold out.

DOWNEY: Yeah, that's for sure. She had me fooled. I thought she really understood us. Now she's one of them.

ALTO: What happened? When she was with us, she'd hang around and have coffee, and she understood how we felt. I mean, we grew up in this system together. That's why I wanted her as my boss. She was the one to stand up for us against administration! Now we just see her in these stupid meetings. This is really a waste of my time.

JENKINS: It's like she's a different person now. You give a person a little power and it goes to their heads. Shh! Here she comes. Shut up and salute.

Ms. Russo had just finished her lunch in her office, which was located on the third floor behind her secretary in back of the waiting room. She thought, "They are right, my office is like an inner sanctum and I am glad to be in it." It was a relief not to run into her administrative cohorts at lunchtime, which was actually easy to do because their offices were on the first floor right off the lobby. Getting away from the 350 nurses she was accountable for was also nice. She hated going to the cafeteria and being deluged with complaints. She wondered why she had worked so hard to get this thankless position.

For Ms. Russo proving the worth of nursing was a constant battle, and she felt like she was fighting it alone. What happened to all her old friends? They were so tight before her promotion and now they sat mute in the management meetings. She used to think she had a great relationship with the physicians, too. Now it was a different story in the administrative meetings. A typical interaction began with Ms. Russo saying, "It is nursing care that patients come to the hospital for." The VP for medicine gave her that patronizing smile and reminded her, "It's the doctors who admit the patients and bring in the money." "Speaking of money," the VP for finance chirped in, "can't you cut back on the outpatient staff? St. Anne's sees the same number of patients with fewer nurses." The VP for special services nodded in agreement and waited for the CEO to speak so he could agree with him because they were buddies from way back. As far as Ms. Russo could see, the only role of the special services VP was to support the big guy.

As Ms. Russo approached the nurse management meeting, she thought, "I hope this meeting ends early. I'll just announce the new discharge plan and the proposed budget cuts and wrap it up. I can't stand being up there, watching the scowls on their faces when we used to be such good friends."

| | | | | | | | | | | | | | | | | | | | | | | | | | | | | | | | | | | | | | | | | | | | | | | | | | | | | | | | | | | | | | | | | | | | | | | | | | |

STRUCTURAL THEORY: ORGANIZATIONAL BEHAVIOR

Kanter's structural theory purports that the structure of the work environment has a significant effect on work behavior. The results of Kanter's research indicated that an individual's work effectiveness is in part a function of the characteristics of her or his position. Positions that afford access to opportunity and power engender effective work behaviors. Kanter defined opportunity as the provision of advancement possibilities as well as the extent to which the job allows the employee to increase competence and skills while being recognized and rewarded for them. Kanter operationalized power as the employee's perception of having access to support, information, resources, and the ability to mobilize them to meet organizational goals.

Opportunity and power were both theorized to be connected with positions. Certain positions within the organization provide access to an opportunity structure, and others do not. People in high-opportunity positions are more motivated to perform, which in turn demonstrates their ability to use their knowledge and skills productively. When individuals perceive they have a chance to grow and develop while contributing to organizational goals, they in turn invest in the organization. Employee investment is manifested behaviorally by commitment, high career aspirations, achievement orientation, risk taking, and high self-esteem. Employees in positions with little chance to gain new knowledge, advancement, or challenge tend to withdraw in response to the organization's lack of investment in them. In response to low opportunity, people tend to limit their career aspirations, are less committed, lack initiative, and devalue their skills.

To maintain some sense of self-esteem in response to not having the opportunity to achieve organizational success, the low-opportunity group redefine the criteria for success and rewards. They redefine success in terms that are more oriented toward achieving success within their peer group. In fact, the alternative criteria for success could run contrary to organizational goals. For example, peer group success might focus on the social aspects of work, such as taking frequent breaks together, getting out on time, or working just enough to maintain a basic level of productivity. Because no intrinsic rewards are perceived as coming from the organization, the peer group designs its own extrinsic reward system to look successful to friends outside work. For example, in our consumer-oriented society, being able to increase purchasing power is rewarding, and buying a new washing machine, barbecue grill, or carpet can be an indicator of success.

In summary, individuals in positions that afford access to opportunity are more productive and in turn invest in the organization. Those who have little access to opportunity are less effective and tend to avoid investing themselves in the organization.

Kanter described positions of power as positions that afforded access to support, information, and resources to enable the individual to accomplish more and pass on resources and information to subordinates. Managers with power tend to delegate and reward talent by supporting subordinates in their growth and development. Those who are thought to be powerful have an easier time obtaining resources and cooperation. They have an easier time forming a team because people like to be associated with people in power. The powerful tend to empower those around them.

In contrast, those who experience powerlessness tend to have a more difficult time getting things done. The powerless tend to do things themselves rather than delegate. They do not have the informal networks they need to cut through red tape to get the job done. Lack of information causes them to hang onto what little information they have. Lacking the critical connections that lead to support leaves the powerless isolated and unable to effect change. This ineffectiveness results in a coercive approach with staff that is manifested as authoritarian, rigid, rules-oriented behavior. Staff then perceives the powerless manager as critical and controlling.

In summary, the powerful who have connections, support, and information networks encourage staff to grow and develop their talents, but the powerless, who have limited influence and restricted information, are threatened by staff development. They become territorial and domain oriented. The area where they have a little influence becomes theirs and only theirs with any infringements being interpreted as a threat. The result is a constrained, rigid, detail-oriented management style that engenders powerlessness in subordinates that mirrors the powerlessness the manager experiences.

The structural theory of organizational behavior is particularly relevant for women. Although women have made some progress as a group, the majority still hold relatively powerless, low-status jobs that offer few opportunities to exert influence on the organization. The structuralist advocates suggest that the individual is not solely at fault if he or she lacks power but rather that segregation in the work force has restricted women's access to powerful positions and that they have had little opportunity for advancement. Although Kanter found that both women and men who are "stuck" in their positions exhibited ineffective work behaviors, women are more likely than men to be in these positions. In fact, Kanter (1979) cited that women managers experience special power failures. For example, they are not part of the old boys' network, they are put in "safe" jobs that do not go anywhere and have little visibility, and women have been viewed as recipients of sponsorship rather than as sponsors themselves.

Women frequently find themselves in supervisory positions managing "stuck" subordinates. Because of the lack of internal support managing a team that is stuck decreases the opportunities to take the kinds of risks that build credibility. It means managing a group that has developed its own criteria for success that are not congruent with the organizational goals. This type of position is incapacitating for women managers.

CASE ANALYSIS

The case at Forest Hospital could readily be interpreted as evidence of the queen bee syndrome in nursing. The Queen Bee Syndrome is used to describe a woman who has made it in a man's world but continues to hold traditional female values. She looks down at her subordinates and thinks, "I came up the hard way; they can, too." Carrying this attitude, she does not offer subordinates any help to grow in their work roles. She typically identifies with those outside nursing. The queen bee syndrome could be said to fit Ms. Russo, but that would be an individual interpretation of her behavior; that is, Ms. Russo has the problem and she must be changed. When the Forest Hospital case is interpreted through a structural perspective, quite a different picture emerges.

Prior to Ms. Russo's VP position, she was on her way up through the ranks. With opportunity to progress along Forest Hospital's career ladder, she felt she had nothing to lose and everything to gain. Her confident attitude was exhibited in her proactive, assertive nursing behaviors that she was not afraid to use with any doctor or administrator. She was known as a rabble-rouser but one who knew what she was talking about. When the VP position opened up, the higher-ups were a little hesitant about recommending Ms. Russo, but the support from the nurses was so strong they gave in and offered her the position. Now they were going to sit back and wait to see what happened.

Once Ms. Russo took the position, she realized she could not go any further in the organization. Nurses did not become the CEO or members of the board. She did not plan on relocating to another city, so this was it. The lack of mobility discouraged Ms. Russo. She became more conservative, hesitant to make changes, and inclined to adopt a cautious, "don't rock the boat" attitude. She felt she had so much responsibility overseeing the nursing department that any change in the status quo was a threat.

In her new position, Ms. Russo went from being at the hub of the grapevine to isolation. With her promotion she left her previous nursing connections and was now faced with the old boys' network, where she was clearly an outsider. Most decisions seemed to her to be made in the racquetball locker room, on the golf course, or during their weekend socializing, none of which involved her. The prevailing attitude of "let's see how she handles this" was not exactly an invitation to join the network. Ms. Russo lacked the critical informal connections needed for empowerment. Even the location of her office isolated her from the other VPs and her own staff.

Ms. Russo responded to her isolation by doing everything herself and not delegating, which only made her appear more controlling. She was trying hard to get in with her new peers, which looked to her subordinates like she was selling out so they backed further away. They thought she was very ungiving and much too rules minded. In fact, the written rules were all she had to go by because no one was sharing any informal information. When she couldn't get into the administrative circle, she responded by being protective of the nursing domain, the only area over which she had some control. This behavior made her appear territorial to her colleagues.

Ms. Russo was left on her own. She could be called a queen bee or her behavior could be interpreted as responding to a position of powerlessness where she was cut off from the critical connections that allow for opportunities to get information, support, and resources, that is, the connections that afford one the opportunity to be a manager "in the know." Ms. Russo was stuck in what Kanter calls a downward cycle of powerlessness and responded with a reluctance to make changes, lack of initiative, lack of risk taking, low motivation, and eventually a lack of self-confidence and self-esteem. From a structural perspective, Ms. Russo's behaviors were not internally motivated, but were a response to lack of access to opportunity and power in the work environment. To alter the downward powerlessness cycle, one would need to change the structure of power and opportunity to change the individual's behavioral response.

RESEARCH

The proponents of the structuralist perspective have utilized the theory in organizational research. Kanter's study is recognized as a seminal piece in organizational research and cited in numerous articles across disciplines, particularly those related to gender and the workplace.

Several investigators note the critical importance of the variables Kanter identified: opportunity, information, support, and resources. Feldman's (1976) studies revealed that employees who are succeeding in their jobs are more likely to be given opportunity to learn new tasks and skills. Success breeds success, and employees need to be in the right position to be able to demonstrate their achievements. Stewart and Gudykunst (1982) found that without jobs that provided opportunities to be visible and influential women were unable to gain access to sources of structural power, and they remained in a cycle of powerlessness. Smith and Grenier (1982) suggested that women have not been able to gain access to centralized critical positions that allow control over resources such as information. Fraker (1984) described the "glass ceiling" that women hit when they attempt to move from middle to upper management. The glass ceiling is a description for the invisible but real barriers women run into when aspiring to reach the top.

Information and feedback are essential empowerment tools. Hackman and Oldman (1980) noted from their study that individuals who had more information about the results of their work are more likely to be internally motivated to perform. Feldman (1976) observed from his study that consistency of feedback makes the need for training and improvement clearer. Without information and feedback, motivation and career aspirations would be depressed.

Being part of a network is an important power strategy. Lincoln and Miller (1979) suggested from their research that friendship networks are not merely a group of friends but rather a system for making decisions, mobilizing resources, and concealing or transmitting information. Lincoln and Miller recognized the need to decrease uncertainty by increasing predictability, which translates into a tendency to keep management groups homogeneous, which in most cases means white, middle class, and male. From Kotter's (1977, 1978) work with power, he recognized the importance of establishing and nurturing informal connections as well as demonstrating visible achievement. One of the critical variables Kotter identified was dependence. A manager can be dependent on superiors, subordinates, and peers as well as on customers, suppliers, and unions. Many of these parties' management does not have direct control over, so they must establish informal connections to assure information, resources, and support. Thompson (1981) and Pfeffer (1981) note how informal alliances help to build coalitions to gain support.

In a recent study of powerlessness utilizing Kanter's theoretical framework, Mainiero (1986) found that women caught in job situations with little opportunity to change were more likely to acquiesce in dependency situations. Too much dependency caused panic, frustration, and a sense of helplessness. In addition it was learned that as women moved into positions with more power their likelihood of acquiescing decreased. Mainiero's work provided support for Kanter's theory that powerless jobs may cause individuals to behave in powerless ways.

The nursing literature, as Farley (1987) observed, is replete with articles related to power but woefully lacking in empirical data. Farley, in a study of power orientations, identified as a significant finding the fact that nursing administrators were unaware of the value of possessing and controlling resources, in particular, information. In the Gorman and Clark (1986) study, Kanter's theoretical framework was utilized to develop a quasi-experimental research project. Through structural intervention, the investigators developed strategies for better utilization of professional knowledge and skills by empowering nurses to do what is needed in patient care settings. Utilizing a structuralist theory, Chandler (1987) tested Kanter's instrument on organizational effectiveness with nurses. The results of the study indicated support for the constructs of opportunity, information, and support. On the scales the nurses distinguished between two types of opportunity—personal and political—and two kinds of support—appraisal and instrumental. Further work on instrument design needs to be done.

Structuralist theory attends to two of the critical variables in the nursing work environment: women and power. With nurse leaders calling for changes in the traditional health care work structure and practicing nurses demanding alterations in the work environment to facilitate empowerment, the time is ripe for moving from an individual focus to utilize a structuralist perspective in nursing practice and research. The structure of power and opportunity affects nurses at all levels and needs to be seriously considered to facilitate nursing empowerment.

REFERENCES

Chandler, G. (1987). The relationship of work environment to empowerment and powerlessness. Unpublished dissertation.

Farley, M.J. (1987). Power orientations and communication style of managers and nonmanagers. *Research in Nursing and Health, 10*(3), 197-202.

Feldman, D.C. (1976). A contingency theory of socialization. *Administrative Science Quarterly, 21* 433-452.

Fraker, S. (1984, April). Why women aren't getting to the top. *Fortune,* 40-45.

Gorman, S.J., & Clark, N. (1986). Power and effective nursing practice. *Nursing Outlook,* 129-134.

Hackman, J.R., & Oldman, G.R. (1980). *Work redesign.* Reading, MA: Addison-Wesley.

Kanter, R.M. (1977). *Men and women of the corporation.* New York: Basic Books.

Kanter, R.M. (1979, July-August). Power failure in management circuits. *Harvard Business Review.*

Kotter, J. (1977, July-August). Power, dependence and effective management. *Harvard Business Review,* 125-136.

Kotter, J. (1978, Winter). Power, success and organization effectiveness. *Organizational Dynamics,* 27-40.

Lincoln, J., & Miller, J. (1979). Work and friendship ties in organizations: A comparative analysis of relational networks. *Administrative Science Quarterly, 24,* 181-199.

Mainiero, L. (1986). Coping with powerlessness: The relationship of gender and job dependency to empowerment-strategy usage. *Administrative Science Quarterly, 31,*633-653.

Pfeffer, J. (1981). *Power in organization.* Mershfield, MA: Pitman.

Smith, E., & Grenier, M. (1982). Sources of organizational power for women: Overcoming structural obstacles. *Sex Roles, 8,* 733-746.

Stewart, L., & Gudykunst, W. (1982). Differential factors influencing the hierarchical level and number of promotions of males and females within an organization. *Academy of Management, 25,* 586-597.

Thompson, M. (1981). Sex differential access to power on sex role socialization? *Sex Roles, 7,* 413-424.

PART IV

MOTIVATE

Chapter 22

Hierarchy of Needs
A.H. Maslow

Alice F. Smith

❙❙ CASE STUDY

The head nurse of a 35-bed medical unit appears more concerned with her own affairs both within and outside the hospital. The employees are neglected and struggle to perform their daily duties in spite of disharmony. The employees work long shifts trying to cover the floor. Often employees work 16 hours a day, sometimes unexpectedly. They also work long stretches at a time without adequate time off for recuperation.

Employees feel inadequate when working with patients and performing other duties. They never have the time to attend in-service education to keep them updated on policies or procedures. Unsafe technique is practiced by most employees because of lack of knowledge or insufficient staff.

The employees frequently bicker and lack a sense of closeness. Some employees are envious of time off given to other employees. A feeling of competition is felt by many. The employees try to talk with their head nurse, but her response is a hurried one of "later we'll talk," or when she listens, she does not follow through with employees' suggestions or her promises.

No employee is encouraged or recognized for doing a job well. All workers lack confidence because they do not know if a task is performed well or when it needs improvement. Tasks are not performed in a timely manner and sometimes are left for the next shift, creating further disharmony.

The head nurse criticizes her employees without offering suggestions for improvement. Employees are highly discouraged during yearly evaluations, and sometimes her comments are ambiguous and leave the employee with a lack of understanding about what the head nurse expects. Employees are not encouraged to improve or to set goals for improvement.

The effect is seen in high employee burnout and turnover. Frequent absenteeism is also seen on this unit, both legitimately and otherwise. Solutions to problems are minimal and slow to evolve. Morale is very low, and the employees lack trust in their leader.

The head nurse resigns her position and her employment in order to accept a part-time position at a health department that allows her to pursue outside interests. The employees are left without a leader. How should a new leader approach the situation?

| | | | | | | | | | | | | | | | | | | | | | | | | | | | | | | | | | | | | | | | | | | | | | | | | | | | | | | | | | | | | | | | | | | | | | | |

HIERARCHY OF NEEDS THEORY

A. H. Maslow wrote and published many books, articles, and journals during his 62 years of life. He is famous for his theory of the hierarchy of needs, which began as an article in the *Psychological Review* in July 1943 (Hill, 1974). It was derived as a theory of motivation. The hierarchy of needs included five basic needs: physiological needs, safety needs, love needs, esteem needs, and the need for self-actualization. Each need acts as an unconscious, biological motivator for each human being.

The physiological needs are the lowest-level need. They have to be satisfied before a person can move on to another need level. These needs include hunger, sex, thirst, rest, and activity. "When these physiological needs are not satisfied the individual becomes totally preoccupied with the object involved" (Miner, 1980, p. 20). These needs are the major motivators. "If all the needs are unsatisfied, and the organism is then dominated by the physiological needs, all other needs may become simply nonexistent or be pushed into the background" (Maslow, 1970, p. 37). The human being, then, is preoccupied with the present need.

If the physiological needs are relatively well satisfied, a new set of needs emerges, categorized as the safety needs (Maslow, 1970). Safety needs include freedom from danger, insecurity, and illness. Anything that may make a person feel safe or secure, such as a job, a satisfying marriage, or good health, is included in the safety needs.

Once the physiological and safety needs are gratified, the love and belongingness need emerges as the motivator. Each human will want to have a sense of belongingness and love. Friendships, family, and groups provide fulfillment of this need. A person will want a place in her or his particular group or family. The love needs in this category do not include sexual needs, which are physiological. A person must give love as well as receive love.

The next category of motivation needs is the esteem needs, which is divided into internal and external esteem needs. Internal esteem needs include feelings of self-respect or self-esteem. The feelings are derived from strength, achievement, competence, confidence, adequacy, independence, and freedom. External esteem needs are derived from sources such as reputation, prestige, status, fame and glory, dominance, recognition, attention, importance, dignity, and appreciation. If these needs are satisfied, a person feels self-confident and adequate. If they are unmet, a person feels inferior and helpless.

The highest-level need is the need for self-actualization. To reach self-actualization, people must realize what they can become and what their potential is and reach a level of self-fulfillment. This need is highly individualized. Self-actualization can begin only when the first four levels of needs are met.

> Self-actualizing people are, without one single exception, involved in a cause outside their own skin, in something outside of themselves. They are devoted, working at something, something which is very precious to them—some calling or vocation in the old sense, the priestly sense. (Maslow, 1971, p. 43)

By definition, self-actualizing people are gratified in all their basic needs (of belongingness, affection, respect, and self-esteem). (Maslow, 1967, p. 93)

"All people have needs for physiological satisfaction, for safety, for love and belonging, for esteem, and for self-actualization" (Paris, 1986, p. 26). These needs are more often unconscious than conscious. The needs exist in an order of prepotency, beginning with the physiological needs as the most powerful needs. The higher needs are no less basic but are weaker. In order for a person to develop in a healthy way, each need must be gratified.

Maslow also recognized other needs that are not a part of the basic five needs. "Science has its origins in the needs to know and to understand (or explain), i.e., cognitive needs" (Maslow, 1966, p. 20). The cognitive need is divided into two parts. The first part is the need to know, which is prepotent to the need to understand, which is the second part.

Aesthetic needs may or may not involve all people. These needs are least known. They include impulses to beauty, simplicity, completion, order, and symmetry and overlap with cognitive needs.

Deficiency needs and growth needs separate the five basic needs. The first four levels of needs are considered deficiency needs, that is, motivated by a deficiency. The highest-level need, self-actualization, is a growth need. This need motivates from growth. "The physiological life of the person, in many of its aspects, is lived out differently when he is deficiency-need-gratification-bent and when he is growth-dominated or 'meta-motivated' or growth-motivated or self-actualizing" (Maslow, 1968, p. 27). When a person is working through the deficiency needs, deprivation results in illness, either physical or psychological. Illness states are avoided when the needs are gratified. Growth needs produce positive health.

Self-actualization is a relatively achieved "state of affairs" in a few people. In most people, however, it's rather a hope, a yearning, a drive, a "something" wished for but not yet achieved, showing itself clinically as drive toward health, integration, growth, etc. (Maslow, 1959, p. 130)

The order of the hierarchy is not fixed. Most people have basic needs in the order previously suggested. There are, however, exceptions. Some people need self-esteem more than love, and the self-esteem need comes before love in their hierarchy. Some people who are chronically at a lower level become deadened or lowered, and the higher-level needs lose importance to these individuals. Conversely, people who have remained at the higher level of needs for a long period of time have forgotten or may have never experienced lower-level needs such as hunger. These needs to them are underevaluated.

Each need presented does not have to be wholly satisfied before moving on to the next level of need. Most normal members of our society are only partially satisfied with most needs at any given time. As these people move up the hierarchy, their percentages of satisfaction decrease.

Needs emerge gradually over a period of time. Needs are not totally satisfied at a given time, and immediately the next need emerges. As a more prepotent need becomes satisfied, the next need begins to emerge.

Self-actualization was elaborated on more than any other of Maslow's theoretical formulations. "At times Maslow comes very close to equating self-actualization with a type of religious conversion" (Miner, 1980, p. 24). Maslow (1971) describes eight ways in which a person self-actualizes.

"First, self-actualization means experiencing fully, vividly, selflessly, with full concentration and total absorption" (Maslow, 1971, p. 45). The person is considered fully human and whole at this point of experiencing. Self is actualizing itself at this moment.

Second, a choice has to be made. Life is filled with choices. The choices result in progression or regression. The progressive choice is the growth choice. The more progressive choices made, the closer an individual comes to self-actualization. Progressive choices move an individual toward self-actualization, and regressive choices move an individual away from self-actualization. "Self-actualization is an ongoing process" (Maslow, 1971, p. 45).

Third, in order for self-actualization to occur, there must be a self to actualize. Self must be allowed to emerge and be listened to. A person should act and react according to the way he or she feels, not according to the expected response.

Fourth, each person should be honest. Looking inside the self for answers is taking responsibility and a great step toward self-actualization.

Fifth, make all the choices previously listed and listen to the self. In order to choose wisely, a person must listen to herself or himself. This is the only way people can know their mission in life or their destiny.

Sixth, self-actualization is the process of actualizing one's potentialities at any time. Self-actualization is not an end state. "Self-actualization means using one's intelligence" (Maslow, 1971, p. 47).

Seventh, moments of ecstasy and peak experiences are moments of self-actualization. Although people may not recognize them, practically everyone has peak experiences.

Eighth, completely knowing who one is, inside and out, and discovering defenses and identifying them are essential to self-actualization. When defenses have been discovered and identified, they must be given up.

Self-actualization does not occur at any given moment. It is an experience any human being can reach, and it is reached at certain points in life. Self-actualization is accomplished little by little until a person realizes she or he has reached self-actualization, knowing oneself, the real self.

CASE ANALYSIS

A head nurse from another unit accepts the open position on this unit because of the challenge it offers. She realizes the basic needs of the employees are not being met. She also realizes that gaining their trust will take time. She is familiar with Maslow's hierarchy of basic needs and decides on a plan to meet her employees' needs.

When scheduling her employees, she is careful not to schedule too many days without a day off and tries to maintain the working day at 8-hour shifts per employee. The employees in turn work their designated time without undue complaints or requests for time off. This allows the employees time to fulfill their need for rest and activity. When this need is met, the next need emerges.

The head nurse decides that monthly in-service education should be held for her employees to update them on the latest safety techniques in patient care and policy items such as fire safety and disaster policy. Keeping employees updated on safety techniques and hospital policies meets their safety needs, encourages self-confidence, and enables them to feel more comfortable in their working environment. The next need begins to emerge.

The employees are encouraged to work together as a team, combining efforts to assist each other as needed when time permits. This creates a sense of "family" or belonging among the employees. Also, a suggestion box is utilized by the employees for complaints and suggestions on ways to solve problems. During quarterly staff meetings, the problems and suggestions are discussed and workable solutions are derived. Differences slowly resolve. The head nurse sets a good example by encouraging and practicing getting along with other employees. Employees learn to compromise and collaborate and make choices best for the group. When the ability to work together, accomplish tasks, and meet goals together is reached, a sense of belonging to this "family" on the medical unit emerges. The next need begins to emerge.

Each employee is encouraged individually by the head nurse and commended for doing good work. The employees are told they are appreciated on a regular basis. Employee-of-the-week recognition is instituted within the unit; all employees vote for an employee they see doing something extra or special during the week. The employee with the most votes is designated employee of the week. This recognition encourages employees to do their best and try to give a little extra. Having others and especially the head nurse recognize when one is doing a good job allows the esteem need to be met. When one is elected as employee of the week, a sense of accomplishment and pride is felt. Not only is one commended by others but also one commends oneself and feels confident in meeting and exceeding requirements for his or her job. The next need begins to emerge.

During yearly employee evaluations, the head nurse encourages each employee to evaluate herself or himself. This evaluation includes listing potentials and setting reachable goals by the next evaluation. Each employee is encouraged to be the best that he or she can be. Employees are allowed to express themselves and are encouraged to give what they feel is necessary for accomplishment. They are encouraged to set goals and try to meet them. They are encouraged to realize their capabilities and strive to meet them.

RESEARCH

The need hierarchy theory has been applied to management of companies and organizations. Research has also been performed to test different aspects of the theory for validity. If it is valid, then managers can learn a lot about managing their employees and their need levels.

Work now can meet the higher-level needs of individuals in today's industrial society. Work is most satisfying and can meet needs for recognition, achievement, and self-actualization. Maslow's theory of motivation states that lower-level needs must be met before higher-level needs can emerge.

In some underdeveloped countries, people are at the lowest level of needs, and the productive capacity of each individual is limited. Although Maslow did not study undeveloped countries, other researchers have. According to Dunnette (1976), "When we examine underdeveloped nations, we are in a sense taking a step back in time from the perspective of the developed Western Nations" (p. 1644). The physiological needs of thirst and hunger have to be met before an individual can be motivated by the next level of need. The worker's intake of calories reflects on the job according to the required energy levels of the job. This does not imply that economic growth in less industrialized countries is slowed by malnutrition. Compensations are made. Labor is cheap, so many more workers are used. Another solution is to work employees for less time and hire more people, which reduces unemployment and allows workers to perform at an optimal level. This increases motivation. They are also earning money to help pay for food to meet their hunger needs.

"The hierarchal concept has received a great deal of attention among those interested in organizations" (Lawler, 1973, p. 29). The hierarchical concept provides a powerful tool, if it is valid, for predicting how the importance of various outcomes will change in response to certain actions by organizations. It suggests what is more important to an employee. It also suggests that a company cannot give an employee enough growth and development. The more valued outcomes are received, the more will be wanted. Need hierarchy suggests that employees will never be satisfied. They will always want to improve, want to make more decisions, want more interesting jobs, and so on.

"In our society there is no single situation which is potentially so capable of giving some satisfaction at all levels of basic needs as is the occupation" (Roe, 1956, p. 31). The occupation satisfies physiological needs by providing money that can be exchanged for food, drink, and pleasures. Safety needs are satisfied in the same manner. Money is received and used for renting apartments or buying houses, clothes, sanitary techniques, and medical expenses. Also, jobs offer security through long-range plans such as insurance and retirement benefits. The occupation offers belonging to a group and functioning as an intrinsic part of a group. Esteem needs are met by the occupation, which offers independence and freedom. Obtaining a job is a symbol of entering adulthood. Just having a job carries a certain measure of esteem. Self-actualization can be satisfied if a person is happy in a job and has a lot of personal involvement in a job. A sense of accomplishment can be achieved from a job. Some jobs meet the need for knowledge and understanding, and some jobs meet the aesthetic needs, as well. A learned job requires new knowledge and a certain amount of understanding. Artistic jobs satisfy the aesthetics.

A self-actualizing person, according to Maslow (1965), is a highly evolved individual who assimilates work into the identity, into the self; that is, work actually becomes a part of the self, part of the individual's self-definition. A good organization tends to improve the person, who in turn tends to improve the organization. According to Maslow (1965), good management can lead to such cycles and result in a utopian or revolutionary technique to improve the world.

According to Miller (1981),

> Understanding people's needs is important in establishing a system of incentives. Originally, security and individual competitiveness were the only two needs that industry directed its efforts toward. Today, much effort is being directed toward tapping needs for self-realization and self-actualization. (p. 25)

Several studies have been statistically analyzed by using Maslow's theory of the hierarchy of needs in the business management arena. According to Alderfer (1972),

> Data bearing on Maslow's theory strongly suggested that this conceptual scheme had difficulties with the middle level (interpersonal) needs. Whatever support for the theory that was found pertained to self-actualization needs. No support was found for predictions bearing on safety, belongingness and esteem needs. (p. 53)

Porter (1964) developed a need satisfaction questionnaire for the management level in business. The questionnaire consisted of 13 items pertaining to the needs of a manager. Managers were tested on a score of 1 to 7, 1 being the lowest degree of fulfillment and 7 being the highest degree of fulfillment. A scale of 1 to 7 was also set up for degree of importance. A satisfaction score was based on the difference between obtained and expected fulfillment. Complete satisfaction was 0, and 6 was complete dissatisfaction. Findings show that higher-level managers obtain more need fulfillment than do lower-level managers. Higher-level managers have been shown to be more satisfied than lower-level managers. "There is a slight but not always consistent trend on the part of the higher-level managers to consider most of the needs as more important to them than do the lower-level managers" (Porter, 1964).

A study by Wahba and Bridwell (1976) on the need hierarchy theory consisted of a review of the research. They found a lack of empirical evidence to validate the theory. They reviewed ten factor-analytic and three ranking studies that tested Maslow's theory. Partial support was found for the concept of need hierarchy. Maslow's deprivation-domination proposition was studied by cross-sectional studies. Self-actualization was the only supported concept.

"Longitudinal studies testing Maslow's gratification/activation proposition showed no support, and the limited support received from cross-sectional studies is questionable due to numerous measurement problems" (Wahba & Bridwell, 1976, p. 212).

A study in Israel by Yinon, Bizman, and Goldberg (1976) was performed on 40 married female students. "The hypothesis is then, that as the need is located higher in Maslow's hierarchy, the level of its satisfaction will be affected more by the relative than by the absolute magnitude of the reward" (Yinon et al., 1976, p. 326). The self-actualization need was excluded, and the hypothesis was confirmed.

Schneider and Alderfer (1973) performed "three studies attempting to achieve convergence between different measures designed to assess need satisfaction in organizations" (p. 489). Study I used 146 registered nurses working in two midwestern hospitals. Porter's (1964) need satisfaction questionnaire was used, along with a questionnaire with a series of self-ratings of effort and performance. Schneider also added a third part containing items to operationalize Maslow's concepts. Poor convergence between the measures of Maslow's concepts resulted.

Study II used a large sample of 217 subjects. The Maslow items constructed by Schneider were revised. The sample included men and women from all jobs in a bank. This showed poor convergence between Maslow and Alderfer's existence, relatedness, and growth measures.

Study III consisted of a sample of 522 employees from 50 agencies of life insurance companies. Some convergence was seen between Maslow and ERG measures and "some meaningful correlation between Maslow measures and the Job Description Index measure of job satisfaction" (Schneider and Alderfer, 1973, p. 489).

Maslow's need hierarchy theory was empirically tested by Rauschenberger, Schmitt, & Hunter (1980). The theory was expressed in Markov chain form.

A Markov chain model is a dynamic probabilistic model, which allows one to investigate the likelihood of movement from a given state (i.e. some defined conditions and/or property of the entity being studied) to any other state over some specified time interval. (Rauschenberger, Schmitt, & Hunter, 1980, pp. 654-655)

The subjects included 547 high school graduates from 11 different high schools in the Midwest urban area. According to Maslow, a person would be dominated at any given time by one of five basic needs. This implies a negative correlation between two needs. "The data closely contradicts Maslow's argument" (Rauschenberger et al., 1980, p. 667). The average correlation was found to be positive. The empirical evidence in this study disconfirms Maslow's theory.

A factor-analytic study was performed by Roberts, Walter, and Miles (1971). The study tested job satisfaction items designed to measure Maslow's need categories. Subjects included 380 managers from six organizations. The Porter (1964) methodology was followed. "Our analysis at best, provides a mixed support for the usefulness of Maslow need categories as a means of structuring the dimensions of job satisfaction" (Roberts et al., 1971, p. 218).

Mitchell and Moudgill (1976) measured Maslow's need hierarchy with a ten-item instrument. Subjects included 247 certified general accountants, 355 chartered accountants, and 290 engineers and scientists from public and private organizations in Canada. The analysis supported that lower needs are more localized and more limited than higher needs. This evidence for a two-way classification is not evidence against a five-way classification, however.

Maslow's need hierarchy was also researched and tested in a longitudinal study by Hall and Nougaim (1968). Subjects included 49 young management-level AT&T employees. Three hypotheses were stated.

Hypothesis I: Within a given year, the satisfaction of a given level of needs will be positively correlated with the strength of the needs at the next higher level (static analysis). Hypothesis II: From one year to the next, changes in the satisfaction of a given level of needs will be positively correlated with changes in the strength of the needs at the next higher level (change analysis). Hypothesis III: After five years of employment, successful managers will show lower need strength and higher satisfaction in the safety needs than will their less successful colleagues. Thus, they will show higher achievement and self-actualization need strength than will the less successful group (success analysis). (Hall and Nougaim, 1968, p. 16)

These managers were tested yearly over a 5-year period. The results concluded that the predicted correlations are smaller than the nonhypothesized relationships in the static analysis hypothesis. Each need correlated with its own satisfaction more strongly than with any other need except affiliation. The concern for safety was decreased in the fifth year among both groups. Both groups increased their concern for achievement, esteem, self-actualization. No strong evidence was found to support Maslow's hierarchy.

Another longitudinal study was conducted by Lawler and Suttle (1972). Data were collected from 187 managers in two organizations. This study, too, was to test the validity of the need hierarchy concept. The Porter (1964) questionnaire was used. The subjects were divided into two groups. The first group completed the questionnaire at the beginning of the study and again in 6 months. The second group completed the questionnaire at the beginning of the study and again in 12 months. The results offered little support for the view of a hierarchical arrangement of needs of managers in an organization. Evidence against the theory is not conclusive. The sample was small and was not randomized across the population.

In 1977, Wanous and Zwany performed a cross-sectional test of need hierarchy. The test was actually studying Alderfer's ERG theory. However, "Maslow himself appeared to advocate a more simplified (deficiency and growth) two category system" (Wanous & Zwany, 1977, p. 78). Others have also taken Maslow's need hierarchy and shortened it into two or three levels. Lawler grouped a lower level of needs from the physiological and safety needs and a higher level from the love, esteem, and self-actualization needs. Also, Maslow focused attention on upward movement in the hierarchy, whereas Alderfer states that movement can occur in either direction.

Campbell (1971) researched the basis of job attitudes. "The question addressed is whether similarities of job attitudes among workers are more closely associated with the nature of the job itself or with the nature of the supervision received" (Campbell, 1971, p. 521). The subjects were 311 workers in southern Michigan. The results were a consistent association of common supervision with attitude similarity. A suggested explanation for this result is Maslow's hierarchy of needs. The highest-order needs and the lowest-order needs are met through the job. The middle needs of belongingness, love, and esteem can be met by people in the work environment, one such person being the supervisor, who has the greatest influence over a worker's job.

According to Salancik and Pfeffer (1977), Maslow's need theory has been tested empirically and the theory has not been supported. Hall and Nougaim (1968) found little evidence for the theory at a two-level or five-level hierarchy. Wahba and Bridwell (1976) concluded that the need hierarchy was only partially supported. The need hierarchy sequence represented a sequence of increasing indefiniteness and ambiguity.

Tuzzolino and Armandi (1981) suggest an organizational need hierarchy. Corporate profitability and survival are the lower-level need categories. Classical economic norms satisfy organizational security, safety, and survival. "Market structure (degree of competitive imperfection), conduct (degree of informational imperfection), and performance manifest levels of affiliative — and status — need satisfaction" (Tuzzolino & Armandi, 1981, p. 23). Self-actualizing needs are satisfied by industry recognition and leadership. Having satisfied prepotent needs, the self-actualizing organization is a socially responsible organization. The motivators are the prepotent organizational needs.

Regardless of the findings in the research studies, organizations still use the need hierarchy as a basis for management. In order for an employer to have an improved attitude toward his job, Sondak (1980) recommends to "present the job so that it works to satisfy the employee's needs" (p. 13). Using work to satisfy needs is the key to motivation. A good manager must be able to determine the needs of his or her employees in order to motivate them. A person can move up or down the ladder according to situational behavior. Understanding situational behavior requires good management skills. Supervisors need to be aware and understand the behaviors and needs of others. In this way, the supervisor can assist the employee to move up the hierarchical ladder to reach her or his level of capability.

Little research has been performed on Maslow's hierarchy of needs by nurses. Davis-Sharts (1986) did perform an empirical test of Maslow's theory of need hierarchy. The hypothesis was "that prior to sleep onset the physiological need for thermoregulation must be satisfied before the psychological need for protection will be satisfied" (Davis-Sharts, 1986, p. 60). The study was a hologeistic comparative study. The results were that thermoregulation behaviors prior to sleep onset, regardless of climate, occurred more frequently than behaviors to provide protection. This empirical evidence supports Maslow's theory. Further research should be done on other needs. More nominal and correlational studies need to be done as well.

Other studies have been performed using Maslow's hierarchy but not necessarily statistical research. Whall (1980) studied nursing theories related to family functioning. She concludes from Maslow that assessing holistically is necessary in order to perceive holistically. The Cartesian position holds that mind and body may be considered separately. The parts then can separately be assessed. This leads to reductionism or that the sum of the parts equals the whole. In contrast, Maslow believes it is better to know through cognitive operations and the senses. In this way mind is not split from body, and a person is perceived as a whole.

King (1981) reviewed motivational theories. Among the first to propose a motivational theory was Abraham Maslow. "Even though it has been the source of considerable controversy since its first appearance, a brief summary may still provide the manager with insight" (King, 1981, p. 35). King states that two basic assumptions must be known to understand the hierarchy. First, when a lower level need is met, a new need emerges. Second, one need dominates, but more than one may be operating at the same time. "Most managers today are primarily concerned with the top two or three needs in the hierarchy. Physiologic and safety needs are generally adequate in the work environment, and so our attention must be directed toward the higher motivational levels" (King, 1981, p. 35). King suggests that managers study motivation theory to find methods that encourage greater efficiency and productivity, not just to understand why people do not produce. Motivation theory is something that should be a part of one's management style. It should become as a natural outgrowth instead of a conscious effort.

Yura (1986) states that human need theory is a framework for the nurse supervisor. Nursing practitioners have focused on conceptual and theoretical frameworks for nursing practice for more than a decade. "Human need theorists view the person as an integrated, organized whole who is motivated toward meeting human needs" (Yura, 1986, p. 46). Need satisfaction (gratification) and need fulfillment deprivation are two significant concepts of human need theory. "In nursing, human needs supply the theoretical substance of the nursing process" (Yura, 1986, p. 48) Needs at all levels must be considered for use by nursing practitioners and supervisors. The territory of nursing is to preserve, foster, maintain, and facilitate the integrity of all human needs. The nurse supervisor, regardless of setting, functions within this context of nursing service.

Fuszard (1984) studied job enrichment and its path to self-actualization for nurses. Maslow's esteem needs and self-actualization needs are discussed. Adequate self-esteem produces confidence and capability, which in turn bring about greater productivity. Chronic poor staffing makes self-esteem impossible in relation to patient care. "Correct placement in and orientation to a job can help the employees achieve mastery, independence, and freedom" (Fuszard, 1984, p. 35). A job well done brings about respect from others. Co-workers and employers recognize jobs well done, also. "This respect from society meets one of the characteristics of a profession" (Fuszard, 1984, p. 36). Once the esteem needs are met, the need for self-actualization emerges. This need can be met at work and at play. It requires growth to meet one's full potential. Work becomes as exciting and pleasurable as play. For self-actualization to occur, people must not only like their job, but do the job well and strive to make it better. A professional wants to meet this level of self-actualization.

Marriner-Tomey (1988) suggests that "Maslow's outline is correct in general, [but] human needs are more complex than a simple listing would indicate" (p. 196). Maslow's hierarchy of needs can be applied directly to patient care, to individual workers, or to groups. The hierarchy can be applied to nursing management at each level. The physiological level of needs should include adequate pay to purchase food and shelter, adequate hours for rest, and adequate breaks during the day for personal and physiological needs. A stable environment is needed for safety. Nurse managers should encourage cohesive work groups to satisfy love needs and to encourage more effective work. Management plays a big role in the esteem needs by giving due praise and other incentives to employees. A nurse manager can contribute to nurses reaching self-actualization by encouraging them to set goals and strive to meet them.

Little research has been done on Maslow's theory of needs hierarchy, especially in the nursing realm. Marriner-Tomey (1988) discussed the theory applied to nursing management. No research was found. The validity of the theory will become more evident as more research of the needs hierarchy is completed.

REFERENCES

Alderfer, C.P. (1972). *Existence, relatedness and growth: Human needs in organizational settings.* New York: Free Press.

Campbell, D.B. (1971). Relative influence of job and supervision on shared worker attitudes. *Journal of Applied Psychology, 55,* 521-525.

Davis-Sharts, J. (1986). An empirical test of Maslow's theory of need hierarchy using hologeistic comparison by statistical sampling. *Advances in Nursing Science, 9,* 58-72.

Dunnette, M.D. (Ed.). (1976). *Handbook of industrial and organizational psychology.* Chicago: Rand McNally College Publishing.

Fuszard, B. (Ed.). (1984). *Self-actualization for nurses: Issues, trends and strategies for job enrichment.* Rockville, MD: Aspen.

Hall, D.T., & Nougaim, K.E. (1968). An examination of Maslow's need hierarchy in an organizational setting. *Organizational Behavior and Human Performance, 3,* 12-35.

Hill, R. (1974). Abraham Maslow: The philosopher who ranked human needs. *International Management, 29*(11), 46-51.

King, B.W. (1981). Motivation theory. *Journal of Emergency Nursing, 7,* 35-38.

Lawler, E.E., III. (1973). *Motivations in work organizations.* Monterey, CA: Brooks/Cole.

Lawler, E.E., III, & Suttle, J.L. (1972). A causal correlational test of the need hierarchy concept. *Organizational Behavior and Human Performance, 7,* 265-287.

Marriner-Tomey, A. (1988). *Guide to nursing management* (3rd ed.). St. Louis: C.V. Mosby.

Maslow, A.H. (1943). A theory of human motivation. *Psychological Review, 50,* 370–396.

Maslow, A.H. (Ed.). (1959). *New knowledge in human values.* New York: Harper & Brothers.

Maslow, A.H. (1965). *Eupsychian management: A journal.* Homewood, IL: Richard D. Irwin and Dorsey Press.

Maslow, A.H. (1966). *The psychology of science: A reconnaissance.* New York: Harper & Row.

Maslow, A.H. (1967). A theory of metamotivation: The biological rooting of the value-life. *Journal of Humanistic Psychology, 7,* 93–127.

Maslow, A.H. (1968). *Toward a psychology of being* (2nd ed.). New York: Van Nostrand Reinhold.

Maslow, A.H. (1970). *Motivation and personality* (2nd ed.). New York: Harper & Row.

Maslow, A.H. (1971). *The farther reaches of human nature.* New York: Viking Press.

Miller, G. (1981). Management guidelines: Understanding needs. *Supervisory Management, 26,* 21-29.

Miner, J.B. (1980). *Theories of organizational behavior.* Hinsdale, IL: Dryden.

Mitchell, V.F., & Moudgill, P. (1976). Measurement of Maslow's need hierarchy. *Organizational Behavior and Human Performance,16,* 334-349.

Paris, B.J. (Ed.). (1986). *Third force psychology and the study of the literature.* Cranberry, NJ: Associated University Press.

Porter, L.W. (1964). *Organizational patterns of managerial job attitudes.* American Foundation for Management Research.

Rauschenberger, J., Schmitt, N., & Hunter, J.E. (1980). A test of the need hierarchy concept by a Markov model of change in need strength. *Administrative Science Quarterly, 25,* 654-670.

Roberts, K.H., Walter, G.A., & Miles, R.E. (1971). A factor analytic study of job satisfaction items designed to measure Maslow need categories. *Personnel Psychology, 24,* 205-220.

Roe, A. (1956). *The psychology of occupations.* New York: John Wiley & Sons.

Salancik, G.R., & Pfeffer, J. (1977). An examination of need satisfaction models of job attitudes. *Administrative Science Quarterly, 22,* 427-456.

Schneider, B., & Alderfer, C.P. (1973). Three studies of measures of need satisfaction in organizations. *Administrative Science Quarterly, 18,* 489-505.

Sondak, A. (1980). The importance of knowing your employee's needs. *Supervisory Management, 25,* 13-18.

Tuzzolino, F., & Armandi, B.R. (1981). A need-hierarchy framework for assessing corporate social responsibility. *Academy of Management Review, 6,* 21-28.

Wahba, M.A., & Bridwell, L.G. (1976). Maslow reconsidered: A review of research on the need hierarchy theory. *Organizational Behavior and Human Performance, 15,* 212-240.

Wanous, J.P., & Zwany, A. (1977). A cross-sectional test of need hierarchy theory. *Organizational Behavior and Human Performance, 18,* 78-97.

Whall, A.L. (1980). Congruence between existing theories of family functioning and nursing theories. *Advances in Nursing Science, 3,* 59-67.

Yinon, Y., Bizman, A., & Goldberg, M. (1976). Effect of relative magnitude of reward and type of need on satisfaction. *Journal of Applied Psychology, 61,* 325-328.

Yura, H. (1986). Human need theory: A framework for the nurse supervisor. *The Health Care Supervisor, 4,* 45-58.

Chapter 23

Existence, Relatedness, and Growth Theory
Clayton P. Alderfer

Darla D. Meyers

┃┃ CASE STUDY

Over a year has passed since Alice Jones, the head nurse of a 35-bed surgical unit, lost her husband in a tragic automobile accident. At the time of the accident, their two boys were 8 and 13 years old. Alice and the two boys were filled with disbelief and grief. A 2-month leave of absence was granted for her to begin to work through the grieving process and add some stability to the boys' home life.

Alice was well respected as a head nurse. Her floor was noted for excellent nursing care and employee attitudes. Morale was never a problem on the unit, and patient complaints were at a minimum. She was enrolled in college seeking a master's degree in nursing; her enthusiasm and quest for knowledge were contagious on her unit, and many of her staff were also enrolled in higher education courses.

At the end of 2 months Alice returned to work. She wore little makeup, her hair was unkempt, and her physical appearance was indicative of depression. Her unit, which was in need of leadership after her absence, became more unsettled in her presence. The leader who always handled crisis situations calmly with no frustration looked as though one display of emotion would make her crack. The staff nurses began protecting her until their frustration with this lack of leadership turned to anger.

Alice was counseled by the director of nursing and encouraged to seek therapy for depression. She began treatment and gradually improved. Although Alice was frequently absent to stay at home with her 8-year-old son for frequent "illnesses," when she was at work, the unit ran smoothly. Alice was functioning well at work, but she had to drop out of school to be available for her sons, who were having trouble at school. Money was not a problem if she continued working, but any decrease in salary would be a financial burden for the family.

At the 1-year anniversary of her husband's death, the school called Alice and stated that her now 14-year-old son was not in class. She went home to find her son drunk in his bedroom. She had suspected alcohol abuse by her son for a month, but she had not dealt with the issue. The next day she reported to work tearful, with no makeup, and generally unkempt. The director of nursing wondered what she should do about the situation.

┃┃┃

ERG THEORY

Existence, relatedness, and growth, Clayton P. Alderfer's ERG theory, conceptualizes basic human needs in three categories. A basic human need is one that requires gratification for its own sake and not as a stepping stone to achieve a higher goal.

Existence needs are desires for materials that are finite in supply, such as food, shelter, and clothing. Pay and fringe benefits in an organizational setting are included in this category. Existence needs are satisfied when individuals have enough, and in sound economies no individual has to be without.

Relatedness needs are desires for mutual sharing of thoughts and feelings with significant others. The sharing and communication are important, not the content of the discussions.

Growth needs are interactions between individuals and the environment to develop intrinsic talents to the individual's potential. Growth needs require change in an individual's capacity.

"Few ideas or theories emerge from a vacuum" (Alderfer, 1972, p. 30). The ERG theory evolved from Maslow's hierarchy of human needs. Contrary to Maslow's idea of prepotency, Alderfer states the need is always present and consciously recognized (Campbell & Pritchard, 1976). Alderfer (1972) lists ten major propositions in the ERG theory that can empirically test hypotheses relating satisfaction to desire.

The major propositions in ERG theory are as follows:

P1. The less existence needs are satisfied, the more they will be desired.
P2. The less relatedness needs are satisfied, the more existence needs will be desired.
P3. The more existence needs are satisfied, the more relatedness needs will be desired.
P4. The less relatedness needs are satisfied, the more they will be desired.
P5. The less growth needs are satisfied, the more relatedness needs will be desired.
P6. The more relatedness needs are satisfied, the more growth needs will be desired.
P7. The more growth needs are satisfied, the more they will be desired.
   These propositions indicate that any desire can have several types of satisfaction (including some outside its particular category) affecting its strength. Any satisfaction also affects more than one type of desire (including some outside its particular category). (Alderfer, 1972, p. 13)

The ERG theory does not assume that all people have the same chronic strength of the needs.

When existence needs are scarce, a person with high needs will be able to obtain a lower proportion of his desires than a person with low needs. When there is no scarcity then everyone can get what he wants and there should be no difference in degree of satisfaction between those with chronic existence needs. . . . To summarize:
P8a. When existence materials are scarce, then the higher chronic existence desires are, the less existence satisfaction.
P8b. When existence materials are not scarce, then there will be no differential existence satisfaction as a function of chronic existence desires. (Alderfer, 1972, p. 18)

People differ in the amount of sharing of thoughts and feelings they want or can comfortably exchange. The ERG theory provides the following propositions to accommodate the various interpersonal states in relatedness needs:

P9a. In highly satisfying relationships, there is no differential relatedness satisfaction as a function of chronic relatedness desires.
P9b. In normal relationships, persons very high and very low on chronic relatedness desires tend to obtain lower satisfaction than persons with moderate desires.
P9c. In highly dissatisfying relationships, then, the higher chronic relatedness desires, the more relatedness satisfaction. (Alderfer, 1972, pp. 19-20)

Self-actualization	Growth
Esteem-self confirmed	
Esteem-interpersonal	Relatedness
Love (belongingness)	
Safety-interpersonal	
Safety-material	Existence
Physical	

FIGURE 23-1   Maslow's hierarchy relating to ERG Theory. *Adapted from Alderfer, C.P. (1972).* Existence, relatedness and growth. *New York: Free Press.*

Growth needs depend on an individual actively seeking ways in the environment to develop his or her talents to their fullest extent; however, if the environment is unresponsive, the individual may be restricted from growth. The following propositions apply to growth needs:

P10a. In challenging discretionary settings, then, the higher chronic growth desires, the more growth satisfaction.

P10b. In nonchallenging, nondiscretionary settings, there will be no differential growth satisfaction as a function of chronic growth desires. (Alderfer, 1972, p. 20)

The above ten propositions lead to different predictions from the ERG theory and Maslow's theory. "The differences concern (1) how the categories of needs are formed, (2) the presence or absence of a strict prepotency assumption, (3) how frustration of higher-order needs affects lower-order desires, and (4) how chronic desires relate to satisfaction (Alderfer, 1972, p. 24). A conceptualization of Maslow's hierarchy as it relates to the ERG theory is displayed in Figure 23-1.

As Alderfer (1972) compiled data for the ERG theory, the three following areas required changes:

1. Determination of the relationship of specific needs within each broad category was needed.
2. Specific conditions affecting the validity of the propositions were found, thereby changing the propositions.
3. Certain propositions that were not found to have consistent empirical support need to be questioned.

When measures of satisfaction and desires were obtained on needs within a category, not all satisfactions had the same size correlation with the desires. The relationship of the satisfaction to the desire varied according to the need category. Existence needs and desires of the same type were more highly correlated with each other than existence needs of different types. An example would be the correlation between satisfaction and desire needs of a monetary nature compared to those of safety.

Relatedness needs among members of the same group were contingent upon the group positions of the persons involved in the relationship and receiving the satisfaction. "Managers (who were group leaders) tended to show higher correlations between satisfaction and desire for significant others outside the work group than employees (who were group members)" (Alderfer, 1972, p. 146). Growth satisfaction in one setting was related to growth desires in another setting when the norms of ongoing behavior patterns of the two settings were comparable (Alderfer, 1972).

Propositions P3 and P5 were dropped from the ERG theory because of lack of consistent empirical support. The following propositions of the ERG theory are the most consistent with the empirical data:

P1. The less existence needs are satisfied, the more they will be desired.

P2. (Revised) When both existence and relatedness needs are relatively dissatisfied, the less relatedness needs are satisfied, the more existence needs will be desired.

P4. (Revised) When relatedness needs are relatively dissatisfied, the less relatedness needs are satisfied, the more they will be desired; when relatedness needs are relatively satisfied, the more relatedness needs are satisfied, the more relatedness needs are satisfied, the more they will be desired.

P6. (Revised) When both relatedness and growth needs are relatively satisfied, the more relatedness needs are satisfied, the more growth needs will be desired.

P7. (Revised) When growth needs are relatively dissatisfied, the less growth needs are satisfied, the more they will be desired; when growth needs are relatively satisfied, the more growth needs are satisfied, the more they will be desired.

P8a. When existence materials are not scarce, then the higher the chronic existence desires, the less the existence satisfaction.

P8b. When existence materials are not scarce, then there will be no differential existence satisfaction as a function of chronic existence desires.

P9a. In highly satisfying relationships, there is no differential relatedness satisfaction as a function of chronic relatedness desires.

P9b. In normal relationships, persons very high and very low on chronic relatedness desires tend to obtain lower satisfaction than persons with moderate desires.

P9c. In highly dissatisfying relationships, then, the higher chronic relatedness desires, the more relatedness satisfaction.

P10a. In challenging discretionary settings, then, the higher chronic growth desires, the more growth satisfaction.

P10b. In nonchallenging, nondiscretionary settings, there will be no differential growth satisfaction as a function of chronic growth desires. (Alderfer, 1972, pp. 149-150)

Miner (1980) states that

the revisions tend to upset the internal logical integrity of the original formulators. Thus, the revised theory is at a lower level of abstraction and tends to approach a set of empirical generalizations. Accordingly, it becomes more cumbersome to use E.R.G. theory for managerial decisions. (p. 40)

CASE ANALYSIS

Before the death of her husband, Alice had satisfied her existence and relatedness needs. Her desires were growth oriented. She was continuing her education and molding her work environment to be receptive to growth. Her growth potentiated the growth of her staff, and the unit was functioning smoothly (relates to ERG proposition 10a, that is, higher chronic growth desires, more growth satisfaction).

The death of Alice's husband made her relatedness needs almost totally deficient. Her spouse and his support were completely withdrawn, and her sons became confused and angry. Family communications were disrupted. After she returned to work, the support of her peers was withdrawn as her lack of functioning persisted. Her relatedness desires and satisfactions were out of control (relates to ERG proposition 4). Alice had to drop out of school, which dissatisfied her growth needs. Depression overtook her life. Maslow (1971) states that life is a process of choices and that there are progression choices and regression choices. A regression choice often moves one toward defensiveness and perceived safety, and a growth choice stretches one toward the unknown.

At this point Alice's supervisor stepped in and directed her toward counseling. The director of nursing accomplished two tasks: (1) she showed Alice that she cared about her as a person by paying her some attention, and (2) therapy was initiated. Campbell (1971) states "the intermediate needs (belongingness, love, and such esteem factors as the desires for prestige, recognition, attention and appreciation) can be met to a great extent only by people, and, in the work environment, especially the supervisor" (p. 524). Counseling also meets relatedness needs as it opens communication, an important aspect of relatedness. Alice subsequently began to function better at work, although at home her children were still exhibiting signs of emotional distress.

Yura (1986) states that

> a supervisor whose human needs are reasonably well met will more likely facilitate the human needs of those being supervised and will be able to identify and use problem solving when the nursing staff overuses the work place and colleagues or coworkers for need fulfillment. (p. 57)

A year passed, her son was in trouble with alcohol, and Alice relapsed. Communication and unresolved relatedness needs in the family surfaced. The director of nursing asked Alice if there was a problem in which she could be helpful. Tearfully, Alice relayed the problems about her children. The director of nursing helped arrange alcohol and drug counseling for the family.

After 3 months of family counseling, Alice is again functioning on her unit as a respected leader. She has been unable to return to school but does have plans for continuing her education in the future. Family problems are not completely resolved but are at a manageable level. Alice voices confidence that her family is healing and her career is again a major focus in her life.

With the relatedness needs of the family healing, Alice is more efficient and productive in her job, which also increases her satisfaction of relatedness desires by the respect of her peers. She is aware of her growth needs although she is still having trouble with her relatedness. School is in her immediate plans, and her career seems to be on a more positive course.

RESEARCH

Earlier research on need hierarchy and need strength addressed job enlargement and Maslow's theory. Alderfer (1967a, 1967b, 1969) researched job enlargement and found that satisfaction with skills and abilities increased with job complexity, but respect from supervisors decreased. Roberts, Walter, and Miles (1971) researched job satisfaction and Maslow's need categories and concluded that the results did not accurately reflect the Maslow category domains.

Schneider and Alderfer (1973) performed three studies comparing Maslow's hierarchy, ERG theory, and the job description index. Maslow's hierarchy showed no patterns of reliability or validity; however, ERG and the job description index did correlate at all need levels.

Alderfer's categories in the ERG theory were supported by Yinon, Bizman, and Goldberg (1976). The hypothesis that the level of satisfaction will be affected more by the relative than by the absolute amount of the new reward as the need is located higher on the hierarchy was upheld. Mitchell and Moudgill (1976) state Maslow's conceptual framework has not yet been validated. Wahba and Bridwell (1976) state that Maslow lacks empirical support but that Alderfer provides impressive evidence.

Salancik and Pfeffer (1977) state that

> need satisfaction models have survived more because of their aesthetics than because of their scientific utility. . . . While need-satisfaction models posit rationality and the possibility of individual action, they do not give humans credit for much adaptability in the pursuit of satisfaction. (p. 453)

Miner (1981) points out the failure of ERG to incorporate the full complexity of individual differences. Alderfer in his "Critique of Salancik and Pfeffer" (1977a) states their study was oversimplified and inaccurate and that the need theory does not contradict the principles of individual differences; rather, it focuses on the differences of need strengths.

Wanous and Zwany (1977) supported the empirical integrity of the ERG categories through cluster and factor analysis. Hierarchy was also demonstrated among the ERG needs.

Rauschenberger, Schmitt, and Hunter (1980) performed empirical testing of Maslow's need hierarchy and Alderfer's ERG theories that disconfirmed both theories. However, the authors suggest further research due to several limitations of their study.

Hypotheses pertaining to relatedness satisfaction and desires from the ERG theory were tested by Alderfer, Kaplan, and Smith (1974). The hypotheses of relatedness satisfactions and desires were supported, and a link was formed between the two methodologies of laboratory and field settings. Alderfer (1977b) confirms that the importance of a reward is relative to the amount of that reward the person has. People who value a reward most typically have a small amount of the reward.

Sims and Szilagyi (1976) supported the growth hypothesis and determined that individuals with a higher need for self-actualization are better candidates for enrichment of their jobs. The higher the occupational level and role ambiguity, the stronger the relationship between feedback and work. Pierce and Dunham (1976) also showed that workers with strong higher-order need strengths or growth strengths respond better to expanded task designs than other workers.

Hackman and Oldham (1976) proposed from their research on motivation through job design relating to growth needs that an individual's needs change to meet the challenge of the situation. An individual confronted with a complex job will develop herself or himself to meet the task.

> The person living in an environment favorable to growth will move steadily up the hierarchy until he is free to devote most of his energies to self-actualization, which is the full and satisfying use of his capabilities in a calling suitable to his nature. (Paris, 1986, p. 27)

Very little nursing research could be found regarding human need theory and no nursing research specific to ERG theory. Yura (1986) stated that "human need theory . . . has considerable utility for the nurse supervisor. It consists of knowledge to assist the nurse supervisor to explain, interpret, and predict the behavior of the nursing staff, coworkers, colleagues, and the self in the work setting" (p. 46).

REFERENCES

Alderfer, C.P. (1967a). An organizational syndrome. *Administrative Science Quarterly, 12,* 440-460.

Alderfer, C.P. (1967b). Convergent and discriminant validation of satisfaction and desires measures by interviews and questionnaires. *Journal of Applied Psychology, 51,* 509-520.

Alderfer, C.P. (1969). Job enlargement and the organizational content. *Personnel Psychology, 22,* 418-426.

Alderfer, C.P. (1972). *Existence, relatedness and growth.* New York: Free Press.

Alderfer, C.P. (1977a). A critique of Salancik and Pfeffer's examination of need-satisfaction theories. *Advances in Nursing Science, 22,* 658-669.

Alderfer, C.P. (1977b). Group and intergroup relations. In J.R. Hackman and J.L. Suttle (Eds.), *Improving life at work.* Santa Monica: Goodyear Publishing. *Administrative Science Quarterly, 24,* 347-361.

Alderfer, C.P., Kaplan, R.F., & Smith, R.K. (1974). The effect of variations in relatedness need satisfaction on relatedness desires. *Administrative Science Quarterly, 19,* 507-532.

Campbell, D.B. (1971). Relative influences of job and supervision on shared worker attitudes. *Journal of Applied Psychology, 55*(6), 521-525.

Campbell, J.P., & Pritchard, R.D. (1976). Motivation theory in industrial and organizational psychology. In M.D. Dunnette (Ed.), *Handbook of industrial and organizational psychology,* Chicago: Rand McNally College Publishing.

Hackman, J.R., & Oldham, G.R. (1976). Motivation through the design of work: Test of a theory. *Organizational Behavior and Human Performance, 16,* 250-279.

Maslow, A.H. (1971). *The farther reaches of human nature.* New York: Viking Press.

Miner, J.B. (1980). *Theories of organizational behavior.* Hinsdale, IL: Dryden.

Miner, J.B. (1981). Theories of organizational motivation. In G.W. England, A.R. Negandhi, & B. Wilport (Eds.), *The functioning of complex organizations.* Cambridge, MA: Oelgeschlarger.

Mitchell, V.F., & Moudgill, P. (1976). Measurement of Maslow's need hierarchy. *Organizational Behavior and Human Performance, 16,* 334-349.

Paris, B.J. (Ed.). (1986). *Third force psychology and the study of the literature.* Cranberry, NJ: Associated University Press.

Pierce, J.L., & Dunham, R.B. (1976). Task design: A literature review. *Academy of Management Review, 1*(4), 83-97.

Rauschenberger, J., Schmitt, N., & Hunter, J. (1980). A test of the need hierarchy concept by a Markoz model of change in needs strengths. *Administrative Science Quarterly, 25,* 654-670.

Roberts, K.H., Walter, G.A., & Miles, R.E. (1971). A factor analytic study of job satisfaction items designed to measure Maslow need categories. *Personnel Psychology, 24,* 205-220.

Salancik, G.R., & Pfeffer, J. (1977). An examination of need-satisfaction models of job attitudes. *Administrative Science Quarterly, 22,* 427-456.

Schneider, B., & Alderfer, C.P. (1973). Three studies of measured need satisfaction in organizations. *Administrative Science Quarterly, 18,* 489-504.

Sims, H.P., & Szilagyi, A.D. (1976). Job characteristic relationships: Individual and structural moderators. *Organizational Behavior and Human Performance, 17,* 211-230.

Wahba, M.A., & Bridwell, L.G. (1976). Maslow reconsidered: A review of research on the need hierarchy theory. *Organizational Behavior and Human Performance, 15,* 212-240.

Wanous, J.P., & Zwany, A. (1977). A cross-sectional test of need hierarchy theory. *Organizational Behavior and Human Performance, 18,* 78-97.

Yinon, Y., Bizman, A., & Goldberg, M. (1976). Effect of relative magnitude of reward and type of need on satisfaction. *Journal of Applied Psychology, 61,* 325-328.

Young, L.C., & Hayne, A.N. (1988). *Nursing administration from concepts to practice.* Philadelphia: W.B. Saunders.

Yura, H. (1986). Human need theory: A framework for the nurse supervisor. *The Health Care Supervisor, 4*(3), 45-58.

Chapter 24

Motivation-Hygiene Theory
Frederick Herzberg

Glenda C. Floyd

‖ CASE STUDY

Linda Johnson, a 40-year-old married woman, applied for a job as a staff nurse in a psychiatric hospital. Her husband is a physician, and she was seeking employment after 5 years as a homemaker. Her verbalized reasons for applying were (1) diversion from the household routine and (2) fear of losing the skills she had acquired.

She graduated from a diploma program and then completed her bachelor's degree in nursing. She had approximately 10 years of nursing experience (5 were in supervision) before applying for this job. She stated that she did not want the responsibilities of a leadership role.

She was selected for the position of staff nurse. However, within a few months she began to show dissatisfaction with the job. Some of the signs of her unhappiness were interrelationship problems. She had disagreements with staff and other departments. When she was dissatisfied, she threatened to resign and became unreasonable with her demands. She turned concerns of staff into a personal confrontation, which caused them to question her ability as a leader. Small occurrences were exaggerated into catastrophic events.

In spite of the negative aspects of Linda's performance, she had some strong leadership abilities. She made thorough and equal assignments, relieved the head nurse, and effectively completed the time assignments. She also gave excellent patient care and had good rapport with patients.

She had obtained certification in psychiatric nursing and frequently attended continuing education programs on her own time. She was very amiable about her work schedule and would work compensatory time for patient care coverage. However, her unscheduled leave use was above average with a pattern of abuse.

Some of Linda's frequent complaints were that she worked too hard, received poor pay and inadequate recognition, and lacked staff respect. The head nurse wondered what could be done to increase Linda's job satisfaction.

‖‖‖

HERZBERG'S MOTIVATION-HYGIENE THEORY

Frederick Herzberg established the motivation-hygiene theory in 1959 following 2 years of literature review on job satisfaction (Miner, 1980). This theory classifies achievement, recognition, the work itself, responsibility, and advancement as job satisfiers because they are more likely to motivate individuals to excel in performance and produce positive attitudes. The items identified as dissatisfiers are company policy, administration, supervision, salary, interpersonal relations with co-workers, and working conditions. These have been labeled as hygiene factors. These hygiene items are nonmotivators because they only prevent dissatisfaction and do not improve attitudes or performance. These are two independent dimensions—one to achieve satisfaction and the other to prevent dissatisfaction (Marriner-Tomey, 1988).

CASE ANALYSIS

The case of Linda Johnson was analyzed according to the motivation-hygiene theory. The causes of the employee's dissatisfaction with her work assignments were carefully reviewed. Some of the problems identified were lack of recognition and needs for increased responsibilities and professional growth. According to Herzberg's theory, if these areas are corrected, the employee should be satisfied and performance should improve.

The first area addressed was responsibility. Linda made the statement, "You mean I went to school for 7 years and I am doing the same work as nurse's aides?" Her assignments and capabilities were reviewed. As a result, her duties and responsibilities were expanded. She was made coordinator for patient teaching and documentation. When this assignment was running smoothly, she was given assistant head nurse functions. She completed time schedules and filled in for the head nurse. In the role of head nurse relief, she provided supervisory coverage in the hospital on weekends and holidays. She was also assigned to the recruitment team that goes to colleges to recruit nurses. She was put on the committee that sets salaries and hires new nurses.

The second area considered was professional growth. Linda was encouraged to join the professional association and the Nursing Honor Society. She became officers in these organizations. She also earned certification in medical-surgical nursing.

The third motivator to Linda was recognition through salary increases. She was given an increase in pay after she proficiently performed the expanded role. She was also paid extra for certification. The next year she was promoted to the head nurse pay level but remained a staff nurse.

Linda has now worked at her present job for 12 years and has become a dynamic leader for staff. She no longer causes confusion with other hospital departments. She encourages staff when they are dissatisfied and has helped two staff members obtain aid for college courses. Linda's leave record has improved. She was taking sick leave as accrued and now she has a month of leave saved.

In this case study, increased responsibility, professional growth, recognition, and salary were major motivators for Linda Johnson. She was financially secure prior to her employment; however, a major part of recognition to Linda was financial rewards.

RESEARCH

Kahn (1961) reviewed Herzberg, Mausner, and Snyderman's *Motivation to Work* and discovered that the most important finding was that satisfiers and dissatisfiers are caused by two different factors, not more or less of the same factor (p. 9).

Numerous studies replicated the original research and found varying support for the motivation-hygiene theory. House and Wigdon (1967) and Dunnette, Campbell, and Hakel (1967) disagreed with the simplicity of the theory and established data that did not support this theory.

In order to study the motivation-hygiene theory explicitly, King (1970) took five distinct versions of the theory and determined that three were invalid and two contained defensive-biases. Gordon, Pryor, and Harris (1974) also identified biases in the storytelling method that prevented respondents from recording negative reactions to motivators and positive reactions to hygienes. Miner (1981) states that

> scorer reliability appears to be good. However, the tendency has been to relate theoretical variables and criterion measures obtained at the same time as part of the same measure. Under these conditions, response bias is almost inevitable and it is apparent that it does occur. Thus, the preferred measure leaves much to be desired in testing the theory. (p. 87)

Schwab and Henemen (1970) tried to validate Herzberg's motivation-hygiene theory by using the storytelling method that was originally used (Herzberg et al., 1959). However, their study tried to eliminate the biases identified in Herzberg's study.

Schwab, DeVitt, and Cummings (1971, p. 294) contend that there is another area of controversy about the two-factor theory. They identify the theory and problem. The theory states that performance effects are more likely to be associated with the satisfiers (hence the term "motivators") than with dissatisfiers. The latter serve merely to maintain performance levels (hence the term "hygienes"). From the view of employee performance, clearly this hypothetical linkage between satisfiers and performance is of more concern than the contention that satisfiers and dissatisfiers differ qualitatively, per se. Indeed, in recommendations for executive action, Herzberg (1966) has stressed the performance implications in his theory.

In order to establish further the relevancy of the motivation-hygiene theory, Grigaliunas and Herzberg (1971) had three hypotheses. This study supported the theory that motivators are more likely to be satisfiers and hygiene factors are most often dissatisfiers.

In 1974 Herzberg and associates expanded the theory to include the mentally ill. This study reviewed the degree of motivational inversion as compared to the degree of mental illness. Inversion is the predisposition to dirve affective experiences of both relief and fulfillment from pain avoidance. A direct relationship between the severity of mental illness and the degree of motivational inversion was supported.

Robert Ford (1973) applied the two-factor theory to job enrichment. He identified work aspects that "maintain" employees as wages, fringe benefits, nice working area, and the like. He called the "use me well" the work motivators (p. 97). To expand the original theory, Herzberg and Zantra (1976) applied it to job enrichment by measuring the quality of job satisfaction. They did job satisfaction surveys at Ogden Air Logistics Center after implementing the Orthodox Job Enrichment Program.

For personal clarification of Herzberg, Mausner, and Snyderman's book *The Motivation to Work* (1959), Kahn (1961) carefully reviewed the book and found areas for skepticism. However, he felt that the book clearly identified a linkage between attitudes and motivation and a distinction between satisfiers and dissatisfiers. He further noted that these findings were probably related to using employee descriptions of job attitudes and the cause and the actions they created. Individuals recorded recognition as the major reason for high job attitude and unfairness for low job attitude. The controversy arises in the individual's personal perception of whether he or she deserves recognition or not. Kahn believes that this research with more objective measures could have a significant impact on large organizations.

The motivation-hygiene theory can be classified into a content or intrinsic category and a context or extrinsic category, according to Wolf (1970). Biases are easily built into studies of these factors because people tend to attribute satisfaction as internal and dissatisfaction as environmental or external (Vroom, 1964). The two-factor theory is plagued with controversial results. Content and context factors can be either satisfiers or dissatisfiers.

Regarding the two-factor theory, Wolf (1970) states, "Herzberg erred by equating 'satisfaction' with 'motivation.' Satisfaction is an end state, while motivation is a force (drive) to achieve an end state. Atkinson and Feather (1966) define a motive as a "disposition to strive for a certain kind of satisfaction'" (p. 90).

Job motivation results from the opportunity to satisfy an active need through certain work behaviors. The satisfaction is greater when an ungratified need is satisfied than when a need is continuously gratified.

Hygiene factors are not motivators because they usually cannot be changed by employee behaviors. They are controlled by management and organizational objectives. Salary has been found to be a satisfier and a dissatisfier. The motivating factor in salary depends on the individual's high expectancy to increase the salary and if the employee sees a direct relationship between pay and performance. When the relationship is not perceived, the employee perceives salary as a dissatisfier because it prevents gratification of other needs (Wolf, 1970).

King (1970, pp. 19-22) established the following five theories based on the two-factor theory to determine if motivators are mainly satisfiers and hygienes are primarily dissatisfiers:

Theory 1. All motivators combined contribute more to job satisfaction than to job dissatisfaction, and all hygienes combined contribute more to job dissatisfaction than to job satisfaction.

Theory 2. All motivators combined contribute more to job satisfaction than do all hygienes combined, and conversely the hygienes contribute more to job dissatisfaction than do the motivators.

Theory 3. Each motivator contributes more to satisfaction than to dissatisfaction (and conversely each hygiene contributes more to dissatisfaction than to satisfaction). (This is essentially a strong version of Theory 1.)

Theory 4. Each principal motivator is mentioned in good critical incidents more frequently than is any hygiene.

Theory 5. Only motivators determine job satisfaction, and only hygienes determine job dissatisfaction.

A hypothesis is validated only when it is supported by at least two different testing methods and where a collection of methods eliminate alternate hypotheses (Garner, Hake, and Eriksen, 1956; Webb, Campbell, Schwartz, & Sechrest, 1966). According to these criteria, Theories 1, 2, and 3 have not been validated. No relevant data were available to support theories 4 and 5. The study was then restricted to Theories 1, 2, and 3 (King, 1970).

Another criticism of Herzberg's two-factor theory was that bias was introduced by relaying the recall of critical incidents (Eiven, 1964) and by the restricting of negative responses to motivators and positive reactions to hygienes (Gordon et al., 1974).

Gordon, Pryor, and Harris (1974) took King's three theories and devised a checklist with a 7-point scale so subjects could indicate levels of satisfaction and dissatisfaction. Questionnaires were administered in the scheduled classes by school staff. Approximately 1 month after the first study, a retest was conducted to establish reliability. King's (1970) Theory 1, which states that there will be more satisfying motivators than dissatisfying and more dissatisfying hygienes than satisfying, was investigated (Gordon et al., 1974). This study revealed more motivation and hygiene satisfiers than dissatisfiers. Theory 2 states that there will be more satisfying motivators than satisfying hygienes, and more dissatisfying hygienes than dissatisfying motivators. Even though motivators were more frequently satisfiers than hygienes, the motivators and hygienes did not differ as a source of dissatisfiers in this study. Theory 3 was rejected because it is a stronger version of Theory 1. More positive than negative responses were given to motivators and hygienes in the study (Gordon et al., 1974).

Two criticisms of Herzberg's theory on job satisfaction—reliability of response classification and analysis and interpretation of individual responses—were reviewed by Schwab and Heneman (1970). To examine intercoder reliability, 85 supervisors were asked to identify times they felt exceptionally good or bad about their present job. These responses were analyzed by two coders who placed responses in sequence of events and identified favorable and unfavorable sequence and thought units.

The analysis tended to conform to previous studies. Close analysis of individual responses shows that over half of the respondents did not follow the two-factor theory. Forty percent gave favorable and unfavorable responses to motivators. Although achievement and recognition were mentioned more as satisfiers than dissatisfiers, more than 25% of participants described them in both the favorable and unfavorable sequence. Four motivators and five hygiene group responses were too infrequent for statistical analysis. The overall study supported Herzberg and associates' original results (1959) and those summarized by Herzberg (1966); because this study erred in predicting individual attitudes more often than not, however, the theory needs modification (Schwab & Heneman, 1970).

To further test the two-factor theory regarding the connection between job satisfaction and performance, Schwab, DeVitt, and Cummings (1971) used the storytelling technique. A questionnaire was given to 124 volunteers from seven geographical offices of a public accounting management consulting firm. Eighty-five questionnaires were included in the study. Participants were asked to identify a time at work in which they felt really good (bad) and describe what happened to cause that feeling. Coders then classified the statements into 16 categories (6 satisfiers and 10 dissatisfiers). Respondents were then asked to rate themselves from extremely productive to extremely unproductive during these times of favorable and unfavorable consequences. Performance effects could not be attributed to motivators or hygienes. There was an attributable difference if the individual perceived the job experience as favorable or unfavorable (Schwab et al., 1971).

Grigaliunas and Herzberg (1971) further studied the relevancy of the motivator-hygiene theory by examining three hypotheses:

Hypothesis 1. The content analysis coding will yield the predicted M-H theory results—the high incidents will consist of significantly more motivator sequences while the low incidents will consist of significantly more hygiene sequences.

Hypothesis 2. The S's rating of the statements will not yield the predicted M-H theory results. Both motivation and hygiene statements, but especially motivator statements, will be rated highly for both high and low incdients.

Hypothesis 3. When only the relevant ratings are used, the predicted M-H theory outcome will result. The high incidents will consist of significantly more motivator sequences while the low incidents will consist of significantly more hygiene sequences. (p. 74)

Hypothesis 1 was validated through research of 43 male and 38 female college students. In the high incidents of satisfaction, 71% were motivator sequences and 29% were hygiene. In the dissatisfiers sequence, 79% were hygienes and 21% motivators. Hypothesis 2 was substantiated when researchers found motivators to be more important than hygienes in determining job satisfaction/dissatisfaction. For hypothesis 3, judges read 76 high and 81 low sequences and rated them on relevancy. They found 67% of satisfiers were motivators and 33% were hygienes. Of the dissatisfiers, 72% were hygienes and 28% motivators.

When the motivation-hygiene theory is applied to the mentally ill, the hygiene factors are considered pain avoidance and the motivation is growth. Herzberg, Mathapo, Wiener, and Wiesen (1974) found a direct relationship between the degree of mental illness and the satisfying aspects of pain avoidance and growth. The greater the disturbance, the more satisfying is pain avoidance; the lesser the mental illness, the greater the satisfaction of growth.

As an outgrowth of the motivation-hygiene theory, the American Telephone and Telegraph Company (AT&T) conducted studies on job enrichment. In one study Ford (1973) identified maintenance factors as hygienes or "treat me well" and motivators as "use me well" (p. 97).

Capable employees were given additional duties with control to execute these responsibilities. This meant that supervisory responsibilities were moved downward. For example, the service representatives became responsible for all parts of customer service. The representative decided when a customer must be contacted and did this without supervisory intervention. Work was also divided into modules, and workers were able to do more than was originally expected. As the employee gained experience, the responsibilities were increased.

Job enrichment decreased employee turnover, decreased job duplication and fragmentation, improved morale, and increased production. These improvements were made by using motivators. Hygiene factors were also used. Employees who were increasing production and assuming additional responsibilities expected to be compensated financially (Ford, 1973).

In 1976, Herzberg and Zantra expanded previous studies on the two-factor theory to include job enrichment strategies in the Ogden project. In this study middle managers were taught to redesign jobs according to the motivation-hygiene principles and implement these changes for job enrichment for employees. This study identified three hypotheses to evaluate the effectiveness of job enrichment. The first one was that employees would report positive changes attributed to job enrichment. The second hypothesis expected emphasis to be on three motivators: responsibility, advancement, and growth. Third was the spread of job enrichment concepts throughout the company (Herzberg & Zantra, 1976).

Many researchers have investigated the validity of Herzberg's motivation-hygiene theory. The theory contends that motivators (achievement, recognition, advancement, and the work itself) are predominantly satisfiers and hygienes (salaries, working conditions, company policy, administration, and relationships) are most often dissatisfiers. Researchers have been about equally divided between support and nonsupport of this theory.

Classifying motivators is difficult without identifying individual needs and the mental status of those individuals being studied. There is a tendency for motivators to be satisfiers more frequently than hygienes; however, studies identified hygienes that were equally satisfying as motivators.

Job enrichment was an outgrowth from the Herzberg theory. Ford's study (1973) at AT&T showed that employees were more satisfied when their abilities were recognized, when duties commensurate with employee's capabilities were assigned, and when duties were combined into modules with added responsibilities.

The current studies that have been conducted in nursing are primarily interested in what motivates individuals to apply for a job, excel in performance, remain on a job. Nursing studies conducted within the past 10 years have concentrated on reviewing motivators as they apply to job turnover (Ulrich, 1978), performance (Lancaster, 1986; Warren, 1978), and job satisfaction (Lenz, 1986; Eason & Lee, 1987).

Ulrich conducted a study in a hospital with turnover rates for registered nurses of 60% to 70% annually. Herzberg's two-factor theory was used to explain nursing management problems. Of the 139 nurses, 47 volunteered for the study. This research supported previous work of Herzberg's that identified intrinsic factors as predominantly satisfiers and extrinsic elements as mainly dissatisfiers. Two extrinsic elements were added as dissatisfiers. These were incurable illness and interpersonal relations with patients and kin (Ulrich, 1978).

Positive achievement occurred 59.1% of the time, whereas negative achievement was noted 23.5% of the time. Responsibility was the one intrinsic item that had more negative responses than positive (21.6 and 6.8). All extrinsic elements except interpersonal relations with peers were negative more than positive (Ullrich, 1978).

According to Ullrich, dissatisfactions with intrinsic and extrinsic factors are associated with turnover rates in nursing. One important part of a decision to leave a job is the individual aspirations of nurses. When these are unmet, there is major dissatisfaction. Therefore, hospital administration must arrange the job environment to meet the nurse's aspirations. Otherwise, there will be dissatisfaction and high turnover rates (Ullrich, 1978).

There is controversy over money being a motivator or hygiene. Lenz (1986) believes that it is a motivator because of its symbolic nature. It represents almost all values people are motivated to pursue. When money is a reward for performance, it is a motivation; however, the leader must determine its importance to individuals.

In today's society, money serves as a measuring device for accomplishments, competence, achievement, and prestige (Lenz, 1986). Merit pay is determined by competence and achievements. This pay is used to compare co-workers' performance and denote approval by leaders.

According to research, the achievement motive is most influential in determining success or failure of an enterprise. In the achievement-motivated individual, money is a measurement of accomplishment. Prestige, although not a true motivator, provides positive reinforcement when an employee excels over a co-worker (Lenz, 1986).

All nursing leaders must be cognizant of providing a motivating environment and identifying motives of subordinates. Money can motivate by reinforcing an employee's motives. Lack of monetary rewards can decrease employee motivation (Lenz, 1986).

Eason and Lee (1987) had 120 baccalaureate nursing students identify the reasons they would take a job. They were asked to rank from most important to least important eight variables: interesting work, good pay; desirable work hours; good benefits, such as vacation time and insurance; job location near home; opportunity available to earn MSN; association with a progressive medical school; and nice, comfortable work area (Eason and Lee, 1987, p. 4).

The findings in this study cannot be applied to the worksite because these were students. However, the highest ranked variable was interesting work. The second most important item was good pay. Then desirable working hours, good benefits, having a job near home, and a comfortable work area were identified.

These results agreed with those in a study reported by Marriner and Craigie (1977) who surveyed nurses regarding job satisfaction. "They identified a sense of achievement, recognition, challenging work, responsibility, pleasant work environment, and agreeable working hours as satisfiers" (p. 350). The above-listed variables are significant in nurse recruitment. Administrators should take these into consideration when establishing recruitment strategies (Eason & Lee, 1987).

Stroking is a method of employee motivation discussed by Davidhizar and Giges (1987). Stroking consists of giving positive reinforcement, encouraging, praising, appreciating, and respecting personnel. Positive reinforcement can be external (monetary) or internal (praise, appreciation, and respect). An employee with a good self-image performs better. Rewarding and encouraging build self-esteem (Davidhizar & Giges, 1987).

A common statement is that a good nurse is rewarded by promotion into an administrative position instead of remaining in patient care. Warren (1978) reported on a study in Presbyterian Medical Center (PMC) in Colorado, which established an earned Staff Nurse II position. In order to achieve the position, a nurse must earn at least 65 approved, validated credits, of which 15 must be by special projects. To maintain this position, the nurse must earn 12 educational credits and participate in one project annually. Certificates are given when credits are earned. This program has enabled nurses to be rewarded with recognition and increased pay and yet remain at the bedside. Paying qualified staff nurses is more economical than training new ones who may not be as qualified to perform the job (Warren, 1978).

Lancaster (1986) identified four preconditions to motivation: a recognizable need, a goal, drive to meet goals, and a reward or payoff. Managers can provide a nurturing environment by helping people feel good about themselves. Some ways to help employees feel good are to emphasize results rather than techniques, match employee talents to job, be interested in an employee as a person, emphasize strengths, and be supportive during change.

There must be clear communication between manager and employee. For employees to establish clear goals, they must understand their manager's organizational goals and expectations. Employees need feedback and reinforcement without threats (Lancaster, 1986).

Managers are responsible for providing opportunities and encouraging employee growth, including effective communication, making expectations clear, helping employees establish specific goals, and identifying performance (Lancaster, 1986).

Recent studies have emphasized motivation without specifically dividing variables into motivators and hygiene factors. Although the emphasis has not been directly related to Herzberg's two-factor theory, these studies supported that motivators (achievement, recognition, the work itself, and advancement) were primarily satisfiers. Contrary to the two-factor theory, most authors identify money as a motivator. However, the symbolic meaning of money as recognition for achievement is consistent with the theory.

Related research is important for nurse managers for recruitment, retention, and job satisfaction. Nurses must be attracted to a facility and then the manager must set the environment for the nurse to achieve the desired goals.

REFERENCES

Atkinson, J.W., & Feathers, N.T. (1966). *A theory of achievement motivation.* New York; Wiley.

Davidhizar, E., & Giges, J.N. (1987). Management stroking motivating employees. *AORN Journal, 46,* 492-496.

Dunnette, M.D., Campbell, J.D., & Hakel, M.D. (1967). Factors contributing to job satisfaction and job dissatisfaction in six occupational groups. *Organizational Behavior and Human Performance, 2,* 143-174.

Eason, F.R., & Lee, B.T. (1987). Job motivators: A ranking of eight variables. *Journal of Nursing Administration, 17*(6), 4, 35.

Eiven, R.B. (1964). Some determinants of job satisfaction: A study of the generality of Herzberg's theory. *Journal of Applied Psychology, 48,*161-163.

Ford, R.N. (1973). Job enrichment lessons from AT&T. *Harvard Business Review, 51*(1), 96-106.

Garner, W.K., Hake, H.W., & Erikson, C.W. (1956). Operationalism and the concept of perception. *Psychological Review, 63,*149-159.

Gordon, M.E., Pryor, N.M., & Harris, B.V. (1974). An examination of scaling biases in Herzberg's theory of job satisfaction. *Organizational Behavior and Human Performance, 11,* 106-121.

Grigaliunas, B.S., & Herzberg, F. (1971). Relevancy in the test of motivator-hygiene theory. *Journal of Applied Psychology, 55,* 73-79.

Herzberg, F. (1966). *Work and the nature of man.* Cleveland: World.

Herzberg, F., Mathapo, J., Wiener, Y., & Weisen, L. (1974). Motivation-hygiene correlates of mental health: An examination of motivational inversion in a clinical population. *Journal of Consulting and Clinical Psychology, 42,* 411-419.

Herzberg, F., Mausner, B., & Snyderman, B.S. (1959). *The motivation to work.* New York: Wiley.

Herzberg, F., & Zantra, A. (1976). Orthodox job enrichment: Measuring true quality in job satisfaction. *Personnel, 53*(5), 54-68.

House, R.J., & Wigdon, L.A. (1967). Herzberg's dual factor theory of job satisfaction and motivation: A review of the evidence and a criticism. *Personnel Psychology, 20,* 369-390.

Kahn, R.L. (1961). Review of the motivation to work. *Contemporary Psychology, 6,* 9-10.

King, N. (1970). Clarification and evaluation of the two-factor theory of job satisfaction. *Psychological Bulletin, 74,*(1), 18-31.

Lancaster, J. (1986). Motivation creating the environment. *AORN Journal, 43*(1), 202-208.

Lenz, C.L. (1986). Money as a motivator. *JONA, 16*(9), 4-5.

Marriner, A., & Craigie, D. (1977). Job satisfaction and mobility of nursing educators in baccalaureate and higher degree programs in the west. *Nursing Research, 26,* 349-360.

Marriner-Tomey, A. (1988). *Guide to nursing management* (3rd ed.). St. Louis: C.V. Mosby.

Miner, J.B. (1980). *Theories of organizational behavior.* Hinsdale, IL: Dryden.

Miner, J.B. (1981). Theories of organizational motivation. In G.W. England, A.K. Negandhi, & B. Wilpert (Eds.), *The functioning of complex organizations.* Cambridge, MA:

Schwab, D.P., DeVitt, H., & Cummings, L. (1971). A test of the adequacy of the two-factor theory as predictor of self-report performance effects. *Personnel Psychology,* 293-303.

Schwab, P.D., Heneman, H.G., III (1970). Aggregate and individual predictability of the two-factor theory of job satisfaction. *Personnel Psychology, 23,* 55-66.

Ullrich, R.A. (1978). Herzberg revisited: Factors in job dissatisfaction. *Journal of Nursing Administration, 8,* 19-24.

Vroom, U.H. (1964). Work and motivation. New York: Wiley.

Warren, J.B. (1978). Motivating and rewarding the staff nurse. *Journal of Nursing Administration, 8,* 4-7.

Webb, E.J., Campbell, D.T., Schwartz, R.D., & Sechrest, L. (1966). *Unobtrusive measures: Nonreactive research in the social sciences.* Chicago: Rand-McNally.

Wolf, M.G. (1970). Need gratification theory: A theoretical reformulation of job satisfaction/dissatisfaction and job motivation. *Journal of Applied Psychology, 54,* 87-94; *70,* 10.

Chapter 25

Achievement-Motivation Theory John Atkinson, David McClelland, and Joseph Veroff

Debbie Reese Hutchinson

❙❙   CASE STUDY

Marie Allison was a nursing manager at the Johnston Medical Center. She had a staff of excellent nurses, two of whom were restless and constantly looking for creative outlets. Marie was concerned that Katherine and Jessica might look for other jobs if she did not challenge their energies appropriately.

Jessica was a BSN graduate who had worked in staff positions in various units within the hospital. She was extremely active in social arenas within the community, always organizing and arranging various functions and activities. She had worked on several projects within the hospital and chaired several committees at various times. Organization of various groups was an area she managed well.

Katherine was a diploma graduate who was constantly involved in one project or another. As soon as one project was completed, another was initiated. She kept a continuing list of ideas that would benefit the unit. Clinical skills were a high priority, as well as continuing education. Katherine sought challenges that would allow her personal responsibility and recognition.

Marie was a diploma graduate who only a few years before accepting the nursing manager position had returned to work after raising her family. She now found that developing her nursing staff to their fullest potential brought her much satisfaction. Faced with the possible loss of two highly skilled and motivated nurses, she went to the nursing administrator for assistance in analyzing her staff's needs.

❙❙

ACHIEVEMENT-MOTIVATION THEORY

The achievement-motivation theory encompasses three forms of motivation:
1. *Need for achievement.* These individuals have a strong desire to achieve, a hope of success as well as a fear of failure. They work toward a specific set of goals and strive toward excellence.
2. *Need for power.* These people desire to have an impact, to be influential, and to

control others. They enjoy having the authority to be in charge and work well in competitive and status-oriented positions.

3. *Need for affiliation.* These individuals have a desire to be liked and accepted by others. They prefer cooperative situations rather than competitive ones and work well in supportive areas (Miner, 1980).

The need for achievement (n-Ach), the need for power (n-Pow), and the need for affiliation (n-Aff) are three social motives that make up the core of achievement-motivation theory. These motives (drives) have been labeled as *social* motives because they are human motivators that most frequently come into play and dominate situations when individuals interact with other people.

Motivation theory "attempts to account for the determinants of the direction, magnitude, and persistence of behavior in a limited but very important domain of human activities" (Atkinson, 1964, p. 241). The word *motivation* comes from the Latin *morvere,* "to move." We most often use this word when referring to a behavior that has been initiated by a drive or a force within an individual. The implication for understanding motivation can be great both personally and professionally. Behavioral interactions of individuals in a society force the individual to assess constantly the motives of others as well as those of her or his own.

In the 1950s and 1960s, prominent motivational researchers studied the achievement motivation in men and concluded that men were motivated to achieve success academically and professionally but specified that their theories did not apply to women. Working under a grant from the Office of Naval Research, McClelland and Atkinson investigated the relationship between how subjects who had gone long periods without food utilized food-related words in stories they wrote in response to various pictures (Atkinson & McClelland, 1948).

David McClelland took this original work and developed the theory that all motives are learned (McClelland et al., 1976). The degree to which the motive may influence behavior varies from individual to individual. McClelland's theory states that as people have different experiences during their lives they learn to associate positive and negative feelings with various events. These events may happen to or around them. High achievement needs (n-Ach) "is an inference as to the extent to which the person's behavior is guided by anticipated or past achievement satisfactions or dissatisfactions (a) in a standardized class of situations (b) within certain limits, as to the specific kinds of past experiences (reinforcements) the person has had in those situations (McClelland, 1975, p. 585). People may develop a strong n-Ach motive when they receive positive reinforcement from their accomplishments; thus they are stimulated to achieve more.

The individuals must know that their performance is being evaluated either by themselves or others "in terms of some standard of excellence and that the consequence of [their] actions will be either a favorable evaluation (success) or an unfavorable evaluation (failure)" (Atkinson, 1964, pp. 240-241).

The person with high n-Ach seeks out certain characteristic situations. They look for situations where they can attain success through their own efforts, accept personal responsibility, and receive personal credit for the outcome. They want to ensure that the chance of success is good. Risks are calculated. If a task is too difficult or the chance of succeeding minimal, the individual may find motive satisfaction low. The entrepreneur role is excellent for the high n-Ach.

The characteristics of a high-need achiever are as follows:

1. Focuses primarily on rewards of success
2. Competes against some standard of excellence such as an objective goal
3. Sets challenging but realistic goals for himself
4. Seeks feedback

5. Takes moderate risks
6. Prefers risk situations where he can affect the odds of succeeding
7. Likes entrepreneurial roles (Rue and Byars, 1977, p. 338).

Children's early orientation to what is expected of them can strongly influence their achievement motivation. As a child grows up, certain families or cultures are more prone to stress achievement, particularly when there can be competition with a predetermined standard of excellence. A family with strong achievement orientation stresses independence of the child at a early age.

Power is another motive that is incorporated into this theory. Power is the motive within that drives an individual to want to influence situations that have a direct impact on other people. The power motive drives people to want to gain recognition for their accomplishments through rewards that are prestigious and that can be publicly acclaimed. Power has long been a fascination for people. The quest for power is entrenched in our history, myths, and religion. David McClelland utilizes these examples in the introduction of his book *Power: The Inner Experience.* He discusses the biblical references to how God is believed to be all powerful and how religions other than Judaism and Christianity are intermingled in the need to control power (McClelland, 1975).

Four major elements are associated with the need for power (n-Power): (1) people whose need for power is high and who consequently can spend a great deal of time thinking about how to make a direct impact on other people; (2) a concern with how to control people and events; (3) a desire to get things accomplished through others; and (4) an interest in enhancing their personal status and reputation. Individuals with high n-Power express their needs through influencing others (McClelland, 1975). Individuals with high n-Power seek leadership positions.

Individuals' resources, assets, and personal attributes provide them with the bases of social power. Concerning the various bases of power, not only having the base(s) of power but also how these characteristics are perceived by others determines the degree of power an individual possesses. This perception can vary from relationship to relationship.

CASE ANALYSIS

When Marie met with her nursing administrator, she asked for assistance in analyzing what she could do to retain her staff as well as utilize their skills to their fullest potential. She received feedback on herself as well as her two nurses' possible motives.

The nursing administrator showed her the achievement-motivation theory and pointed out that her concern and desire to support her staff placed her as having strong affiliation needs. Jessica preferred to work in situations where she could maintain control and liked being influential. This preference could be associated with a strong need for power. Katherine had a strong desire to be successful and liked recognition for the projects she undertook and successfully completed. A strong need for achievement could be her associated need.

The hospital was about to initiate a new program for a clinical ladder. This concept for the nursing staff would give administrators a new way to reward the nursing staff in clinical practice for their efforts and willingness to accept professional peer review.

Marie went back to her unit and recommended that both nurses pursue the clinical ladder program. She discussed the achievement theory with them and ways that they could utilize this to benefit themselves both professionally and personally. Both nurses started the clinical ladder procedure. They found that this option offered challenges, recognition in status, and monetary gain. The nurses could see their efforts being rewarded and were motivated toward further accomplishments.

Katherine finished her bachelor in nursing degree shortly after completing the clinical ladder. She organized a new program at the facility and returned to school for her master's. Jessica became the nursing manager of one of the largest and more powerful nursing units in the facility. Marie continued her role as a nursing manager working with and encouraging her staff to seek their own individual pathways.

RESEARCH

Veroff and Veroff performed studies regarding "the desire for power in terms of influence and control" (Veroff & Veroff, 1972, p. 279). They utilized the Thematic Apperception Test (TAT) as their assessment technique and found that the power motive could be interpreted as a concern about weakness. Sex and education played a major role in the scores of the individuals. Men who attended school only until grade school had higher power motive scores than their counterparts who obtained higher education, but women had higher power motive scores with higher educational levels.

Veroff and Veroff felt that men scored the way they did because of the feelings of inferiority men of lower educational standings have in contrast to men with higher education. Race was another issue with black men (n = 38) scoring 61% above the median and white men (n = 538) scoring only 48% above the median in the sample. The scores are in relation to the need for power scores (Veroff & Veroff, 1972, p. 281).

Although women scored high on the power need, many have higher education and work in influential positions. They may derive their high needs scores from their nonconformity to the "traditional" woman's role. Single women as well as married women without children scored higher than mothers.

Women who have high n-Power view themselves as resourceful—a resource for the family by producing the children, the food, and emotional support (McClelland, 1975). The male with high n-Power is pictured as the aggressive, assertive protector of the family. "The male high in n-Power has an emotionally assertive approach to life, whereas the female high in n-Power focuses on building up the self which may be the object of that assertiveness" (McClelland, 1975, p. 51).

Expounding on McClelland and Atkinson's theories of motivation, Winter (1973) states that "there are said to be two achievement-related motives—Hope of Success (approach) and Fear of Failure (avoidance)" (p. 42). He feels an individual will respond according to their related hopes and fears.

The quest for power can be both an internal and external force for all humankind. In these days, with the threat of nuclear war ever present, David McClelland points out to us that "the need for understanding the psychology of power is even greater today, when man's capacity for destroying himself and the universe has reached a new level of seriousness" (McClelland, 1975, p. 4).

Affiliation is the third motive associated with the achievement-motivation theory. Examples of humankind's need to belong, to be loved, and to be socially acceptable have been with us for many years. Maslow sees the need for affiliation as being basic to the nature of man. Until this need is met, Maslow feels a person cannot go on to achieve status and self-actualization. Individuals with a high need of affiliation (n-Aff) have a strong need for social interaction and a need to belong and to be well liked. Affiliation has been the least studied of the three motives.

The major researchers in this area have been Shipley and Veroff and later Atkinson. They found individuals with high n-Aff also had a high need for security. Boyatzis took into consideration that there may be two types of affiliation, "hope of affiliation" (approach) and "fear of rejection" (avoidance) (cited in Beck, 1978, p. 355).

Affiliation is interpreted differently in correlation to sex. Many researchers have associated female achievement behavior with need for social approval (affiliation) rather than with achievement motivation. Stein and Bailey in their study "The Socialization of Achievement Orientation in Females" (1973) state that research on this "suggests that social skill and interpersonal relations are often important areas of achievement (i.e. attainment of excellence) for females" (p. 348).

A person with high n-Aff may face a difficult task as a manager because decisions must be made that will not be favorable for everyone. Professional roles that require good interpersonal skills tend to suit the individual with high affiliation needs.

Management is a process or form of work involving directing, guiding, and facilitating the efforts of a group of people toward meeting organizational goals or objectives. A manager must understand his or her own behavior and the behavior of others and utilize this knowledge to build a sound management foundation.

Nursing is a predominantly female profession. When McClelland and Atkinson did the original studies, they were funded by the Navy during a time when very few women (even nurses) were in the armed forces. Miner discussed the variety of research done on women in his book *Theories of Organization Behavior* (1980) and related that attempts to apply the theory to women did not meet with much success. The reason could be related to the testing techniques, the goals that women value, and the culturally prescribed sex roles of women today (Miner, 1980).

Nursing has long been considered a traditional career choice for women who wish to make marriage and children their major occupation. In the past decade an emphasis on and an increase in professionalism in nursing has brought about a new respect for the professional nurse.

> In the nursing organization, administrators and supervisors are beginning to realize that if . . . professional nurses are not permitted to express their competence motives in the care of patients, the departments as a whole will suffer the consequences. (Alexander, 1978, p. 102)

When we know the type of motivation and the needs regarding these motives that the individual may have, we can make certain predictions.

> For example, knowledge of n-Achievement scores will enable us to predict how well a group of people will do in a laboratory task, but knowledge of n-Affiliation scores will not. Knowledge of n-Affiliation scores will enable us to predict something about popularity where knowledge of n-Achievement scores will not. (McClelland, 1955, p. 42)

Managers could benefit from understanding what each motivator's characteristic needs are.

Successful managers need to have this understanding of their personal motives and their employees' motives. Managers may find themselves more successful if they have stronger needs for power than for affiliation and achievement. Achievers need to feel the personal satisfaction of accomplishment, and in large organizations many tasks must be delegated. High need affiliation managers must struggle with making decisions that are not favorable to everyone. Part of the success of the high need for power individuals comes from expressing their needs through their concern for influencing people. This drive helps to make them successful.

Cornell (1987) discusses the need for organizations to utilize nurses with strong needs towards entrepreneurship and turn those drives into "intrapreneurship" for the organization. A person with a strong achievement need can make a good intrapreneur in a business or organization. However, Cornell states that intrapreneurship flourishes best in an environment where people are allowed to give their best and where a reward system is built in.

The high need achiever can do well professionally if placed with the organization in an intrapreneur role, but several factors should be taken into account. This type of individual may militate against strong control from administration or the parent company. Such individuals need to succeed through their own efforts and receive appropriate credit. Bureaucratic constraints and authority relationships make the high n-Ach uncomfortable.

Managers can utilize individuals with high need for achievement in certain areas and find them more productive than individuals with low n-Ach.

1. Situations of moderate risk offer a challenge yet provide a good chance for goals to be accomplished.
2. Situations where knowledge of results will be provided give the necessary feedback to people regarding their achievements.
3. Situations where individual responsibility is provided enable achievement-oriented persons to ensure that they receive the proper credit for their accomplishments (Korman, 1974).

A manager can take certain measures to facilitate the high achiever, such as joint goal setting, allowing personal responsibility, and frequent appraisals. Courtemanche (1986) discusses the importance of nurses knowing what power is, what it can do, and how to utilize power effectively. Alexander (1978) points out that "as professional nurses become more involved in complex patient care, community health care and research, an understanding of the achievement motive will be important" (p. 102). She related that the power motive is present but has been insufficiently researched to determine its true effects.

Management concerns revolving around individuals' affiliation needs can be utilized to produce more effective performances. An individual with a low affiliation need may not be responsive to others because whether others like them or not is of little concern to them. Someone with a high n-Aff may be overly concerned with how others perceive them, whereas an individual with a moderate n-Aff may become a very effective manager. Although working together productively remains important, individuals with the various need levels can often be placed in an area that produces the most beneficial results.

We have reached an age of specialization that far exceeds any previous period. We have an increased number of highly trained and educated professionals entering the health care profession, and nurses must strive to improve their understanding and practice in working effectively with other professionals. "The traditional content factors in motivation such as money, security, and status and the more sophisticated factors such as power, competence, and achievement play important roles in work motivation" (Alexander, 1978, pp. 101-102).

Nurses are now teaching assertiveness skills and placing new emphasis on the important roles that nurses play in the health care industry. Clinical ladder programs, continuing education, and modification of higher degree programs to accommodate the professional nurse allow the high achievers avenues to excel.

Power can be interpreted as knowledge. Nurses have the capacity to increase the power of their peers, themselves, and their clients through education. Nursing management can provide information to their staff, and in turn the staff can provide information to their clients. This continuing exchange of knowledge provides an increase in everyone's power base.

Achievement-motivation theory has been utilized very little in nursing management. The concept is one that could be expounded on for nursing, particularly with educators now evaluating both female and male responses. Goals are something the health care profession is continually addressing. The utilization of individuals' needs to benefit the overall institution or industry cannot help but benefit all parties involved.

REFERENCES

Alexander, E.L. (1978). Nursing administration in the hospital health care system. St. Louis: C.V. Mosby Company.

Atkinson, J.W. (1964). *An introduction to motivation.* New York: American Book.

Atkinson, J., & McClelland, D.C. (1948). The projective expression of needs. 11. The effect of different intensities of the hunger drive on thematic apperception. *Journal of Experimental Psychology,* 643-658.

Beck, R.C. (1978). *Motivation: Theories and principles.* Englewood Cliffs, NJ: Prentice-Hall.

Cornell, D. (1987). Management brief—Intrapreneurship in nursing. *Nursing Management, 8,* 20-23.

Courtmanche, J. (1986). Powernomics: A concept every nurse should know. *Nursing Management, 7,* 39-41.

Korman, A. (1974). *The psychology of motivation.* Englewood Cliffs, NJ: Prentice-Hall.

McClelland, D.C. (1955). Some social consequences of achievement motivation. In M.R. Jones (Ed.), *Nebraska Symposium.* Lincoln, NB: University of Nebraska Press.

McClelland, D.C. (1975). *Power: The inner experience.* New York: Irvington Publishers.

McClelland, D.C., and Atkinson, J.W. (1976). *The achievement motive.* New York: Irvington Publishers.

Miner, J.B. (1980). *Theories of organization behavior.* Hinsdale, IL: Dryden.

Rue, L.W., and Byars, L. (1977). *Management—theory and application.* Homewood, IL: Richard D. Irwin.

Shipley, T.E., Jr., and Veroff, J. (1952). A projective measure of need for affiliation. *Journal of Experimental Psychology, 43,* 349-356.

Stein, G.A., and Bailey, M.M. (1973). The socialization of achievement orientation in females. *Psychological Bulletin, 5,* 345-356.

Veroff, J., and Veroff, J. (1972). Reconsideration of a measure of power motivation. *Psychological Bulletin, 4,* 279-291.

Winter, D. (1973). *The power motive.* New York: Collier MacMillan Publishers.

Chapter 26

Expectancy Theory
Victor Vroom

Sharon Holcombe Servais

❙❙ CASE STUDY

Over a 2-year period, a large emergency center experienced high turnover in nursing management. The nurses who left were mid-management, responsible for the day-to-day operations of the center. Each of three managers was responsible for one of three 8-hour shifts. Over this 2-year period, five managers resigned from the three positions. Early in this period, applicants for the positions were plentiful. The attractive salary served as the primary motivator for those pursuing advancement. In reviewing the professional age of the nurses who applied and occupied these positions, it was found that four of the five had practiced nursing less than 3 years. As staff members observed the fast turnover of managers, other prospective applicants from within the ranks grew fearful of applying for these positions. Late in this 2-year period, one position was vacant for 4 months.

The following observations were made. First, money was no longer a motivator. The general response among the staff nurses was "There's no amount of money to pay me to take that job!" Additional incentives, including specialty certification reimbursement, opportunity to attend management seminars, and flexible work hours, were also marketed to attract nurses to apply for this salaried position. All incentives were attached to a monetary reward.

Second, during the period of difficulty in recruiting this manager, behaviors were observed among the individuals most likely to be promoted, the alternates. These alternates were in charge of the shift in the absence of the supervisor. One alternate stood out from the rest in that she was in charge of this shift each time she worked. She demonstrated behaviors that indicated her distaste for the role she was filling by default. Her behaviors showed lack of teamwork, verbalization of negative feelings about coming to work, and inability to make any decision without consulting the director. It was suspected that these behaviors developed in this nurse and within the group of alternates because each feared he or she would be promoted into the open position.

Concerning the events surrounding specific turnover issues of the five managers who left the positions, a close look at the demographics of this department is revealing. The median age of the nurses was 30. The average age was 26. It would follow that internal hiring would come from a group of younger nurses. In this center, nurses over 30 who remained in staff positions did not aspire to management. Internal hiring was another issue. Promoting from within had traditionally served as a positive motivator. In this center, experience from hiring outside into management roles had proven hazardous because of increased orientation time and the lack of comparable centers within the area from which it recruits. Traditionally, higher success rates

245

had occurred with internal promotions. Therefore, if internal hiring was practiced, nurses in early stages of professional development would be the applicants.

One other variable comes into play in this situation. Traditionally, emergency care facilities are very clear on departmental goals and purposes. These mission statements include concepts such as acute management of life-threatening conditions, interim stabilization prior to transfer to inpatient care areas, and providing effective triage of patient conditions so as to meet the needs of each category of patients in a timely manner. The final half of this 2-year period was very stressful to the mission of the department. Availability of inpatient beds was diminished. Nursing shortages and high patient acuity had reduced the prompt availability of inpatient beds. Areas such as the post-anesthesia care unit and the emergency center were forced to hold critical patients for up to 48 hours because of this dilemma. The mission of the emergency center was challenged. Not only was caring for long-term intensive patients difficult in this setting but also the nurses could not effectively (by their standard of emergency care) manage the emergency patients. This series of events cast a negative appearance on the management roles. The staff viewed management as a daily course of crisis intervention. The existing managers spent the majority of their day begging for inpatient beds and calling in additional staff to care for the intensive patients and little time developing themselves or their own staff. What could be done to make promotion appealing?

| | | | | | | | | | | | | | | | | | | | | | | | | | | | | | | | | | | | | | | | | | | | | | | | | | | | | | | | | | | | | | | | | | | | |

EXPECTANCY THEORY

Victor Vroom formalized the association of personality and environment into expectancy theory of work and motivation. The hedonistic concept of minimizing pain and maximizing pleasure is the basis for this theoretical framework. Vroom (1960) in his doctoral dissertation (p. 73) stated

$$\text{Performance} = \text{Ability} \times \text{Motivation}$$

This equation suggests that managers should strive to develop employees and motivate employees simultaneously. He also concluded that achievement of the ultimate effect of motivating employees depends on their aptitude and ability. This conclusion further demonstrates the dynamic role managers can play in selection and training to have an outcome of high employee motivation.

Further development of this theory by Vroom (1964) provided a second mathematical statement describing performance.

$$\text{Motivation} = \text{Expectancy} \times \text{Instrumentality} \times \text{Valence}$$

Descriptively, this formula states that the basis of a person's motivation toward job performance is the ideas he or she has about the outcome of job performance and the associated value placed on the outcome. Central to the theory is expectancy, the association between the action and the outcome. Instrumentality describes the type of outcome yielded by way of the action. The value placed on the desirability of the outcome is valence. Examples lend better understanding to these associations. First, consider a nurse manager who rewards good performance with an extra weekend off. Perhaps the nurse prefers to work weekends so she can attend classes during the week. The valence for the reward in this situation is negative; therefore, this reward would not serve as a motivator for the desired outcome. A contrast to this situation is the nurse who does not like to work weekends. The valence of the reward of an extra weekend off is positive, so this performance-outcome system would serve to motivate the nurse to high performance.

Another application can be made to demonstrate further the multiplicative relationship of Vroom's formula. In a situation where instrumentality is zero (no association between performance and reward), motivation would also be zero, regardless of the expectancy or valence. To illustrate this, consider a system where *all* nurses received a raise every year, regardless of performance. The raise cannot serve as a motivator because there is no association between the performance and the reward. Associations between performance and outcome should be made very clear by managers in order to motivate employees.

CASE ANALYSIS

Marriner-Tomey (1988) simplifies the expectancy theory when she states that "motivation is dependent on how much someone wants something and her estimate of the probability of getting it" (p. 234). If this process is applied to the case presented earlier, the outcome can be determined.

Fortunately for this center, the current managers were well prepared and maintained a strong team approach to the situation. This group of upper management had filled nursing roles for more than 5 years and possessed strong motivational abilities. Had the latter not been true, the entire center would have suffered.

Management theory provides many models to utilize in dealing with employee behavior. As displayed previously, Vroom's expectancy theory (1964) provides the framework for resolving this situation. The categories mentioned correspond to forces that provide the manager with the ability to anticipate and redirect employee behavior. The forces are expectancy, instrumentality, and valence. Expectancy is the perceived probability that an action will yield achievement of some goal. Instrumentality is the perception that performance of some goal will lead to a reward. Valence is the value assigned, by the employee, to the perceived reward. Several key factors derived from the case study are categorized according to Vroom's framework in Table 26-1.

In the case study, there was no immediate solution to changing the staff's attitude toward the management position. An organized approach was applied. The responsibilities of the remaining managers were redistributed so that all shifts had consistent management. Another level of management just below mid-management was created for those who were not quite ready for promotion but still were aspiring to management. This group of six nurses (two from each shift) was organized. Common objectives and expectations for the group were developed. A monthly meeting was established to allow them opportunity to interact and learn through management presentations done by upper management. This new program allowed them to slowly gain confidence and regain a positive valence toward promotion.

Through this 6-month process, an increase from 30% to 90% board certification occurred. These individuals, knowing specialty certification was required of all top management, independently pursued the certification process. The initial restructuring commitment was for 1 year. At the end of 6 months, two senior staff nurses expressed desire for promotion.

Departmental restructuring played a large role in restating work distribution. No changes in inpatient bed availability were anticipated. The emergency center was recategorized to allow for an area to meet the needs of nonacute patients in a timely manner, which increased positive patient feedback. This measure also allowed the emergency center to remain available for high acuity patients. A pool of part-time staff was developed and staff from the pool came in when

TABLE 26-1   Case Study Actions Analyzed Using Vroom's Framework

Actions/Behavior	Outcome	Instrumentality	Valence
Perform well as alternate manager	Promotion to manager	High	Negative
Demonstrate inability to make decisions or achieve teamwork from staff	No promotion to manager	High	Positive
Promotion to manager	Increase in pay	High	Positive (early) Negative (latent)
Promotion to manager	Additional management benefits	High	Positive (early) Negative (latent)
Promotion to manager	Fail as manager	Low (early) High (latent)	Negative
Promotion to manager	Performance of nothing but negative duties such as calling in help, shifting patients	High	Negative
Promotion to manager	Continue to practice emergency nursing along with managing	Low	Positive
Increased managerial function, decrease nursing function	Sense of competency	Low	Negative

critical patients were being held for extended periods. This streamlined the call-in process to decrease the amount of time managers spent calling in nurses.

Upper management played a strong supporting role. When senior staff nurses were in charge, one manager carried a beeper as a security blanket for the senior staff nurse. This precaution gave the senior staff nurses feelings of support and provided them with immediate feedback when problems arose beyond their managerial confidence level.

The final measure involved forced feedback. The nurses participated in patient callback 24 hours after their emergency center visit. The staff received positive reinforcement from patients. This feedback is often lacking in emergency settings, but this measure ensured it.

All of these measures were instituted to alter expectancy (a certain outcome would follow effort in the form of recognition and feedback), instrumentality (an association of effort to reward would exist in the form of promotion, available staff for call-ins, internal satisfaction from individual patient callbacks), and valence (the value assigned to the reward by improving the image of the manager by educating the senior staff nurses and recognizing that nurses at various levels of professional maturity have differing professional values).

At the 9-month period in this developmental project, an assessment was performed. No turnover in management or mid-management had occurred. The survey asked these nurses to rank the reasons they continued to work in the emergency center. Six nurses completed the survey, which identified educational opportunities, income, and chance to use ability as the top three ranked reasons to stay in the center. This assisted management in identifying job characteristics valued by the nurses. The survey also asked about expected reward versus actual reward. A summary of this information revealed these nurses received most of their motivation from their peers and colleagues and received most of their rewards from working hard and receiving monetary gain from pay increases and educational offerings. These data provided a management map for structuring performance outcome issues for the remaining 3 months. Management established a positive valence for promotion and identified an individually patterned reward system for each member of middle management.

RESEARCH

The importance of theory application and research can never be overemphasized. The application of theories to practice demonstrates that behavior is very similar and predictable across disciplines. A general review of generic research here is followed by a review of expectancy theory application to the practice of nursing.

Miner (1980) identifies Georgopoulos, Galbreath and Cummings, Porter and Lawler, and Graen as researchers whose work has developed and broadened the expectancy theory. A historical progression of this work will expand on Vroom's work.

Georgopoulos, Mahoney, and Jones (1957) asked the simple question of why some workers tend to be high producers while others with similar background, engaged in the same activity under comparable conditions, demonstrated varied output. The basic hypothesis they developed is:

> If a worker sees high productivity as a path leading to the attainment of one or more of his personal goals, he will tend to be a high producer. Conversely, if he sees low productivity as a path to the achievement of his goals, he will tend to be a low producer. (p. 346)

This hypothesis depends on two situations. First, needs must be high enough, and second, no other appealing paths are available to the worker. Georgopoulos and associates (1957) specifically identify path-goal perception, level of need, and level of freedom as determinants of productivity behavior. Sociopsychological variables, such as group norms, account for the remainder of the variance in individual performance.

The Georgopoulos study supported the hypothesis. The relationship between motivation and performance was documented. The results demonstrated opportunity for the manager to control facilitating and inhibiting forces to give the employee freedom to act; however, the high producer–low producer question was still subject to study.

Galbraith and Cummings (1967) identified three conditions necessary for the organizational reward system to impact employee behavior. First, the reward must be desirable to the employee. Second, the employee must associate variation in performance with variation in the amount of reward received. Finally, given desirability and association of reward, benefits such as organizational environmental factors and other controlling factors must be varied by the employer to produce variation in employee performance.

Lawler and Porter (1967) expanded the mathematical formula developed by Vroom. Miner (1980, p. 139) describes this formula as

Performance = f(Ability × Motivation)

That is, performance is a function of ability times motivation. Lawler and Porter (1967) identified factors that determine effort.

1. Value of rewards or valence
2. Probability that rewards depend on effort
3. Effort or motivational energy
4. Abilities or the individual's currently developed power to perform, including intelligence, skills, and personality traits

5. Role perceptions or the activities and behaviors the individual feels he or she should engage in to perform their job successfully

6. Performance or the amount of successful accomplishment

Miner (1980) describes the most recent feedback loop described by Porter and Lawler. Miner (1980) states that when "performance results in reward, the perceived effort-reward probability is increased" (p. 139). He also states that "when satisfaction is experienced after receiving a reward, it tends to influence the future value (valence) of that reward" (Miner, 1980, p. 139). His additional feedback loop enhances self-esteem and boosts expectancy. The additive effect results in greater performance.

Graen (1969) extends Vroom's expectancy theory to consider role concepts in defining differences between first level (being a "good" nurse) and second level (being rewarded for being a "good" nurse) outcomes. Graen (1969) defines a *work personality* "as a person's preferences for various consequences of attaining work roles and his dispositions for perceiving and evaluating various instrumentality and expectancy relationships" (p. 2). He also defines the *work role* "as a set of behaviors expected by the organization and considered appropriate of an incumbent of a position within the organization" (p. 2). The employee is motivated to behave (possess work personality) as expected for his or her work role. The attraction to the work role depends on perceived attraction of various role outcomes (valence specific to work role) and perceived relationship between work role and outcome (instrumentality specific to work role). The goal of relating these factors mathematically is to predict job satisfaction. Graen also participated in research of leadership turnover through instrumentality and equity theories (Dansereau, Cashman, & Graen, 1973).

Research can be grouped into studies of organizational design and its effect on motivation as well as the study of the use of motivational strategies to achieve job satisfaction. Organization design includes the job itself, on-the-job interactions, and policies that define or limit the job. Job satisfaction includes growth needs, work satisfaction, and satisfaction with career.

A quality of a job where expectancy theory is applied is the presence of clear, well-defined job expectations. The question then is raised as to the presence of a well-defined setting. Well defined does not imply rigidity. Motivation theory equates high satisfaction to high performance.

Lawler (1974) describes organization characteristics that allow for individual differences. These organizations allow for flexibility in self-placement choices, choice of hours worked, fringe benefit choices, style of supervision, and training offered. The employer matches the employee to the job and its setting. Research supports the concept that individuals respond differently to organizational policies and practices. Organizational design can maximize the motivating potential of a job by identifying individual reward systems.

Pinder (1976) questions the ethics of job redesign. He questions the evolution of motivation into manipulation and advises careful application of academic theories to real-world practices because the theories have not been thoroughly tested. By comparing two plants — one organized as to outcome and reward and one not — Dachler and Mobley (1973) demonstrated that organizational characteristics in the form of boundaries produced stronger performance-outcome contingencies. The expectancy model specified contingencies between performance and outcome that led to enhanced organizational effectiveness.

Kopelman and Thompson (1976) were able to expand the theory's domain into multicompany application. They found that certain boundary conditions (entry level and intrinsic versus extrinsic reward) affected the ability of expectancy theory to predict motivation. In another study, however, Reinharth and Wahba (1975) found inconsistencies between companies. They demonstrated more accuracy by using environmental and demographical predictors of work motivation than the actual expectancy model components. These efforts were all attempting to validate the predictive ability of expectancy theory.

Mitchell (1973) compared the effects of motivation through the structured expectancy theory using participative techniques or task-motivated techniques of management. His findings demonstrated the participative approach is successful in achieving motivation because participation increases the likelihood that employees will work for valued outcomes. In selection of personality variables in the employee to achieve high levels of motivation, five studies demonstrated the effects of existing inherent motivational traits, which weighted the overall valence component of the theory application. In other words, many variables affect valence, which reduces the overall predictive abilities of the theory. Wahba and House (1974), Matsui, Kagawa, Nagamatsu, and Ohtsuka (1977), Broedling (1975), Szilagyi and Sims (1975), and Lied and Pritchard (1976) all demonstrated that selecting employees for certain outcome was not purely independent of individual personality traits such as self-esteem, perceptions of one's own abilities, and internal-external traits.

Organizational policy controlling pay policies have also been shown to influence motivational levels. The argument for open pay policies (Miner, 1974) reveals that openness results in the increased instrumentality of pay policies in motivating employees. This argument is cloaked with caution from the standpoint that equity must exist or a perceived inequity in pay among employees could serve as a demotivator, as shown by Lawler (1968) and Klein (1973).

Lawler (1971) indicates that theory and research provide evidence that pay can motivate good performance, but certain conditions should exist. For pay to motivate, it must

1. Create a belief among employees that good performance will lead to high pay
2. Contribute to the importance of pay
3. Minimize the perceived negative consequences of performing well
4. Create conditions such that positive outcomes other than pay will be related to good performance (p. 45)

The need also exists to mention the concern that contingent financial rewards reduce intrinsic motivation, as shown by Pritchard, Campbell, and Campbell (1977). Arnold (1976) showed that extrinsic rewards do not affect or enhance intrinsic motivation when intrinsic motivation is high. Other attempts at quantifying intrinsic motivation were made by Farr, Vance, and McIntyre (1977), which led to further study of the appropriate method to study motivation-reducing variables such as individual differences and situational effects.

Although Miner (1981) calls expectancy theory a theory for the scholar and not the practitioner, one finds much truth in the basic premise that motivation is conscious and based on the pleasure-maximization principle (Mitchell, 1974). Perhaps the theory requires additional application instead of study to reveal the secrets of the associations between expectancy, instrumentality, and valence.

Nursing literature provides applications of this theory into practice. The same framework will be used to organize this research: organizational design and job satisfaction.

Organizational design can include the institution, setting, manager, interactions, policies, and so on. Looking at the manager first sets the stage for the organizational climate. The complexity of the nurse manager role requires much flexibility. Douglass (1984) believes nurses who have the potential to be flexible in their leadership styles can meet the flexibility required by the manager role. She applies Vroom's concepts that "Managers can develop the ability to select and use different leadership styles . . . in accordance with their analysis of the needs of the leader, follower, and work situation" (Douglass, 1984, p. 28).

Also applied to nursing practice is the Vroom and Yetton decision-making model. This model describes the participative problem-solving process that supports Vroom's expectancy theory in allowing employees to communicate rewards. Stevens (1985) described this model in her book *The Nurse as Executive*. La Monica and Finch (1977) applied this model to nursing education and practice. Their findings demonstrated involvement of all variables (the manager, the followers, environment, and their goals) in the process to assure the decisions reflect an awareness of how the variables integrate into a participative system. The leader in the application of this concept must again demonstrate flexibility of leadership style.

Institutional policy compliance is a prevalent issue in the practice of nursing. Shea (1986) applied expectancy theory to the completion of nursing care plans. A model was developed for use in examining nursing care plan behavior. Institution-specific variables were proposed to be subject to alteration and manipulation to increase nurse compliance with requirements. The nurse must see a benefit from the behavior to motivate compliance. Wong, Wong, and Mensah (1983) studied the effects of expectancy theory as applied to nursing students. Strategies were identified to enhance the student's need value by rewarding them for certain performances with desirable rewards. Lack of motivation for learning is the problem that stimulated this investigation. Wong and associates (1983, p. 116) state, "Teacher's moods, feelings, general philosophies and their use of learning theories indeed influence the students they teach." This is not unlike the management application. The mood, feelings, and professional behaviors of the manager all influence the employees' behaviors. The manager must be very familiar with personal philosophies and personal motivators in order to deal effectively with unmotivated employees.

Job satisfaction is essential in this day of critical nursing shortages. Nursing research shows promise for improving retention. Birkenbach and Vander Merwe (1983) were unable to use expectancy theory measures to predict turnover; however, expectancy concepts did influence turnover through identification of variables that influenced commitment and job satisfaction. Seybolt (1980) studied nurses at different stages in professional development. He found that different facets of the work role environment influence job and career satisfaction at different stages in the nurse's career. Seybolt (1986) designed a model of work role design that identifies characteristics of work that enable managers to predict premature turnover. Performance-outcome linkage, a component of expectancy theory, involves the employees' perception that they will receive certain valued outcomes if they perform at high levels. The most useful component of this application is the variability of desired reward across staff nurse stages of professional maturation. Seybolt (1986) states, "The work-role-design factors which explained the most variance in career satisfaction are autonomy, the amount of supervisory positive feedback, and the lack of role dissension" (p. 30). Singularly these factors influence turnover at different professional stages. Through extensive research of varied experience levels of nurses, Benner (1984) describes benefits people wish to gain from their work. Yankelovich (1974) identifies psychological benefits people strive to gain from their work.

1. Opportunity to advance to more interesting, varied, and satisfying work that pays better and wins more recognition than the individual's current job
2. Desire to do a good job at whatever one is doing
3. Yearning to achieve self-fulfillment through one's idea of "meaningful work"

This analysis supports the findings in other applications. In earlier work, Seybolt, Pavett, and Walker (1978) studied nurses in a large university hospital. The findings again documented that nurses' motivation to have a position was "dominated by a frustration of their needs for growth and development on the job" (Seybolt et al., 1978, p. 9).

Pavett (1983) applied expectancy concepts to a group of staff nurses. She observed an impact on performance and motivation when frequent positive feedback from supervisors and co-workers is given. Krizek (1987) applied Seybolt's work role design model to emergency nurses in a predictive fashion in an attempt to prevent turnover. She suggested environmental construction and manipulation as a measure to improve retention as professional needs change.

All of these studies where specific needs are identified are amenable to expectancy theory application.

Sullivan and Decker (1985) describe a nurse manager's approach to expectancy theory usage in staff motivation. They suggest that the nurse manager ask of each staff member, "What does this staff member believe about her or his ability to do the work (expectancy), the probability that the work will lead to outcomes (instrumentality), and the desirability of those outcomes (valence)?" (p. 109).

Finally, the issue of pay is discussed. Alexander (1978) reminds us that Vroom's model clearly supports the assumption that money influences satisfaction. She describes clinical supervisors who express satisfaction in salaries, but cautions that such reports should not be misinterpreted to decrease the importance of salaries. Seybolt (1986) does not discuss salary in his latest analysis of premature employee turnover. He places most of the emphasis on needs for growth and development in settings where competing hospitals paid similarly.

Walker and Thomas (1982) studied the application of expectancy theory to the compliance of an individual with preventive health care practices. The results supported the general theoretical model but named social norms, personality characteristics, and personal habits as potential additions to the theory to increase its predictive ability. Once a significant predicted model is refined, work role design can play a greater role in motivation.

The literature identifies a clear active role to be played by managers in preventing turnover through application of the expectancy model. Nursing is a good profession to study management theory because of high career mobility and few outside variables such as job shortage and lack of penalty for short-tenure positions.

The possibilities of predicting and preventing nursing turnover are exciting. Once the turnover issue is reduced, this identical model can address issues of job satisfaction. Further application of the expectancy model to specialty units is also needed. By design, specialty units are nursing centered, which allows for nursing manipulation to provide an environment amenable to retention. Study of these units utilizing expectancy theory in controlling turnover is needed. Application of the expectancy model to nursing accelerates the professionalization. Successful management is often judged by the motivation and achievement of employees. Future study should reflect the success of a nursing unit in terms of financial viability, retention, and overall customer satisfaction because of a performance-outcome model. This final application exemplifies the ultimate performance test of the professionalization of nursing.

REFERENCES

Alexander, E.L. (1978). *Nursing administration in the hospital health care system.* St. Louis: C.V. Mosby.

Arnold, H.J. (1976). Effects of performance feedback and extrinsic reward upon high intrinsic motivation. *Organizational Behavior and Human Performance, 17,* 275-288.

Benner, P. (1984). *From novice to expert.* Menlo Park, CA: Addison-Wesley.

Birkenbach, X.C., & Vander Merwe, R. (1983). An evaluation of the utility of expectancy theory in studying turnover in with nurses. *South African Journal of Psychology, 13*(3), 87-93.

Broedling, L.A. (1975). Relationship of internal-external control to work motivation and performance in an expectancy model. *Journal of Applied Psychology, 60*(1), 65-70.

Dachler, H.P., & Mobley, W.H. (1973). Construct validation of an instrumentality-expectancy-task-goal model of work motivation: Some theoretical boundary conditions. *Journal of Applied Psychology Monograph, 58,* 397-418.

Dansereau, F., Cashman, J., & Graen, G. (1973). Instrumentality theory and equity theory as complementary approaches in predicting the relationship of leadership and turnover among managers. *Organizational Behavior and Human Performance, 10,* 184-200.

Douglass, L.M. (1984). *The effective nurse leader and manager* (2nd ed.). St. Louis: C.V. Mosby.

Farr, J.L., Vance, R.J., & McIntyre, R.M. (1977). Further examinations of the relationship between reward contingency and intrinsic motivation. *Organizational Behavior and Human Performance, 20,* 31-53.

Galbraith, J., & Cummings, L.L. (1967). An empirical investigation of the motivational determinants of task performance: Interactive effects between instrumentality-valence and motivation-ability. *Organizational Behavior and Human Performance, 2,* 237-257.

Georgopoulos, B.S., Mahoney, G.A., & Jones, N.W. (1957). A path-goal approach to productivity. *Journal of Applied Psychology, 41,* 345-353.

Graen, G. (1969). Instrumentality theory of work motivation: Some experimental results and suggested modifications. *Journal of Applied Psychology Monograph, 53*(2), 1-24.

Klein, S.M. (1973). Pay factors as predictors to satisfaction: A comparison of reinforcement, equity, and expectancy. *Academy of Management Journal, 16,* 598-610.

Kopelman, R.E., & Thompson, P.H. (1976). Boundary conditions for expectancy theory predictions of work motivation and job performance. *Academy of Management Journal, 19,* 237-258.

Krizek, M.B. (1987). Emergency nursing recruitment and retention: Meeting the challenge of another nursing shortage. *Emergency Nursing Reports, 2*(7), 1-6.

La Monica, E., & Finch, F.E. (1977). Managerial decision making. *Journal of Nursing Administration, 7,* 20-28.

Lawler, E.E. (1968). Equity theory as a predictor of productivity and work quality. *Psychological Bulletin, 70,* 596-610.

Lawler, E.E. (1971). Using pay to motivate job performance. In B.M. Staw (Ed.), *Psychological foundations of organizational behavior.* Santa Monica, CA: Goodyear.

Lawler, E.E. (1974). The individualized organization: Problems and promise. *California Management Review, 17*(2), 31-39.

Lawler, E.E., & Porter, L. (1967). Antecedent attitudes of effective managerial performance. In V.H. Vroom & E. Deci (Eds.), *Management and motivation.* New York: Penguin.

Lied, T.R., & Pritchard, R.D. (1976). Relationships between personality variables and components of expectancy-valence model. *Journal of Applied Psychology, 61,* 463-467.

Marriner-Tomey, A. (1988). *Guide to nursing management* (3rd ed.). St. Louis: C.V. Mosby.

Matsui, T., Kagawa, M., Nagamatsu, J., & Ohtsuka, Y. (1977). Validity of expectancy theory as a within-person behavioral choice model for sales activities. *Journal of Applied Psychology, 62*(6), 764-767.

Miner, J.B. (1980). *Theories of organizational behavior.* Hinsdale, IL: Dryden.

Miner, J.B. (1981). Theories of organizational motivation. In G.W. England, A.R. Negandhi, & B. Wilpert (Eds.), *The functioning of complex organizations.* Cambridge, MA: Oelgeschlarger, Gunn, & Hain.

Miner, M.G. (1974). Pay policies: Secret or open? And why? *Personnel Journal, 53,* 110-115.

Mitchell, T. (1973). Motivation and participation: An integration. *Academy of Management Journal, 16,* 670-679.

Mitchell, T.R. (1974). Expectancy models of job satisfaction, occupational preferrence and effort: A theoretical, methodological, and empirical appraisal. *Psychological Bulletin, 81,* 1053-1077.

Pavett, C.M. (1983). Evaluation of the impact of feedback on performance and motivation. *Human Relations, 36,* 641-654.

Pinder, C.C. (1976). Concerning the application of human motivation theories in organizational settings. *Academy of Management Review, 2,* 384-397.

Pritchard, R.D., Campbell, K.M., & Campbell, D.J. (1977). Effects of extrinsic financial rewards on intrinsic motivation. *Journal of Applied Psychology, 62*(1), 9-15.

Reinharth, L., & Wahba, M.A. (1975). Expectancy theory as a predictor of work motivation, effort expenditure, & job performance. *Academy of Management Journal, 18,* 520-537.

Seybolt, J.W. (1980). The impact of work role design on the career satisfaction of registered nurses. *Proceedings, Academy of Management,* 42-46.

Seybolt, J.W. (1986). Dealing with premature employee turnover. *Journal of Nursing Administration, 16*(2), 26-32.

Seybolt, J.W., Pavett, C., & Walker, D.D. (1978). Turnover among nurses: It can be managed. *Journal of Nursing Administration, 8,* 4-9.

Shea, H.L. (1986). A conceptual framework to study the use of nursing care plans. *International Journal of Nursing Studies, 23*(2), 147-157.

Stevens, B.J. (1985). *The nurse as executive* (3rd ed.). Rockville, MD: Aspen.

Sullivan, E.J., & Decker, P.J. (1985). *Effective management in nursing.* Menlo Park, CA: Addison-Wesley.

Szilagyi, A.D., & Sims, H.P. (1975). Locus of control and expectancies across multiple occupational levels. *Journal of Applied Psychology, 60*(5), 638-640.

Vroom, V.H. (1960). *Some personality determinants of the effects of participation.* Englewood Cliffs, NJ: Prentice-Hall.

Vroom, V.H. (1964). *Work and motivation.* New York: Wiley.

Wahba, M.A., & House, R.J. (1974). Expectancy theory in work and motivation: Some logical and methodological issues. *Human Relations, 27*(2), 121-147.

Walker, L.R., & Thomas, K.W. (1982). Beyond expectancy theory: An integrative motivational model from health care. *Academy of Management Review, 7,* 187-194.

Wong, J., Wong, S., & Mensah, L. (1983). A conceptual approach to the development of motivational strategies. *Journal of Advanced Nursing, 8,* 111-116.

Yankelovich, D. (1974). The meaning of work. In J. Rosow (Ed.), *The worker and the job: Coping with change.* Englewood Cliffs, NJ: Prentice-Hall.

Chapter 27

Equity Theory
J. Stacy Adams

Joycelyn K. Blackmon

I| CASE STUDY

Originally built in 1930, a 500-bed acute care hospital located in an urban area of a southern city has undergone considerable renovation and construction in the past few years. With the addition of a new cancer research center, outpatient surgery center, and infectious disease unit, the institution is now considered the leading hospital in the city. The hospital has an excellent reputation for providing personalized patient care and often sponsors seminars for members of the community as well as its own health care workers. Approximately 75% of the hospital's income is supplied by private insurance payments, and fiscal management is not a problem.

The hospital is considered a pleasant place to work by most of the employees. Salaries are competitive, and needed supplies and equipment are usually available. The atmosphere is friendly, but employees address each other by "Mr." or "Mrs." on the job. Personnel are rewarded for their support to the hospital; effort is made to promote from within, although several outsiders have been hired in the past few years. Nursing management has always prided itself on the cohesiveness of its nurse managers. The nursing department frequently sponsors management seminars for nurses citywide. There is a nursing education department; employees are encouraged to attend continuing education seminars and meetings.

Management style is traditional, with communication flowing from the top down. Employees do, however, have the opportunity to discuss problems and suggestions with their immediate superior.

The supervisor of the infectious disease unit has held that position for 11 months. She obtained her baccalaureate degree in nursing 4 years prior to her employment and obtained a rich medical-surgical background during her employment as a staff nurse at a local hospital. Since her employment, she has attended a number of seminars dealing with management, infectious disease, and the treatment and care of the AIDS patient. The previous supervisor, who practiced a laissez-faire style of management, had been there 2 years. In the past, the patient census was usually low, and the turnover rate of staff nurses on the unit was low.

Recently, with the growing number of AIDS patients being admitted to the unit, the supervisor has had increasing problems with maintenance of an adequate staff. The turnover of nurses on her unit has been high, and she cannot hire and train enough personnel to complete the desired staffing pattern adequately. As a result, she often neglects her managerial responsibilities in order to perform patient care. On many nights she has had to complete paperwork at home. Along with the decrease in the level of productivity of her staff, she has been receiving frequent complaints from attending physicians regarding delays in initiating and maintaining the extensive nursing care plans required by the gravely ill AIDS patients. She has become angry and frustrated with her situation. In addition, this nurse's spouse has begun to express fears that the fatal disease can be brought home to endanger the family.

She has a close friend who owns a car-rental agency. Sensing her friend's declining morale, this person has offered her an upper-level management job in the rental agency with a salary equal to that of the hospital. After prolonged deliberation, the infectious disease supervisor is considering resignation.

| | | | | | | | | | | | | | | | | | | | | | | | | | | | | | | | | | | | | | | | | | | | | | | | | | | | | | | | | | | | | | | | | | | | | | | |

EQUITY THEORY

Equity theory was developed by J. Stacy Adams in 1963 while he was employed as a research psychologist at General Electric. Adams has acknowledged that equity theory owes a strong intellectual debt to the prior formulations of Leon Festinger concerning cognitive dissonance (1957) and George Homans's 1961 work dealing with distributive justice. It is a theory involving a relationship or exchange in which a person gives something and receives something in return. What the person gives is called an "input" and what he receives is called an "outcome." According to Miner (1980), "the major motivating force considered is a striving for equity, but some degree of inequity must be perceived before this force can be mobilized" (p. 107). Adams (1965) stated,

> The term inequity is used instead of injustice first, because the author has used this term before, second, to avoid the confusion of the many connotative meanings associated with the term justice, and third, to emphasize that the primary concern is with the causes and consequences of the absence of equity in human exchange relationships." (p. 276)

Several conditions must exist for inequity to occur. It is necessary for an exchange to take place whereby the person gives and receives. On the person's side of the exchange, the contributions brought into the exchange, for which he or she expects a return, are inputs the contributor perceives and are not necessarily viewed as such by the other party in the exchange. For an attribute to have the potential of being an input, the attribute must be recognized by either the possessor or both members of the exchange. Whether an attribute having the potential to become an input actually does so depends on the possessor's perception of its relevance to the exchange (Adams, 1965). Examples of inputs are age, education, experience, skill, seniority, ethnic background, social status, and job performance.

On the opposite side of the exchange are the individual's receipts or outcomes. As with inputs, these outcomes are as perceived by the individual involved in the exchange, and they must be recognized as being relevant to the exchange. If the recipient or both parties in the exchange recognize the existence of a reward, it has the potential to become an outcome. If the receiver considers the reward relevant to the exchange and it has useful value to her or him, it becomes an outcome. Examples of positive outcomes include pay, rewards intrinsic to the job, job status, fringe benefits, and status symbols. However, outcomes may have a negative valence such as poor working conditions, job insecurity, and monotony. As with inputs, inequity exists if only the giver perceives the reward as an outcome (Adams, 1965).

Normative expectations of what constitute "fair" correlations between input and outcomes are learned during the socialization process (Adams, 1965). A reference person or group is used to evaluate the equity of the individual's exchange relationship. The reference person or group must have one or more attributes comparable to those of the comparer (Miner, 1980). When a person perceives that his or her outcomes and input are significantly different in relation to those of others, feelings of inequity result (Miner, 1980).

Adams (1965) introduced two terms of reference to facilitate discussion, "Person" and "Other."

> Person is any individual for whom equity or inequity exists. Other is any individual with whom Person is in an exchange relationship, or with whom Person compares himself when both he and Other are in an exchange relationship with a third party, such as an employer, or with third parties who are considered by Person as being comparable, such as employers in a particular industry or geographic location. (p. 280)

Other is frequently a different individual, but may be Person in a previously held job or different social role. The terms may also be applied to groups when dealing with a class as a whole (Adams, 1965).

Adams (1965) supplied the definition of inequity as follows: "Inequity exists for Person whenever he perceives that the ratio of his outcomes to inputs and the ratio of Other's outcomes to Other's inputs are unequal" (p. 280). He elaborates, "this may happen either (a) when he and Other are in a direct exchange relationship or (b) when both are in an exchange relationship with a third party and Person compares himself to Other" (p. 280). The perception by Person of the values of outcomes and inputs is what must be addressed, not the actual inputs and outcomes per se (Adams, 1963a).

Inequity may result for Person not only when she or he feels relatively underpaid (underreward) but also when he or she feels relatively overpaid (overreward). The magnitude of inequity felt is related to the amount of discrepancy between the ratios of outcomes to inputs (Adams, 1965). When Person and Other are in an exchange relationship, Other will experience inequity if Person does; however, Other's experience will be the opposite of that of Person. This assumption depends on the factors that Person's and Other's perceptions of outcomes and inputs are equivalent and the outcome-input ratio discrepancy attains threshold level (Adams, 1965).

The presence of inequity results in dissatisfaction. Two general postulates were presented by Adams (1965). First, the presence of inequity in Person creates tension in her or him (which is proportional to the magnitude of inequity present). Second, the tension created in Person motivates him or her to reduce or eliminate it. The strength of the motivation is proportional to the tension created. "In short, the presence of inequity will motivate Person to achieve equity or to reduce inequity, and the strength of the motivation to do so will vary directly with the magnitude of inequity experienced" (Adams, 1965, p. 283).

Several methods to reduce inequity have been postulated. The first involves altering inputs. Person may either increase or decrease inputs, depending on whether the inequity is favorable or unfavorable. Input alteration is often used when there is variation from the perceived inputs of Other, as opposed to discrepancies in outcomes (Adams, 1965). If the inequity is unfavorable to an individual, lowering inputs can be expected; when inequity is favorable, increased inputs are likely (Miner, 1980). Altering outcomes is another method of inequity reduction. Again, Person may either decrease or increase her or his outcomes, depending on whether the inequity is favorable or unfavorable. Increasing outcomes may help to reduce unfavorable inequities. Reducing outcomes in order to achieve equity is not usually employed (Miner, 1980).

Less effective ways of reducing inequity have been discussed. Person may cognitively distort his or her inputs and outcomes, the direction being the same as if Person had actually altered the inputs and outcomes. Because reality heavily influences individuals, a significant amount of distortion is generally difficult to attain. Minimizing exposure to the inequity-producing situation (leaving the field) is another way of reducing or eliminating the inequity. Common forms are transfer, absenteeism, or separation from the job. These actions are considered fairly radical means of coping with existing inequity, used only when the magnitude of inequity is sizable and the availability of other means is decreased.

The last two methods of reducing inequity involve Other (or the reference source). Person may attempt to alter or cognitively distort Other's inputs and outcomes or try to force Other to leave the field. In the final method, Person changes the object of comparison and then experiences inequity when she or he and Other are in an exchange relationship with a third party. This method is difficult to accomplish if Person has been comparing himself or herself to Other for a considerable amount of time (Adams, 1965).

Adams (1965) stated the propositions about conditions that determine the choice of modes by Person as follows:

(a) Person will maximize positively valent outcomes and the valence of outcomes.
(b) He will minimize increasing inputs that are effortful and costly to change.
(c) He will resist real and cognitive changes in inputs that are central to his self-concept and to his self-esteem. To the extent that any of Person's outcomes are related to his self-concept and to his self-esteem, this proposition is extended to cover his outcomes.
(d) He will be more resistant to changing cognitions about his own outcomes and inputs than to changing his cognitions about Other's outcomes and inputs.
(e) Leaving the field will be resorted to only when the magnitude of inequity experienced is high and other means of reducing it are unavailable. Partial withdrawal, such as absenteeism, will occur more frequently and under conditions of lower inequity.
(f) Person will be highly resistant to changing the object of his comparisons, Other, once it has stabilized over time and, in effect, has become an anchor. (pp. 295-296)

Marriner-Tomey (1988) provided a simpler explanation of the equity theory. She indicated that the studies done by Adams and others "found that employees assess fairness by considering their input and the psychological, social, and financial rewards in comparison with those of others" (p. 235). The tension created by perceived inequity serves as a motivational force to reduce the inequity. The amount of motivational strength used to reduce the inequity will be proportional to the cognitive dissonance experienced. The ways for an individual to reduce tension are to change input or outcome, cognitive distortion of input and outcome, comparison change, or separation. In summary, "the manager should be attentive to the perceived equity of the reward system" (p. 236).

CASE ANALYSIS

Tension acts as a motivating force to reduce perceived inequity. Unfortunately, in this case, the nurse is considering reducing her inequity by leaving the field. A number of interventions might have been done by the nurse manager to provide a positive outcome from nursing's viewpoint.

The supervisor, once she felt the inequity, could have asked for an increase in pay that would alter her outcome; therefore, equilibrium might be established. She could also have requested additional hospital staff to be reassigned to her unit, which would decrease her input and that of her staff. Without a supplemental staff, seeing the lowering of job efforts as a viable solution would be difficult for her. The supervisor might have also changed her reference source from that of her co-workers to comparing herself with supervisors in units such as hers.

The nurse supervisor could have used another application of the equity theory regarding her staff. The desired outcomes of her employees could have been investigated concerning recognition for contributions to high-risk nursing, as well as the possibility of incentive pay, in order to reduce inequity and slow the turnover rate. Because pay is not always the reward desired, emphasis on the employees' skill and compassion might have been pursued and publicized.

Finally, if administration and the director of nurses were cognizant of equity theory, they could have applied the same principles to avert the loss of a valuable member of their organization.

RESEARCH

There has been a significant amount of research into the equity theory of motivation. Adams and Freedman (1976) stated that by 1973 more than 170 different authors had conducted research on equity.

The studies of Walster, Berscheid, and Walster (1973) expanded the concepts of the equity theory to include four propositions. Miner (1980) considered these proposals part of the theory of equity because Adams (Adams & Freedman, 1976) acknowledged and endorsed them. Miner (1980) cited the proposals as such:

> Proposition I. Individuals will try to maximize their outcomes (where outcomes equal rewards minus costs). The term reward refers to positive outcomes and the term cost refers to negative outcomes.
> Proposition IIA. Groups can maximize collective reward by evolving accepted systems for "equitably" apportioning rewards and costs among members. Thus, members will evolve such systems of equity and will attempt to induce members to accept and adhere to these systems.
> Proposition IIB. Groups will generally reward members who treat others equitably and generally punish (increase the costs for) members who treat others inequitably.
> Proposition III. When individuals find themselves participating in inequitable relationships, they become distressed (the more inequitable the relationship, the more distress). Anger and guilt are two of the major forms of distress.
> Proposition IV. Individuals who discover that they are in an inequitable relationship attempt to eliminate distress by restoring equity. The greater the inequity, the more distress, and the harder they try to restore equity. There are two ways equity may be restored. A person can restore actual equity by appropriately altering his own outcomes or inputs or the outcomes or inputs of others. A person can restore psychological equity by appropriately distorting the perceptions of his own or others' outcomes or inputs. (p. 112)

The five studies done by and in association with Adams in the 1960s dealt with the predicted effects of overreward inequity. Experiment I (Adams, 1963a) concluded that overreward inequity produced an increase in productivity. Experiment II done by Arrowood but reported by Adams (1963a) addressed the hypothesis that productivity was increased due to job insecurity rather than feelings of inequity. The experimental results validated the conclusions of Experiment I, therefore rejecting the idea that increased production was a result of job insecurity. Experiment III (Adams & Rosenbaum, 1962) was designed to test the effects of inequity motivation on workers paid by the hour versus those paid on a piecework basis. The study indicated that productivity increased in the overreward inequity hourly paid subjects but decreased in those subjects paid per piece who felt overpaid. Experiment IV offered further support of the equity theory. This study concluded that hourly workers increased inputs on a quantitative basis, whereas pieceworkers increased them on a qualitative basis (Adams, 1963b). Experiment V (Adams & Jacobsen, 1964) supported the conclusions of the previous experiments: "Overpayment by an employer need not necessarily increase his labor costs, provided he is primarily interested in quality, as opposed to production volume" (p. 24).

Andrews (1967) further tested Adams's theory of inequity by conducting a study involving piece rate workers. The results of this study were consistent with earlier studies showing an increase in work quality. Zedeck and Smith (1968) conducted research on the theory dealing with inequity thresholds of overreward. Lawler (1968) questioned the role of inequity as a causal influence on motivation. He suggested that perceived equity be treated as one of the factors that influence the attractiveness of rewards.

Pritchard, Dunnette, and Jorgenson (1972) stated that "effects on overall job satisfaction showed that employees under both overreward and underreward conditions were less satisfied than employees made to feel equitably paid" (p. 75). The major finding of Moore and Baron (1973) was that significant effects on quality and quantity of work behavior were produced by variations in manipulated perceptions of qualifiedness, whereas variations in the amount of anticipated compensation resulted in changes of work quality only.

Research done by Lawler and O'Gara (1967) addressed equity theory through the context of personality types. They found that individuals who lacked self-assurance normally responded by increased productivity. Tests conducted on professional employees in a division of the Federal Public Health Service revealed that "those in the inequity subsample displayed greater dissonance, less favorable work-related attitudes and a higher propensity to terminate voluntarily their employment" (Finn & Lee, 1972, p. 291).

Reward allocation research conducted by Leventhal, Weiss, and Long (1969) concluded that intentionally overrewarded subjects of a dyad were motivated to both reciprocate and restore equity. Those subjects overrewarded by chance were motivated only to restore equity. Other reward allocation research studies were designed to test equity theory motivation in conjunction with conflict reduction (Leventhal, Michaels, & Sanford, 1972) and equity motivation versus waste production (Leventhal, Weiss, & Buttrick, 1973). Cook (1975) summarized that individuals must have well-defined perceptions concerning the rank of the evaluations that are the basis for reward allocation in order for equity motivation to be mobilized. Larwood, Kavanagh, and Levine (1978) noted the importance of individual differences in exchange selection.

Adams and Freedman (1976) contended that equity theorists must confront four problem areas. First, researchers must learn more about equity- and inequity-produced emotions such as contentment, anger, shame, and feelings of betrayal and their relationship to behavior. Second, they should study the equity process individuals use. Third, they must study methods of equity and inequity manipulations that people use to get things they want. Finally, they must make equity theory more precise with the development of methods of quantitative measurement. An extensive annotated bibliography on equity is provided in this work.

Mulkowsky (1977) conducted a comparative study of equity theory factors relating to municipal and voluntary hospitals' nurse supervisory personnel. This study revealed that municipal hospital nurse supervisors displayed greater dissatisfaction with job input to outcome ratios than those supervisors in voluntary institutions. It also revealed that a more autocratic supervisory style was exhibited by the supervisors in the municipal setting than by those supervisors in the voluntary hospitals. This research merits attention because it was the first study empirically tested in the context of hospital organization on equity theory job elements. Mulkowsky stated,

> The present research appears to provide validation of the theory for non salary elements: specifically municipal hospital nurse supervisors are less satisfied with recognition from supervisors, the opportunity for advancement, and their physical working conditions than nurse supervisors from voluntary hospitals. (p. 5848-B)

Marriner (1981) reported the results of research into factors considered important in determination of salary in nursing academia. The questionnaire used in her study was composed of three parts. The first part requested an anecdotal account of the person's perception of equity, how it was determined, and how inequity (if perceived) was handled. The second part consisted of factors rated in importance of determination for faculty salaries at the baccalaureate, master's, and doctorate levels. Demographic information was revealed in the third section.

Approximately 50% of nursing faculty members, primarily young married women with master's degrees, at a university responded to the questionnaire. The following results were found:

> The majority of participants indicated that they are satisfied with their job but dissatisfied with their pay. The majority are dissatisfied with their pay in relationship to the quantity and quality of their work. They are equally divided in relationship to satisfaction or dissatisfaction with pay as related to peers. Most do not know how their pay compares to that of faculties at other institutions. (p. 39)

The study also revealed that more than half of the subjects felt underpaid, a third felt equitably paid, and only 2% believed that they were overpaid. Reference sources most cited were nursing school peers, comparable persons outside the school, and previous salary. Recommended criteria for determining salary were educational preparation, experience, evaluations, school responsibilities, comparison with peers, and participation in professional activities.

Employees with 1 to 3 years of service at this institution had the highest percentage of dissatisfaction with pay. There appeared to be a significant increase in percentage of pay satisfaction in those persons who had been employed at the institution for 3 to 7 years. A high percentage of nursing faculty with more than 7 years of service showed dissatisfaction with pay.

Marriner concluded that "although the majority of faculty members felt dissatisfied with their pay, most indicated they were satisfied with their jobs" (p. 40). This conclusion suggests that job satisfaction may be found through sources other than income. Various factors appear to be considered in faculty salary determination; faculty members generally believe that the qualities they possess are important in this determination.

This work was important because it was the first conducted to learn what nurse academicians felt were the factors important in determination of salaries, perceptions of being equitably or inequitably paid, and course of action taken once inequity was perceived.

Buccheri (1981) presented results of a study conducted to examine the perceived levels of job satisfaction and supervisory support. The study was a cross-sectional survey involving 203 registered nurses employed at nine adult psychiatric units on the West Coast. The conceptual framework of this research was based on Likert's work (1967) on supportive relationships and Adams's equity theory of job satisfaction. The participating nurses were divided into four categories: staff nurse, clinical nurse specialist, middle management, and top management. The three instruments used to collect data were the Job Satisfaction Scale, the Supervisor Scale, and the Supervisor Support subscale of the Work Environment Scale.

The results of this study revealed that all ten members of top management displayed high job satisfaction. In the middle-management category, 64% showed high job satisfaction. The majority (59%) of the staff nurses expressed low job satisfaction. There was a positive relationship between nurses' satisfaction with their jobs and their perceptions of their supervisors as being supportive of them. Buccheri concluded that "nurses want their supervisors to facilitate their professional skills by being supportive of their needs for influence, recognition, and communication" (p. 23).

With the exception of the preceding studies, not much nursing research has involved equity theory. This theory can undoubtedly provide many insights for the nurse manager. Applying the "overreward hypothesis" should be useful when dealing with employees to improve work productivity. The manager should also realize that those employees who experience feelings of underreward often display anger and their productivity may decrease. Future research is needed to develop a monitoring system designed to use equity theory as a means of improving the quality of nursing care delivered.

REFERENCES

Adams, J.S. (1963a). Toward an understanding of inequity. *Journal of Abnormal and Social Psychology, 67,* 422-436.

Adams, J.S. (1963b). Wage inequities, productivity, and work quality, *Industrial Relations, 3,* 9-16.

Adams, J.S. (1965). Inequity in social exchange. In L. Berkowitz (Ed.), *Advances in experimental social psychology* (vol. 2). New York: Academic Press.

Adams, J.S., & Freedman, S. (1976). Equity theory revisited: Comments and annotated bibliography. In L. Berkowitz & E. Walster (Eds.), *Advances in experimental social psychology* (vol. 9). New York: Academic Press.

Adams, J.S., & Jacobsen, P.R. (1964). Effects of wage inequities on work quality. *Journal of Abnormal and Social Psychology, 69,* 19-25.

Adams, J.S., & Rosenbaum, W.B. (1962). The relationship of worker productivity to cognitive dissonance about wage inequities. *Journal of Applied Psychology, 46,* 161-164.

Andrews, I.R. (1967). Wage inequity and job performance: An experimental study. *Journal of Applied Psychology, 51,* 39-45.

Buccheri, R.C. (1981). Nursing supervision: A new look at an old role. *Nursing Administration Quarterly, 11,* 11-25.

Cook, K.S. (1975). Expectations, evaluations, and equity. *American Sociological Review, 40,* 372-388.

Festinger, L.A. (1957). *A theory of cognitive dissonance.* Evanston, IL: Row Peterson.

Finn, R.H., & Lee, I.M. (1972). Salary equity: Its determination, analysis, and correlates. *Journal of Applied Psychology, 56,* 283-292.

Homans, G.C. (1961). *Social behavior: Its elementary forms.* New York: Harcourt, Brace.

Larwood, L., Kavanagh, M., & Levine, R. (1978). Perceptions of fairness with three alternative economic exchanges. *Academy of Management Journal, 21,* 69-83.

Lawler, E.E. (1968). Equity theory as a predictor of productivity and work quality. *Psychological Bulletin, 70,* 596-610.

Lawler, E.E., & O'Gara, P.W. (1967). Effects of inequity produced by under payment on work output, work quality, and attitudes toward the work. *Journal of Applied Psychology, 51,* 403-410.

Leventhal, G.S., Michaels, J.W., & Sanford, C. (1972). Inequity and interpersonal conflict: Reward allocation and secrecy about reward as methods of preventing conflict. *Journal of Personality and Social Psychology, 23,* 88-102.

Leventhal, G.S., Weiss, T., & Buttrick, R. (1973). Attribution of value, equity, and the prevention of waste in reward allocation. *Journal of Personality and Social Psychology, 27,* 276-286.

Leventhal, G.S., Weiss, T., & Long, G. (1969). Equity, reciprocity, and reallocating rewards in the dyad. *Journal of Personality and Social Psychology, 13,* 300-305.

Likert, R. (1967). *The human organization: Its management and value.* New York: McGraw-Hill.

Marriner, A. (1981). Factors of importance in determination of faculty salaries. *Journal of Nursing Education, 20,* 34-41.

Marriner-Tomey, A. (1988). *Guide to nursing management* (3rd ed.). St. Louis: C.V. Mosby.

Miner, J.B. (1980). *Theories of organizational behavior.* Hinsdale, IL: Dryden.

Moore, L.M., & Baron, R.M. (1973). Effects of wage inequities on work attitudes and performance. *Journal of Experimental Social Psychology, 9,* 1-16.

Mulkowsky, G.P. (1977). A comparative study of equity theory factors relating to municipal and voluntary hospitals nurse supervisory personnel. *Dissertation Abstracts International, 38,* 5848-B. (University Microfilms International-ISSN 0419-4217).

Pritchard, R.D., Dunnette, M.D., & Jorgenson, D.O. (1972). Effects of perceptions of equity and inequity on worker performance and satisfaction. *Journal of Applied Psychology Monograph, 56,* 75-94.

Walster, E., Berscheid, E., & Walster, G. (1973). New directions in equity research. *Journal of Personality and Social Psychology, 25,* 151-176.

Zedeck, S., & Smith, P.C. (1968). A psychophysical determination of equitable payment: A methodological study. *Journal of Applied Psychology, 52,* 343-347.

Chapter 28

Intrinsic and Extrinsic Motivation
Edward L. Deci

Carol Lavonne Harn

I | CASE STUDY

A 500-bed, acute care, not-for-profit community hospital has undergone considerable renovation and reconstruction over the past few years. It is considered the most successful hospital in the city, which also contains a number of proprietary hospitals.

The hospital has an excellent reputation for guest relations and marketing. Over the past 2 years, all employees have attended classes that focus on development of interpersonal skills and customer relations.

The hospital is a teaching hospital that admits a large number of indigent patients via the various ambulatory care centers. The hospital receives some reimbursement from county, state, and federal funds; however, 70% of the hospital's income is still derived from private insurance payments. Physicians are still viewed as the consumers; therefore, recruitment and retention of private physicians continue to be a strong fiscal focus for the hospital. In most cases, patients go to the hospitals their physicians recommend.

The internal setting for this case is a 40-bed neurological floor. Patients are admitted from a 50-county referral area and are transferred internally from the neurological intensive care unit.

This floor has undergone two changes in the position of nurse manager in the past year. The first nurse manager graduated from this hospital's diploma program and had worked at the hospital for the past 30 years. Her style of management was very autocratic and controlling. The floor was organized in a traditional, centralized manner. Her management style allowed one-way communication—from the top down. The outcomes on this floor were positive in two ways: patient care was good and the physicians were satisfied. Staff members, however, often discussed the nurse manager's controlling style and their lack of understanding about the rationale for her mandates. Most employees were not highly motivated and often performed to avoid punishment or the wrath of the nurse manager.

When this nurse manager retired, a new nurse manager, who preferred a laissez-faire style, was selected. (Her choice of management style was not known at the time of employment.) She was a very hard worker and enthusiastic; however, she quickly burned out and was employed less than a year. During her tenure, outcomes began to deteriorate and become very negative. Patient and physician complaints increased. Systems were disorganized, and employee morale began to decline. Realizing the need for stability, nursing administration promoted an assistant nurse manager who had a proven track record for being able to manage effectively. This nurse manager position was her first, and she was still a novice to management.

This third nurse manager initially seemed to be making progress despite the presence of a variety of management problems. By the time she had been employed 6 months, however, the quality of patient care was rapidly declining. Patient complaints were significant to the point that several physicians requested that their patients no longer be admitted to the neurological floor. Complaints focused on general nursing care and more specifically on interpersonal relationships. Patients described employees as abrupt and discourteous and said they felt they were imposing on the nursing staff.

Further, patients were not shielded from the internal problems of the floor. They were often told of shift rivalry and generally became sounding boards for frustrated employees. Patients also related that continuity and communication were lacking. Patients felt they had become victims in the whole situation, and they were threatening to go to other hospitals.

The turnover rate for nursing staff steadily increased, and staff throughout the hospital began to ask not to be pulled to the neurological floor. General hallway conversations concerned the low morale on the neurological floor. Employees began calling in sick more often and seemed to be doing just enough to get by.

The nurse manager was still trying to be optimistic; however, she seemed to be getting weary. She was not delegating and was trying to do everything herself. She received very little cooperation from her staff. Physicians demanded that the nurse manager take immediate action to improve the nursing care or they would take their patients to other hospitals. The nurse manager was receiving frequent visits from the director and the supervisor. The encounters were filled with complaints and newly identified problems.

Ancillary departments such as the laboratory and x-ray departments became very vocal about the quality of nursing care on the neurological floor. The nurse manager also received overt negative feedback from her charge nurses, who were threatening to resign.

Two days before her scheduled vacation, the nurse manager resigned. She said the situation was out of control, and she had been unable to motivate her employees to correct the problems. Then she acknowledged that she felt depressed and defeated and could no longer even motivate herself. What could a nurse manager do to change such a situation?

| | | | | | | | | | | | | | | | | | | | | | | | | | | | | | | | | | | | | | | | | | | | | | | | | | | | | | | | | | | | | |

INTRINSIC AND EXTRINSIC MOTIVATION

A number of very complex management problems are identified in the preceding case study. All the problems could be viewed as motivational challenges and opportunities. Edward L. Deci presented a formal theory that deals with intrinsic and extrinsic motivation. The entire field of motivation can broadly be divided into the two areas of intrinsic and extrinsic motivation.

Deci says that intrinsically motivated behaviors are involved with the human need for being competent and self-determining, which falls into two behavioral categories. One category deals with a person's need to conquer challenges. People are motivated to reduce uncertainty, dissonance, or incongruity. This reduction activity in turn produces intrinsic motivation (Deci, 1975a, p. 57).

A second category involves a person's need to seek challenges when none is present. People seek challenging situations that optimally use their abilities and strengths. They choose their activities in order to satisfy themselves. They try to achieve goals that give them a high degree of psychological value and offer them a sense of competence and self-determination (Deci, 1975b).

An activity is intrinsically motivating if there is no obvious external reward for the activity.

Extrinsic motivation is associated with receiving external rewards. Deci says that the extent to which people engage in activities that are not linked to external rewards reflects their intrinsic motivation toward such activities (Deci, 1975b).

Intrinsic motivation can also be separated from extrinsic motivation by realizing that intrinsic motives are based on the physiology of the central nervous system. The basis here deals with one's need to feel competent and self-determining. Deci says this is a very appropriate way to view human behavior.

The end state for intrinsically motivated behavior, then, is an affective state that falls under a general framework. A series of motivated behaviors starts with stimulus inputs to the central nervous system. The stimulus inputs initiate awareness of potential satisfaction. The awarenesses are motives or representations of future states (Deci, 1976).

Motives or drives cause people to act. This action is the result of intrinsic motivation. Intrinsic motivation constantly directs people's interaction with their environment.

In 1975, Deci did work with the cognitive evaluation theory and its effect on intrinsic motivation. Basically, he says that intrinsic motivation can be affected by a change in perceived locus of causality. When a person is intrinsically motivated, the perceived locus of causality is within the particular person. However, when people receive extrinsic rewards, the perceived locus of causality shifts from internal to external. People perceive they are performing in order to receive rewards, and their intrinsic motivation for that activity decreases (Miner, 1980).

A second process involving rewards can have an impact on intrinsic motivation. Rewards that let people know they are competent can have a positive impact; rewards that tell people they are not competent or worthwhile can have a negative impact and decrease intrinsic motivation (Miner, 1980).

Deci's theory says that all extrinsic rewards have two aspects: a controlling aspect and an informational aspect. The controlling aspect of the rewards causes the behavior-reward interaction, thereby decreasing intrinsic motivation. The informational aspect communicates to people their effectiveness in an activity. This information is communicated in a way that either increases or decreases intrinsic motivation on the activity.

Deci's research deals with the effects of external rewards on intrinsic motivation. He says that motivating people extrinsically has the unintended consequence of decreasing intrinsic motivation.

Deci also believes there is a high degree of correlation between a person's psychological health and a person's intrinsic motivation. People naturally need to feel good about themselves to have a greater sense of psychological well-being. Experiences that decrease intrinsic motivation and leave people feeling incompetent and non-self-determining on a prolonged basis can cause a decrease in psychological well-being (Deci, 1976).

Deci basically interprets his findings as follows:

> Intrinsic motivation appears to be affected by two processes: a change in perceived locus of causality and a change in feelings of competence and self actualization. Intrinsic motivation decreases when a person's behavior becomes dependent on extrinsic rewards such as money or the avoidance of punishment. It also decreases when a person receives negative feedback on his performance on an intrinsically motivated activity. But it increases as a result of positive feedback and interpersonal supportiveness. (Miner, 1980, p. 157)

Several opinion articles review Deci's work. The studies and articles deal primarily with Deci's research methodology; however, they all agree with the findings that the addition of extrinsic rewards often may be counterproductive and cause a decrease in intrinsic motivation.

CASE ANALYSIS

Deci's theory of intrinsic and extrinsic motivation relates to the nursing case study presented. To understand the importance of Deci's theory, we should first realize the difference between keeping a person on the job and motivating the person to perform effectively on the job.

To recruit and retain employees in this particular case situation, the nurse manager should make sure the salary and benefits are equitable and that working conditions are satisfactory. If an employee's basic needs are not met, they will not remain employed. However, just satisfying needs will not ensure high levels of intrinsic motivation or job performance. The nurse manager cannot be shortsighted and think that just paying staff more money will resolve the problems. Deci's work proves that extrinsic rewards alone may actually reduce rather than enhance intrinsic motivation.

The nurse manager should find a balance between intrinsic and extrinsic rewards if intrinsic motivation is to be stimulated and sustained. Employees should relate well to the work that is to be done. Designing intrinsically motivating jobs is essential. This objective cannot be accomplished unless the leader uses a participative approach to management.

The nurse manager should allow workers to participate in decisions that affect the nature of their jobs. This participation allows the staff to feel competent and self-determining, as proposed by Deci. Under proper conditions, participative management provides encouragement to staff to direct their creative energies toward resolution of the internal problems.

Some techniques of participative management the nurse manager could use would be surveying the staff and asking for their input, having open forums on all shifts, and allowing employees to do their own time schedules. Another important step should be to decentralize decision making on the floor and to change the traditional communication structure from one of top down to one of bottom up. All these efforts take careful planning to create an intrinsically oriented system. These activities require massive reeducation of all staff and some overt risk taking on the part of the nurse manager.

Staff should also be involved in peer evaluation and self-evaluation. The system of peer evaluation allows employees to help set standards and therefore have more ownership in the resolution of problems. Peer evaluation creates a climate that is conducive to professional practice.

Deci says that a person's intrinsic motivation increases as a result of positive feedback and decreases with continual negative feedback. A vicious circle of negative feedback is in place in this case study. The employees are performing poorly and receiving negative feedback from all sources — peers, subordinates, supervisors, even patients. The nurse manager should interrupt this cycle and begin a system of positive feedback and interpersonal supportiveness.

Part of this system could be to encourage satisfied patients to write letters and make return visits to the floor. Physicians should be asked to bring negative feedback to the attention of the nurse manager privately and to give positive feedback publicly. Supervisors should search for opportunities to provide positive reinforcement to employees during rounds. Application of McGregor's theory Y approach in addition to Deci's theory would be appropriate (Marriner-Tomey, 1988).

Deci also says employees need to feel competent in order to have increased intrinsic motivation. These nurses' feelings of competence could be strengthened if the nurse manager provides continuing education and in-service classes, establishes clearly defined performance expectations, holds informative staff meetings, has an effective system for downward communication, markets advancement of the clinical ladder program, and encourages nurses to become certified in medical-surgical or neurological nursing.

The nurse manager could also give additional merit increases or pay to those employees who function above the standard. In some ways this action would be making rewards contingent upon performance; however, Deci says this should work if properly planned and administered.

The case study presents numerous motivational challenges; however, strategic planning and use of Deci's theory provide a framework for assessing, planning, intervening, and evaluating the problems. Deci says,

> Individuals in the organization will be more motivated and satisfied; they will have a greater sense of self-worth and self-control. And the organization will be better able to meet its own goals because the members of the organization will be performing more effectively. (Deci, 1976, p. 72)

RESEARCH

Deci and his associates performed extensive research to investigate the question: "What happens to a person's intrinsic motivation for an activity when he is rewarded extrinsically for performing the activity?" (Deci, 1976, p. 67).

The first studies Deci reported in the literature were in 1971, and they supported the hypothesis that if extrinsic rewards are given to subjects for performing an intrinsically motivating activity, their intrinsic motivation for the activity decreases (Deci, 1971).

In the first study Deci observed hundreds of college students solving Soma puzzles in a laboratory setting. These puzzles were made up of seven pieces; each piece looked as though it were made up of three or four 1-inch cubes. The puzzle could be organized into millions of configurations; however, subjects were asked to replicate a configuration the researcher had drawn on paper. The puzzles were known to be intrinsically motivating to college students (Deci, 1975).

Each subject in the experiment received four puzzles to solve and was allocated 10 minutes for each one. The only difference between the experimental and control subjects was that $1.00 was paid to the experimental group for each puzzle they solved. The extrinsic reward (money) was contingent upon performance. Between the timed puzzle-solving periods, the researcher left the room, and the subjects had 8 minutes of free time to do as they wanted. More puzzles, magazines, and other distractions were available in the room.

The results were consistently the same. The students who had been paid spent less of their free time solving puzzles. They were not as willing to perform the activity without reward as were those who had not been paid. "To some extent, the paid subjects had become dependent on external rewards (money), and their intrinsic motivation has decreased" (Deci, 1976, p. 68).

In another puzzle experiment conducted by Deci, experimental subjects were told that a buzzer would sound when they had used the allocated time to solve the puzzle. The subjects were then performing both because of intrinsic motivation and to avoid a punishment (buzzer). The control subjects were not threatened with a buzzer. The results of the experiment demonstrated decreased intrinsic motivation to solve puzzles in their free time among subjects who were in the experimental groups. Deci concluded that "threat of punishment was the crucial element in decreasing intrinsic motivation in this experiment" (Deci, 1976, p. 68).

All Deci's studies were consistent with his propositions about decreases in intrinsic motivation and shifts in perceived locus of causality.

Another process that affects motivation involves feedback. Deci discovered the effects of feedback during the puzzle experiments. Male subjects who received positive verbal reinforcement while solving the puzzles spent more free time working on puzzles than subjects who were not reinforced. Deci therefore concluded that positive reinforcement enhances a person's internal feelings of self-worth, thereby increasing intrinsic motivation (Deci, 1972).

Deci, Casio, and Krusell (1973) also examined the effect of negative feedback on intrinsic motivation. The results of a number of studies indicate that negative feedback leads to decreased intrinsic motivation (Deci et al., 1973).

In summary, Deci found that intrinsic motivation was affected by two processes:

> A change in perceived locus of causality and a change in feelings of competence and self-actualization. Intrinsic motivation decreases when a person's behavior becomes dependent on extrinsic rewards such as money or the avoidance of punishment. It also decreases when a person receives negative feedback about his performance on an intrinsically motivated activity. But it increases as a result of positive feedback and interpersonal supportiveness. (Deci, 1976, p. 70)

An extensive computer search did not reveal any nursing studies done on intrinsic and extrinsic motivation. The topic of motivation was addressed in most of the nursing administration books and journals reviewed; Deci's theory was discussed only in Marriner-Tomey's book (1988). Interestingly, the topic of motivation was not even addressed in a number of nursing management books.

Clearly, more work and scientific studies need to be done in areas of motivation. A logical starting point could be to survey the American Organization of Nurse Executives (AONE) at their annual meeting because the majority of nurses are employed in hospitals. The AONE members could identify questions they have about motivation.

In the past, certification has been an intrinsically rewarding activity for nurses; it seems to have given them a strong sense of personal worth. Deci's research suggests that extrinsic rewards may decrease their intrinsic motivation for the activity of obtaining certification. If his theory holds true in nursing, a change in the perceived locus of causality and a change in nurses' feelings of competence and self-actualization may occur. Fewer nurses may actually seek certification if they perceive the activity to be driven by extrinsic rewards. A good way to test the theory in practice would be to compare the numbers of nurses obtaining certification before and after the reward implementation and to question the nurses about their motives for obtaining certification.

The nursing literature mentions decentralized management as a satisfier for nurses; however, studies that pinpointed decentralized management as increasing intrinsic motivation were not located. Research is needed in this area in order to prepare models for nurse managers.

In summary, Deci set forth some concrete propositions regarding intrinsic and extrinsic motivation that could be very useful in nursing. The nursing shortage should challenge us to determine factors that intrinsically motivate nurses to enter and remain in nursing.

REFERENCES

Deci, E.L. (1971). Effects of externally mediated rewards on intrinsic motivation. *Journal of Personality and Social Psychology, 18*, 105-115.

Deci, E.L. (1972). The effects of contingent and noncontingent rewards and controls on intrinsic motivation. *Organizational Behavior and Human Performance, 8*, 217-229.

Deci, E.L. (1975a). *Intrinsic motivation.* New York: Plenum.

Deci, E.L. (1975b). Notes on the theory and metatheory of intrinsic motivation. *Organizational Behavior and Human Performance, 15*, 130-145.

Deci, E.L. (1976). The hidden costs of rewards. *Organizational Dynamics, 4*(3), 61-72.

Deci, E.L., Casio, W.F., & Krusell, J. (1973). Cognitive evaluation theory and some comments on the Calder and Staw critique. *Journal of Personality and Social Psychology, 31*, 81-86.

Marriner-Tomey, A. (1988). *Guide to nursing management* (3rd ed.). St. Louis: C.V. Mosby.

Miner, J.B. (1980). *Theories of organizational behavior.* Hinsdale, IL: Dryden.

Chapter 29

Goal-Setting Theory
Edwin Locke

D. Jean Holley

I I   **CASE STUDY**

During a routine utilization review, a nurse discovered that in the previous 4 weeks three patients on a 35-bed surgical unit had developed decubitus ulcers during their hospitalization. The information was given to the nursing quality assurance committee. A chart review showed no preventive measures for decubitus ulcer were documented on these elderly, immobile patients after their orthopedic surgery. Further investigation through an interview with the head nurse from the surgical unit revealed that several recent changes had occurred on her unit that could have contributed to this omission of basic nursing care. The hospital had recently affiliated with an aggressive orthopedic surgeon, and the patient population had increased by one-third and changed in nature. Decubitus ulcer prevention had rarely been needed because 95% of the patients had been ambulatory the day after surgery. The orthopedic patients recently were often older and in poor nutritional status. Nursing assistants had been given little direction in caring for patients with total joint replacements and were fearful to turn them. The hospital had been unable to recruit experienced RNs to meet the patient increase, so novice RNs and technical, task-oriented nurses had been hired. The changes in the unit had met with resistance from the nursing staff, and poor attitudes and low motivation were evident.

| | | | | | | | | | | | | | | | | | | | | | | | | | | | | | | | | | | | | | | | | | | | | | | | | | | | | | | | | | | | | | | | | | |

GOAL-SETTING THEORY

Edwin Locke's theory is by far the most researched of the goal-setting theories. "As far back as the 1930's American psychologists . . . performed extensive studies of 'level of aspiration' (quantitative goal setting), but they were more interested in the causes of aspiration level than in its effects" (Locke, 1975, p. 466). Locke's work was based on Kurt Lewin's view of the individual's level of aspiration and the success or failure of the individual's performance (Lewin, 1935). Thomas Ryan, a professor of Locke's at Cornell, also influenced Locke's development of a goal-setting theory through his work "on the significant role that intentions play in human behavior" (Miner, 1980, p. 170). Locke had access to Ryan's work long before it was published in 1970 and often cited his early research.

Ryan's (1958) theory of motivation which states that "a very large proportion of behavior is initiated by tasks [goals, intentions] and a very large proportion of tasks lead to the behavior specified by the

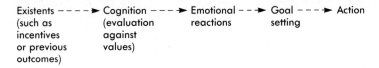

Existents - - - -► Cognition - - - ► Emotional - - -► Goal - - - -► Action
(such as   (evaluation   reactions   setting
incentives   against
or previous   values)
outcomes)

FIGURE 29-1 A theoretical model illustrating the effect of variables in Locke's theoretical formulations. *From Locke, E.A., Cartledge, N., & Knerr, C.S. (1970). Studies of the relationship between satisfaction, goal setting and performance.* Organizational Behavior and Human Performance, 5, *136.*

tasks. . . . A task is a necessary condition for most kinds of behavior [p. 79]." (Locke, Bryan, & Kendall, 1968, p. 104)

Locke's basic theory states that high goals, if they are accepted, have consistently been shown to produce high performance even if the goals are not met (Locke, 1966b; Locke & Bryan, 1966a), and specific goals increase performance over no goals or "do your best" instructions (Bryan & Locke, 1967; Locke, 1968). Locke believes "that the immediate, direct motivational determinant of task performance is the individual's goal" (Hamner & Harnett, 1974, pp. 227-228). "In addition the theory states that a person's goals mediate how performance is affected by monetary incentives, time limits, knowledge of results (i.e., performance feedback), participation in decision making and competition" (Latham & Yukl, 1975a, p. 824). Monetary incentives, time limits, and knowledge of results appear to be important to performance only to the extent that they affect goal setting (Locke, 1967). The effect of decision making or participation in goal setting on production has not been adequately studied. There appears to be a negative effect or no effect except with uneducated workers (Mento, Steel, & Karren, 1987; Latham et al., 1978; Latham & Yukl, 1975b). Job satisfaction from goal setting "is a function of the difference between actual performance and performance goals, and also a function of the difference between actual performance and performance of a reference person" (Hamner & Harnett, 1974, p. 217).

Locke developed his theory through laboratory experiments with college students as subjects. Although Locke was criticized for his lack of field study and use of student samples, recent field studies have been supportive of his early research (Locke, 1986; Brass, 1987).

Goal setting has been more effective in certain situations and with certain people. An ideal situation has noncomplex tasks that can be measured accurately and has strong manager support (Latham & Yukl, 1975a). Highly interdependent or unstructured tasks with the potential for outside influences may make goal setting more difficult to evaluate. Increased effort may not translate into increased performance (Buller & Bell, 1986). Frequent feedback is essential to change of attitudes and sustained increase in performance (Locke, 1975). Although difficult goals increase performance, goals that are viewed as impossible affect performance negatively. Individuals who view themselves as low achievers may not respond to extremely high goals.

Locke, Cartledge, and Knerr (1970) have developed a theoretical model to illustrate the effect of variables in Locke's theoretical formulations (Figure 29-1).

The existents can positively affect the goal acceptance and the goal-setting level if the individual's comparison of his or her values and existing standards results in a motivational emotional reaction. The emotions of dissatisfaction and satisfaction could be motivational. Anticipated existents and emotion also result in goal setting. The goal setting, however, is the most immediate determinant of the action taken (Miner, 1980).

Hirst (1987) also developed two models (Figures 29-2 and 29-3) that illustrate the effect of goal setting on the cognitive understanding of the task, which enables the individual's

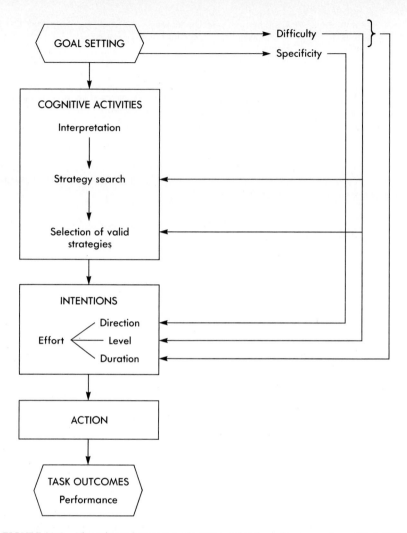

FIGURE 29-2 The relation between goal setting and task performance. *From Hirst, M.K. (1987). The effects of setting budget goals and task uncertainty on performance: A theoretical analysis.* The Accounting Review, 62(4), 776.

intentional effort to produce the action that will cause a task outcome or performance. Goal difficulty and specificity of the goal affect the cognitive activities, and specific, difficult tasks increase the appropriateness of effort direction, the level of effort intensity, and the duration of the effort. Task uncertainty or incompleteness of knowledge inhibits the ability to formulate valid strategies and results in wasted effort.

Despite its limitations and the need for further refinement through research, Miner (1981) finds the goal-setting theory to be appropriate for use in organizations. "Locke et al. (1981) determined that 84% of the laboratory and field studies they examined supported the goal difficulty hypothesis, while 96% of the studies (both lab and field) supported the goal specificity/difficulty hypothesis" (Mento et al., 1987, p. 74). Goal setting for individuals is not related to the expectancy theory because there are no hedonistic assumptions, and Locke

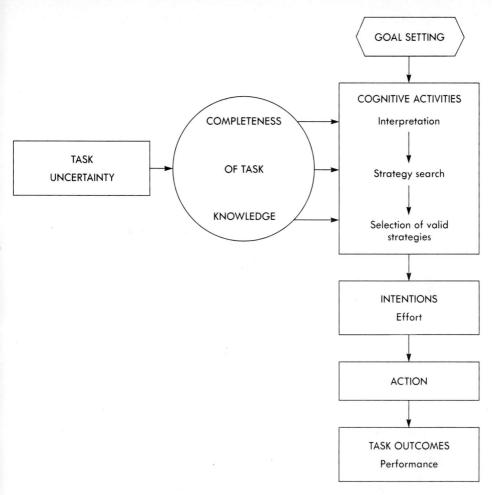

FIGURE 29-3 The effects of task uncertainty on the relation between goal setting and task performance. *From Hirst, M.K. (1987). The effects of setting budget goals and task uncertainty on performance: A theoretical analysis.* The Accounting Review, 62(4), 778.

(1975) makes this point very clear. Although management by objectives (MBO) has different beginnings (Drucker, 1954), goal setting is the basis for objective setting, which expands beyond Locke's work (Carroll & Tosi, 1973). Whether goal setting is a theory or a motivational technique is not clear (Locke, 1975), but "Locke (1978) has argued persuasively that goal setting is either implicitly or explicitly recognized as a component process for virtually every theory of and approach to motivation" (Mento et al., 1987).

CASE ANALYSIS

The quality assurance committee, which had two representatives from the surgical unit, decided to use goal setting as a means of encouraging preventive decubitus care for high-risk patients. The tasks were simplified and standardized, and knowledge of the task was taught. The goals were specific, and feedback or knowledge of results would be reported monthly.

First, 100% of patients admitted to the surgical unit were to be evaluated by an RN during their admission assessment for decubitus ulcer risk (that is, unable to ambulate, in poor nutritional status, incontinent, with poor skin turgor). All those with a high decubitus ulcer risk would be given a routine treatment consisting of turning every 2 hours, beginning a Sween care kit and/or Granulex treatment to the bony prominence and perineal area, use of a convoluted foam mattress or air mattress, and encouraging fluids and adequate nutrition. A "decubitus care" stamp for the nursing care plan Kardex was to be used as a reminder. Nursing assistants would be trained in the proper technique for turning orthopedic patients. Each patient admitted with a decubitus ulcer or who developed one was to be reported for investigation by the committee. A random sampling of 10% of all charts would be monitored for compliance, and monthly reports would be given to the quality assurance committee and to the surgical unit head nurse, who would review these reports with her staff monthly.

"Decubitus ulcer preventive care" was used as the task rather than "prevention of decubitus ulcers" in order to eliminate influences from the patient's condition or the environment that could cause the goal to become impossible. Goal acceptance was expected as the value of this task was evident. This goal was difficult but attainable and should have resulted in enough success to increase job satisfaction.

RESEARCH

Locke began a program of detailed research to develop his theory of goal setting and has established a valid scientific basis for field study and implementation in managerial settings. The majority of the research done both in the laboratory and in the field have measured performance and its relationship to goal setting but not the controlling properties of goal setting (Campbell & Pritchard, 1976).

Locke (1966b; 1968b) began his early studies on the relationship between the level of the intention and the level of the actual performance and found a consistently linear relationship; that is, output increases as the standard becomes harder. These studies usually had preset goals, and the subjects were usually college students. Difficult and specific goals produced even higher effort and reduced boredom (Bryan & Locke, 1967; Locke & Bryan, 1967). Task difficulty when combined with specific goals also increased performance as long as the individual's ability was adequate for the task (Campbell & Ilgen, 1976; Frost & Mahoney, 1976; Shalley & Oldham, 1985). Field study (Latham & Baldes, 1975) with loggers agreed with Locke's theory and saved the logging company a large amount of money. Goal setting was even able to decrease absenteeism as well as increase productivity (Latham & Kinne, 1974) in another study of loggers.

Goal setting continues to be a popular subject for dissertations among psychology and business students. Frederick (1985) found that for ill-structured, problem-solving tasks, general goals were more effective than specific goals. Through laboratory studies, Lant (1987) and Park (1986) found that previous performance (failure or success) affected goal setting, and that goal difficulty was still the best predictor of behavior.

The effect of knowledge of results on motivation and performance was studied by Fryer (1964) and reanalyzed by Locke (1966a), who found that if goals were set, knowledge of results led to higher performance, unless the goals set were low. Locke (1967) and Locke and Bryan (1966b) decided, based on a study using math problems, that knowledge of results affected the subject's performance by influencing her or his intentions or goals. This decision was substantiated by Locke and Bryan (1968) in a complex computation test. Locke (1968a) recognized that some types of feedback taught subjects how to be more effective and some feedback motivated them.

Cummings, Schwab, and Rosen (1971), in a study of simple addition, found that the knowledge of results needed to be complete and correct to be significant in its influence on goals and performance. Dissertations by Bass (1988) and Rudd (1986) are supportive of Locke's findings. Whereas Franklin (1986) found that feedback also improved quality, not just performance, Prospero (1987) in his dissertation did not find significant improvement in quality or quantity of a collating task "when moderately difficult specific goals and accurate nonevaluative feedback were present" (Prospero, 1987, p. 905B).

The task-goal attributes and their effect on performance have also attracted much research. Locke, Bryan, and Kendall (1968) discovered that money incentives did indeed affect goal setting but did not otherwise affect performance in a laboratory setting using a variety of tasks. The possibility exists that the low financial reward was less effective, which would explain the low potency of these incentives. However, these conclusions were supported by Terborg's (1976) results in a study involving hiring 60 subjects for 1 week and measuring their performance after the effect of higher goal setting due to financial rewards was subtracted.

Ivancevich and McMahon (1977) concluded after a field study that the level of higher-order needs in an individual determines which task goal attributes will increase the goals that are set and therefore the performance. Technicians with high higher-order need strengths respond to goal challenge, feedback, and clarity, whereas technicians with low higher-order need strengths found goal acceptance to be crucial to their performance. Howard (1982) recognized that goal acceptance is crucial to task performance on the organizational level. Steers (1975) in a field study with supervisors found similar results with need for achievement being the specific higher-order need addressed in a field study; also, peer competition was found to be unhelpful with low achievers and responsible for poorer performance by high-need-to achieve supervisors. These results are compatible with Steers and Porter (1974) in their evaluation of relevant research. They suggest that management discover which task-goal attributes are meaningful to which employee and provide these in relationship to the employee's task goals.

Participation in goal setting has not been shown to improve performance consistently, especially in a laboratory setting. Latham and Yukl (1975b) found that black, uneducated workers did have slightly higher goals and performance when they assisted in the setting of their goals, but more educated workers produced more when goals were set for them. The self-set goals were lower than the assigned goals for a study of scientists and engineers (Latham, Mitchell, & Dossett, 1978). In a lab experiment of scheduling classes, participation in goal setting enhanced goal acceptance, goal satisfaction, and performance. The presence of a role model increased the effectiveness significantly (Earley & Kanfer, 1985). In another study involving Tinkertoys, Shalley, Oldham, and Porac (1987) found no positive effect for participatory goals and possibly an adverse reaction on subjects' intrinsic motivation. Researchers continue to study this complicated and unclear issue (Gier, 1986; Sauers, 1986) and continue to get conflicting results. More study is needed before participation theory can reliably guide management.

Locke's view of job satisfaction as it relates to goal setting is fairly narrow. He tested his theory that the emotion *satisfaction* is related to the subject's perception of the discrepancy between his or her intended or valued performance and the actual performance by using a questionnaire with college students who had just received their exam grades. Those with personally acceptable grades viewed themselves as satisfied and the others were dissatisfied. However, the dissatisfied subjects were then likely to do well on the next exam (Locke, 1969; 1970; Miner, 1980). Locke also showed that the importance of the goal had the power to increase or decrease satisfaction (Miner, 1980). Locke (1966b) feels that the effect of achievement or failure on an individual depends on whether the individual is motivated "by positives, for example, the desire for achievement . . . or by negatives, for example, the desire to avoid failure or criticism" (Locke, 1976, p. 1342). In a simulated work-environment study, White, Mitchell, and Bell (1977) found that goal setting with evaluation expectancy and social cues from co-workers did not increase overall job satisfaction. It did, however, decrease boredom and increase job pressure and performance.

Field studies seem to show an initial increase in satisfaction related to an increase in performance and goal setting. Overall, participating in goal setting did not increase job satisfaction except in uneducated black workers (Latham & Yukl, 1975b). In a study with sales personnel, Ivancevich (1976) found an increase in motivation and job satisfaction after goal-setting training, but the results dropped after 6 months. In another study involving skilled technicians and supervisors, Ivancevich (1977) again found initial improvements in performance and job satisfaction after goal setting that began to dissipate in 6 to 9 months. Goal setting appeared to be more effective in increasing production but less effective in increasing job satisfaction in a study involving temporary jobs (Umstot, Bell, & Mitchell, 1976). Batten (1986) found that hard goals elevated self-perception, and McIntire (1986) felt that task-specific self-esteem caused the setting of higher goals and, therefore, higher performance. More research is needed to investigate the cause of these results before they can be fully evaluated.

Characteristics of the supervisor can determine the degree that goals are accepted but hard goal setting is motivational (Oldham, 1976) whether the goals are accepted or not (Oldham, 1975). Recent studies have begun to look at the effect of goal setting on complex tasks. Edminister and Locke (1987) found that weighted goals could influence the complex task of lending officers in a simulated situation. Timely feedback could also have affected the increased productivity of these managers. Goals can encourage the development of strategies, but success depends on the ability of the manager to develop appropriate strategies (Koys, 1983; Chesney, 1986). Novak (1982) developed weighted goals for farmers in South Carolina that had strategy suggestions in them. Creativity occurs more often without specific goals and structure if creative potential is present in the subject (Duchon, 1983).

Interdependent tasks, that is, those that depend on the actions of others for success, do not seem as strongly responsive to goal-setting except in short laboratory studies such as Hamner and Harnett (1974) presented involving bargaining. Baumler (1971) used a business game to measure level of interdependence and performance. When interdependence was minimal, performance was improved, but as interdependence increased, it became detrimental to performance. In a study of hard rock miners, team building and goal setting were examined. Team building did not appear to improve performance significantly, whereas goal setting did show some improvement, but the study was actually inconclusive because performance or production might not accurately reflect effort in a complex job with uncertain environmental influences. This experiment shows the difficulty of field studies; the miners distrusted the new management and were not all cooperative.

A study in a new area, cultural influence of management techniques, was published by Shenkar and Ronen (1987). The attitudes toward work goals held by managers in the People's Republic of China were examined and compared to their religious heritage of Confucianism and their strong commitment to Maoism. The results were largely predictable, but the study reinforces the need to recognize the worker's value system in order to predict behavior.

Research in the area of nursing management is just beginning (Batey & Fine, 1986). Nursing has borrowed management styles from other disciplines and published "advice" for the nurse manager as Anderson (1986) and Falasco, Ferguson, Pierce, Price, Schneider, and Schneider (1986) have done, but these concepts have not been tested in a largely female health occupation such as nursing. As Brown (1986) exhorts us, "it is imperative that each nurse administrator recognize the significance of administrative research in order to substantiate forward movement in the practice environment" (p. iv). Stull (1986) did a significant study concerning the effect of goal setting (specific and general) and feedback (specific) on performance. Performance did increase if either goal setting or feedback was specific, but not when both goal setting and feedback were general. The control group also improved, but this may have been due to role modeling by the experimental group, who worked closely with the control group. The experiments appeared to support Locke's theory. Specific feedback influences the setting of specific intrinsic goals if general goals have been given.

The opportunity and the mandate are before nursing scholars to research goal setting in nursing management. An evaluation tool such as the one developed by Schwirian (1978) should be studied and modified to develop a means for specific evaluation of goal-setting effectiveness. Tools to evaluate performance can enable nurse managers to reinforce the caring areas of nursing and set specific goals with their employees. Nurses still need to study the effect of financial rewards on goal setting and on performance ("Consider This," 1986). Nurses can study and compare the fear of penalty theory (Wilson, 1987) or the desire for award theory as the most effective motivator to increase performance. Umstot, Bell, and Mitchell (1976) wrote a proposition that job enrichment and goal setting combined could provide a work environment with job satisfaction and higher performance. Research on this proposition in a nursing setting would provide valuable understanding in these days of nursing shortage.

Nurses guide patients to set goals and assist in the achievement of those goals daily. The nursing profession has set goals to achieve autonomy and professional recognition (Gunn, 1986). Nurses have a basic understanding of goal setting, and research is the way nurses can expand knowledge of solutions to management questions. Florence Nightingale years ago wrote that "all the results of good nursing care may be spoiled or utterly negated by one defect: petty management" (Brown-Stewart, 1987). Nursing management must correct the ambiguity of job requirements by specific goal setting in order to recruit and keep nurses (Brown-Stewart, 1987). First, however, nurses must gain knowledge, not by just repeating Locke's or others' tests, but by developing fresh, new theories and testing them in the work place (Henry & Christman, 1986).

REFERENCES

Anderson, D. (1986). A different approach to traditional nursing goals. *RN, 49*(10), 98.

Bass, R.I. (1988). The effects of goal-setting, goal distance and performance feedback on intrinsic motivation. *Dissertation Abstracts International, 48,* 2128B.

Batey, M.V., & Fine, R.B. (1986). On the scene: Research as a component of graduate study in nursing administration at the University of Washington School of Nursing. *Nursing Administration Quarterly, 11*(1), 27-29.

Batten, D.B. (1986). Goal-setting and self-perception. *Dissertation Abstracts International, 47,* 2208B.

Baumler, J.V. (1971). Defined criteria of performance in organizational control. *Administrative Science Quarterly, 16,* 340-349.

Brass, D.J. (1987). Findings from industrial-organizational behavior, and human resource management [Review of *Findings from industrial-organizational behavior and human resource management.]* Administrative Science Quarterly, 32, 464-465.

Brown, B. (Ed.). (1986). From the editor: Research in the field of nursing. *Nursing Administration Quarterly, 11*(1), iv-v.

Brown-Stewart, P. (1987). Thinly disguised contempt: A barrier to excellence, *JONA, 17*(4), 22-27.

Bryan, J.T., & Locke, E.A. (1967). Goal setting as a means of increasing motivation. *Journal of Applied Psychology, 51,* 274-277.

Buller, P.F., & Bell, C.H. (1986). Effects of team building and goal setting on productivity: A field experiment. *Academy of Management Journal, 29,* 305-328.

Campbell, D.J., & Ilgen, D.R. (1976). Additive effects of task difficulty and goal setting on subsequent task performance. *Journal of Applied Psychology, 61,* 319-324.

Campbell, J.P., & Pritchard, R.D. (1976). Motivational theory in industrial and organizational psychology. In M.D. Dunnette (Ed.), *Handbook of industrial and organizational psychology.* Chicago: Rand McNally College.

Carroll, S.J., & Tosi, H.L. (1973). *Management by objectives: applications and research.* New York: Macmillan.

Chesney, A.A. (1986). An examination of the relationship among goals, strategies, and performance: A simulation study. *Dissertation Abstracts International, 47,* 3479A.

Consider this. (1986). *JONA, 16*(9), 4-5.

Cummings, L.L., Schwab, D.P., & Rosen, M. (1971). Performance and knowledge of results determinants of goal setting. *Journal of Applied Psychology, 55,* 526-530.

Drucker, P.F. (1954). *The practice of management.* New York: Harper & Row.

Duchon, D.J. (1983). Creativity and goal setting. *Dissertation Abstracts International, 44,* 2867A.

Earley, P.C., & Kanfer, R. (1985). The influence of component participation and role models on goal acceptance, goal satisfaction, and performance. *Organizational Behavior and Human Decision Processes, 36,* 378-390.

Edminister, R.O., & Locke, E.A. (1987). The effects of differential goal weights on the performance of a complex financial task. *Personnel Psychology, 40,* 505-517.

Falasco, P.R., Ferguson, M.J., Pierce, L.L., Price, V.J., Schneider, M.J., & Schneider, J.M. (1986). Nursing supervision: A contemporary model. *Nursing Management, 17*(10), 76.

Franklin, R.L. (1986). Moderated goal setting in quality control. *Dissertation Abstracts International, 47,* 1400A.

Frederick, E.A. (1985). The influence of goal specificity and task structure on management problem solving. *Dissertation Abstracts International, 47,* 1400A.

Frost, P.J., & Mahoney, T.A. (1976). Goal setting and task process: An interactive influence on individual performance. *Organizational Behavior and Human Performance, 17,* 328-350.

Fryer, F.W. (1964). *An evaluation of aspiration as a training procedure.* Englewood Cliffs, NJ: Prentice-Hall.

Gier, J.A. (1986). The effects of strategy development on assigned and participatively set goals. *Dissertation Abstracts International, 47,* 4022.

Gunn, I.P. (1986). Nursing innovations help reach traditional goals. *Nursing and Health Care, 7,* 359-362.

Hamner, W.C., & Harnett, D.L. (1974). Goal setting performance and satisfaction in an interdependent task. *Organizational Behavior and Human Performance, 12,* 217-230.

Henry, B., & Christman, L. (1986). New organization theories for future nursing administration research. *Nursing Administration Quarterly, 11*(1), 73-80.

Hirst, M.K. (1987). The effects of setting budget goals and task uncertainty on performance: A theoretical analysis. *The Accounting Review, 62,* 774-784.

Howard, R.H. (1982). Organizational goal congruence: Its potential effect on the acceptance of an innovation. *Dissertation Abstracts International, 43,* 2384A.

Ivancevich, J.M. (1976). Effects of goal setting on performance and job satisfaction. *Journal of Applied Psychology, 61,* 605-612.

Ivancevich, J.M. (1977). Different goal setting treatments and their effects on performance and job satisfaction. *Academy of Management Journal, 20,* 406-419.

Ivancevich, J.M., & McMahon, J.T. (1977). A study of task-goal attributes, higher order need strength, and performance. *Academy of Management Journal, 20,* 552-563.

Koys, D.J. (1983). Managerial goal setting and strategy development: A model of their effects on behavior and performance. *Dissertation Abstracts International, 44,* 1902A.

Lant, T.K. (1987). Goals, search, and risk taking in strategic decision making. *Dissertation Abstracts International, 48,* 1831A.

Latham, G.P., & Baldes, J.J. (1975). The "practical significance" of Locke's theory of goal setting. *Journal of Applied Psychology, 60*(1), 122-124.

Latham, G.P., & Kinne, S.B. (1974). Improving job performance through training in goal setting. *Journal of Applied Psychology, 59,* 187-191.

Latham, G.P., Mitchell, T.R., & Dossett, D.L. (1978). Importance of participative goal setting and anticipated rewards on goal difficulty and job performance. *Journal of Applied Psychology, 63,* 163-171.

Latham, G.P., & Yukl, G.A. (1975a). A review of research on the application of goal setting in organizations. *Academy of Management Journal, 18,* 824-845.

Latham, G.P., & Yukl, G.A. (1975b). Assigned versus participative goal setting with educated and uneducated woods workers. *Journal of Applied Psychology, 60,* 299-302.

Lewin, K. (1935). *A dynamic theory of personality* (D.K. Adams & K.E. Zener, Trans.). New York: McGraw-Hill.

Locke, E.A. (1966a). A closer look at level of aspiration as a training procedure: A reanalysis of Fryer's data. *Journal of Applied Psychology, 50,* 417-420.

Locke, E.A. (1966b). The relationship of intentions to level of performance. *Journal of Applied Psychology, 50,* 60-66.

Locke, E.A. (1967). Motivational effects of knowledge of results: Knowledge or goal setting? *Journal of Applied Psychology, 51,* 324-329.

Locke, E.A. (1968a). Effects of knowledge of results, feedback in relation to standards, and goals on reaction-time performance. *American Journal of Psychology, 81,* 566-574.

Locke, E.A. (1968b). Toward a theory of task motivation and incentives. *Organizational Behavior and Human Performance, 3,* 157-189.

Locke, E.A. (1969). What is job satisfaction? *Organizational Behavior and Human Performance, 4,* 309-336.

Locke, E.A. (1970). Job satisfaction and job performance: A theoretical analysis. *Organizational Behavior and Human Performance, 5,* 484-500.

Locke, E.A. (1975). Personnel attitudes and motivation. *Annual Review of Psychology, 26,* 457-480.

Locke, E.A. (1976). The nature and causes of job satisfaction. In M.D. Dunnette (Ed.), *Handbook of industrial and organizational psychology.* Chicago: Rand McNally College.

Locke, E.A. (1978). The ubiquity of the technique of goal-setting in theories of and approaches to employee motivation. *Academy of Management Journal, 3,* 594-601.

Locke, E.A. (Ed.). (1986). *Generalizing from laboratory to field setting.* Lexington, MA: D.C. Heath.

Locke, E.A., & Bryan, J.F. (1966a). Cognitive aspects of psychomotor performance: The effects of performance goals on level of performance. *Journal of Applied Psychology, 50,* 286-291.

Locke, E.A., & Bryan, J.F. (1966b). The effects of goal-setting, rule learning, and knowledge of score on performance. *American Journal of Psychology, 79,* 451-457.

Locke, E.A., & Bryan, J.F. (1967). Performance goals as determinants of level of performance and boredom. *Journal of Applied Psychology, 51,* 120-130.

Locke, E.A., & Bryan, J.F. (1968). Goal setting as a determinant of the effect of knowledge of score on performance. *American Journal of Psychology, 81,* 398-406.

Locke, E.A., Bryan, J.F., & Kendall, L.M. (1968). Goals and intentions as mediators of the effects of monetary incentives on behavior. *Journal of Applied Psychology, 52,* 104-121.

Locke, E.A., Cartledge, N., & Knerr, C.S. (1970). Studies of the relationship between satisfaction, goal setting and performance. *Organizational Behavior and Human Performance, 5,* 135-158.

Locke, E.A., Shaw, K.N., Saari, L.M., & Latham, G.P. (1981). Goal-setting and task performance: 1969–1980. *Psychological Bulletin, 90,* 125-152.

McIntire, S.A. (1986). Task-specific self-esteem and goal setting as predictors of training performance. *Dissertation Abstracts International, 47,* 3566B.

Mento, A.J., Steel, R.P., & Karren, R.J. (1987). A meta-analytic study of the effects of goal setting on task performance: 1966–1984. *Organizational Behavior and Human Decision Processes, 39,* 52-83.

Miner, J.B. (1980). *Theories of organizational behavior.* Hinsdale, IL: Dryden.

Miner, J.B. (1981). Theories of organizational motivation. In G.W. England, A.R. Negandhi, & B. Wilpert (Eds.), *The functioning of complex organizations.* Cambridge, MA: Oelgeschlarger, Gunn, & Herin.

Novak, J.L. (1982). Incorporating multiple decision criteria in an assessment of the feasibility of row crop irrigation in South Carolina: A goal programming approach. *Dissertation Abstracts International, 42,* 3381A.

Oldham, G.R. (1975). The impact of supervisory characteristics on goal acceptance. *Academy of Management Journal, 18,* 461-475.

Oldham, G.R. (1976). The motivational strategies used by supervisors: Relationships to effective indicators. *Organizational Behavior and Human Performance, 15,* 66-86.

Park, A.K. (1986). An initial test of the theory of constructive failure: The relationship between goal difficulty, goal source, and response following failure. *Dissertation Abstracts International, 47,* 2516A.

Prospero, G.D. (1987). The effect of accurate, nonevaluative feedback and moderately difficult, specific goals on the reliability of performance on two self-paced tasks. *Dissertation Abstracts International, 48,* 905B.

Rudd, J.R. (1986). The effects of feedback frequency and goal setting on data processing performance. *Dissertation Abstracts International, 48,* 589B.

Ryan, T. (1958). Drives, tasks and the initiation of behavior. *American Journal of Psychology, 71,* 74-93.

Ryan, T. (1970). *Intentional behavior: An approach to human motivation.* New York: Ronald.

Sauers, D.A. (1986). Assigned versus participative goal setting: An attributional analysis. *Dissertation Abstracts International, 47,* 4446A.

Schwirian, P.M. (1978). Evaluating the performance of nurses: A multidimensional approach. *Nursing Research, 27,* 347-351.

Shalley, C.E., & Oldham, G.R. (1985). Effects of goal difficulty and expected external evaluation on intrinsic motivation: A laboratory study. *Academy of Management Journal, 28,* 628-640.

Shalley, C.E., Oldham, G.R., & Porac, J.F. (1987). Effects of goal difficulty, goal-setting method and expected external evaluation on intrinsic motivation. *Academy of Management Journal, 30,* 555-563.

Shenkar, O., & Ronen, S. (1987). Structure and importance of work goals among managers in the People's Republic of China. *Academy of Management Journal, 30,* 564-576.

Steers, R.M. (1975). Task-goal attributes, n achievement, on supervisory performance. *Organizational Behavior and Human Performance, 13,* 392-403.

Steers, R.M., & Porter, L.W. (1974). The role of task-goal attributes in employee performance. *Psychological Bulletin, 81,* 434-452.

Stull, M.K. (1986). Staff nurse performance: Effects of goal setting and performance feedback. *Journal of Nursing Administration, 16*(7, 8), 26-30.

Terborg, J.R. (1976). The motivational components of goal setting. *Journal of Applied Psychology, 61,* 613-621.

Umstot, D.D., Bell, C.H., & Mitchell, T.R. (1976). Effects of job enrichment and task goals on satisfaction and productivity: Implications for job design. *Journal of Applied Psychology, 61,* 379-394.

Umstot, D.D., Mitchell, T.R., & Bell, C.H. (1984). Goal setting and job enrichment: An integrated approach to job design. In B. Fuszard (Ed.), *Self-actualization for nurses: Issues, trends, and strategies for job enrichment.* Rockville, MD: Aspen.

White, S.E., Mitchell, T.R., & Bell, C.H. (1977). Goal setting, evaluation apprehension, and social cues as determinants of job performance and job satisfaction in a simulated organization. *Journal of Applied Psychology, 62,* 665-673.

Wilson, J.S. (1987). Have a problem employee? Use this plan. *Nursing, 17*(4), 121-123.

Chapter 30

Management by Objectives

Glenda G. Ridley

│ │   CASE STUDY

Ms. Silva is the nursing administrator for a hospital with a decentralized nursing service organized into eight units, each managed by a director of nursing. She has recently become aware of the need to change the employee appraisal system from the current standardized rating scale to a criteria-based performance evaluation. For some time Ms. Silva has been considering ways to improve motivation and to provide opportunities for the nurse managers and their staff to set goals to guide their practice and performance.

Revision of the appraisal system proved to provide the opportunity to include a process whereby the managers and staff could engage in the establishment and evaluation of goals and objectives as a component of the appraisal process. As this project must affect all units, Ms. Silva has decided the most effective way to implement the change would be to involve all of the nurse directors in the planning process. She wonders how she should proceed.

│ │

MANAGEMENT BY OBJECTIVES

Management by objectives (MBO) is a managerial concept that is both logical and simple, yet difficult to explain in simple terms or in only one dimension (Raia, 1974). Various authors have described the concept as a philosophy, a process, and/or a system that can be used for management of organizations, personnel, resources, and/or change. Miner (1980) points out that different authors define the steps of MBO differently, just as its utilization by different companies varies.

Basically, MBO is a series of steps whereby goals are identified, objectives are set to work toward the goals, and performance and/or achievement is reviewed or appraised.

Application of the MBO concept has evolved through three distinct phases: (1) performance appraisal, the phase during which programs are primarily focused on evaluating the performance of managers with emphasis on developing objective criteria and standards of performance for individuals in a given job description; (2) planning and control, the phase in which objectives are tied to plans, providing for control through budgets with performance appraisal continuing to be an essential element; and (3) integrative management system, a phase designed to integrate the key processes and activities of management, including development of overall organizational goals and plans, problem solving and decision making, compensation, manpower planning, and management training and development (Raia, 1974).

MBO was first introduced by Peter Drucker (1954) as a philosophy of management. In his discussion on the functions of management, he points out that management has three functions: (1) managing a business, (2) managing managers, and (3) managing workers and work. For a business to remain viable, all three must exist. Management must also provide recognition of individual strengths and responsibilities, common direction, establishment of teamwork, and harmonizing of "the goals of the individual with the common weal. The only principle that can do this is management by objectives" (Drucker, 1954, p. 136).

Odiorne (1979) defines MBO as

> a process whereby the superior and subordinate managers of an organization jointly identify its common goals, define each individual's major areas of responsibility in terms of the results expected, and use these measures as guides for operating the unit and assessing the contribution of each of its members. (p. 53)

MBO is a cycle, beginning with the organization's common goals or setting of organizational measures of performance; shaping or changing the organizational structure in relation to the goals; setting down goals and measures for the subordinate by the superior; proposal of goals and measures for his or her job by the subordinate; agreement by the superior and subordinate on the goals and measures; periodic audit, continuing review, and annual review of subordinate results, independently and jointly; and review of organization performance that reflects the organization's goals where the cycle continues (Odiorne, 1979).

McGregor (1957) described the MBO approach to performance whereby the subordinate establishes short-term performance goals for himself or herself and formulates specific plans to accomplish the goals prior to the superior entering the process. "The superior's role is to help the man relate his self-appraisal, his 'targets,' and his plans for the ensuing period to the realities of the organization" (McGregor, 1957, p. 91). The focus of this approach is on the broad areas of the subordinate's job responsibilities and analysis of accomplishments in relation to targets. It places responsibility on the individual to develop her or his own potential.

Raia (1974) describes MBO as a philosophy, a process, and a system of management. As a philosophy, it is "results-oriented," emphasizes accomplishments and results; reflects a proactive rather than a reactive style of management; focuses on change and improvement of both individual and organization effectiveness; and encourages participation at all levels in the management of the organization.

As a process, Raia (1974) describes the steps as

> (1) the formulation of clear, concise statements of objectives; (2) the development of realistic action plans for their attainment; (3) the systematic monitoring and measuring of performance and achievement; and (4) the taking of the corrective actions necessary to achieve the planned results. (p. 11)

As a system of management, MBO facilitates planning and control, organization and assignment of work, problem solving, decision making, motivation, self-control, manager development, compensation, performance appraisal, and other functions of management (Raia, 1974).

Mali (1975) defines *managing by objectives* as "a strategy of planning and getting results in a direction that management wishes to take while meeting the goals and needs of its participants" (p. 3). He presents four basic elements and five phases of MBO. The elements are

1. *Objectives.* Events or accomplishments planned or expected to happen
2. *Time strategy.* Scheduling of activities of each manager to achieve both short- and long-term results

3. *Total management.* Formulized effort to involve and coordinate the contributions of each manager toward a common goal
4. *Individual motivation.* Personal involvement in the process

The five phases are

1. *Isolating the objective.* Identification of needed results
2. *Setting the objective.* Formal process relating resources to involvement of those who are to deliver results
3. *Validating the objective.* Assures that needed resources are ready and willing to reach a desired goal
4. *Implementing the objective.* Implementation of activities to reach objective
5. *Controlling and reporting status of the objective.* Schedule for reporting progress toward completion of the objective (Mali, 1975)

Although authors differ in their description of MBO and its applications, all programs include goal setting, performance, and measurement of results, and all focus on achievement of goals developed and measured through participatory management processes (Kirk, 1981). The terms "goal" and "objective" are sometimes used interchangeably, with both terms representing a process of change. The term "goal" generally is used to refer to the expected outcome or desired result, and "objective" to refer to activities that will lead to the achievement of the goal (Kirk, 1981).

The keys to MBO are clearly articulating goals as meaningful expected outcomes and writing objectives that are clear, concise, and measurable.

Mali (1975) states that "the effective use of MBO by the manager requires a balance of special skills in the areas of objective setting, objective implementing, and measuring and correcting" (p. 221).

CASE ANALYSIS

The nurse administrator in the case presented could use the concept of MBO for two separate management functions — planning and performance appraisal. Ms. Silva could arrange a meeting to define the change, outline the goal and objectives, develop a plan of action, and establish a system for monitoring their progress. The revision of the performance appraisal system could provide opportunities for the nurse managers and their staff to set goals and objectives to guide their practice and performance by incorporating this into the procedure for employee performance evaluation.

Together Ms. Silva and her directors could develop the plan shown on page 284.

In planning the change, the principles of MBO would be applied: (1) a goal would be established describing the final result or expected outcome; (2) objectives would be defined that outlined the activities required for achieving the goal, assigned responsibility, and established a time schedule for action; (3) review mechanism would be established; and (4) the plans would be developed and mutually agreed upon using participatory management, a style consistent with MBO.

The decision to include the process for incorporating mutually established goals and objectives as part of the appraisal system would be consistent with one of the more widely acclaimed applications of MBO. However, the nurse administrator must be sure her directors and other staff receive effective training in MBO prior to implementation of the revised appraisal system. Although the MBO approach has many advantages to guide and motivate staff growth and performance, if not used appropriately, it can become a meaningless, even costly, paper exercise; instead of being a motivator, it can become a demotivator, a burden rather than a helpful tool.

Performance Evaluation

Goal

Evaluate the performance of each staff member at the end of the working test period and at least annually thereafter, based on criteria that reflect standards of performance defined in each employee's job description and that provide an opportunity for the manager and the staff member to establish goals and objectives to guide the individual's performance and growth.

Objectives	Responsibility	Target date
1. Revise job descriptions to include standards of performance.	Directors and staff	6 months
2. Revise appraisal format to provide for evaluation based on job description and individual goals and objectives.	Nurse administrator and directors	6 months
3. Train staff in revised system to include goal setting and writing objectives.	Inservice staff	Months 7 and 8
4. Implement revised system for performance evaluation.	Nurse administrator, directors, and staff	Month 9

Implementation monitoring

1. Progression of plan will be reviewed each month at the nursing administration staff meeting.
2. Implementation of the plan will be reviewed after 6 months by the directors and nurse managers.

Studies discussed in the next section show that top management must support the MBO process and even be involved in the implementation. For the program to be successful at this hospital, Ms. Silva is going to have to play an active part in training and in the implementation of the program. Equally important, the nurse managers must receive effective training.

RESEARCH

According to Odiorne (1979), the origins of the MBO idea is uncertain. Some attribute its beginnings to biblical times, to early philosophers, and to organizers of giant corporations such as Andrew Carnegie or Pierre du Pont (Odiorne, 1979). Odiorne (1979) suggests that Alfred P. Sloan, Jr., along with his associates Donaldson Brown and Albert Bradley of General Motors in the early 1920s, perfected the major elements of MBO. Drucker reported to his biographer that he first heard the term *management by objectives* from Sloan (Odiorne, 1979). However, Peter Drucker is generally considered the theoretician of management by objectives because of his 1954 book, *The Practice of Management,* in which he first uses the expressions "management by objectives" and "self-control" (Odiorne, 1979).

Ivancevich (1972) and Carroll and Tosi (1973) state that only a few research studies on MBO have been conducted, whereas Odiorne (1979) states that, "without a doubt, MBO is one of the best tested, most thoroughly researched techniques of recent times" (p. 14).

Some of the research studies in the literature are summarized here. First is the series of studies conducted at General Electric by Meyer, Kay, and French (1965). The focus of these studies was on alternative methods of performing the appraisal interview and on the effects of a new MBO program adopted for some managers in the company. Results from the first study were used in developing the Work Planning and Review (WPR) program. Results from the second study showed that managers in the WPR group were much more likely to have taken specific actions to improve performance than those using the traditional appraisal approach (Carroll & Tosi, 1973).

Raia (1974) summarizes the results of studies compiled at the Purex Corporation in 1963 and 1964. Purex was looking at the effectiveness of the MBO program they had introduced in 1961. Findings in the first study were generally favorable, showing improved productivity at their manufacturing plants, accompanied by improved morale and increased motivation. The study also showed that the operating managers had an additional administrative burden and that the lower levels of management were not participating meaningfully. The findings from the second study a year later supported those of the first. Productivity remained high. "Success was generally attributed to the fact that MBO improved management planning and control on the job and provided motivation to improve" (Raia, 1974, p. 160). However, several additional problems were identified, including distortion of managerial philosophy, evidence of overemphasis on production goals at the expense of others, and the failure of the program to provide tangible benefits for the individual manager. Gradually the program at Purex lost its identity as a driving force (Raia, 1974).

Ivancevich, Donnelly, and Lyon (1970) compared two different methods of implementing MBO to the manager's sense of job satisfaction (Ivancevich, 1972). In the program where top-level administrative staff handled the implementation and training activities, more improvement was shown in need satisfaction scores, with the most improvement in middle management.

Ivancevich (1972) reported on a study conducted at two firms (Palos and South Deering) and looked at job satisfaction changes of MBO participants. The findings from this study support the need for active participation by top management, which can have a significant effect on the overall job satisfaction of managers.

> The crucial point is that some form of reinforcement of what was learned and practiced in the training sessions is necessary. Without some degree of reinforcement the effects of training if any, are diluted or eliminated completely. (Ivancevich, 1972, p. 135)

Kirchhoff (1975) stated that research in the field had not actually measured the existence of MBO in the organization. He presented the Managerial Style Questionnaire (MSQ) designed to measure goal use. From his study using the instrument, he concluded that MBO training and goal setting do not ensure goal use and that the MSQ is an effective diagnostic tool for MBO in an organization (Kirchhoff, 1975).

Carroll and Tosi (1973) have also summarized case studies reported from British companies. In one case, reported by Preston (1968), the findings included the need for communication of organizational objectives along with company policy to the lower levels of management, cash savings attributed to the MBO program, and implication that MBO helped to identify problems in the organization and improve the overall developmental climate (Carroll & Tosi, 1973).

In a second study, Wickens (1968) reports that MBO has been successful in many British firms but has failed where it has not been institutionalized (Carroll & Tosi, 1973). In a factory studied by Wickens, MBO was not successful because of organizational problems such as conflicting objectives set with no procedure to resolve the conflicts, a rapidly changing market that caused changes in the priority of problems and objectives, lack of integration with other organizational components, and reorganization of management (Carroll & Tosi, 1973).

From data collected at Black and Decker, Carroll and Tosi (1973) reported findings suggesting positive results from an MBO program that included "judgements of success in achieving assigned goals, changes in attitudes and relations with the superior, attitudes toward the MBO approach, and changes in motivational level" (p. 129).

In addition to the studies cited, numerous other management studies addressing different aspects of MBO have been reported, along with volumes of publications concerning MBO or some variation of MBO. Raia (1974) states that "like almost everything else in the world, 'management by objectives' comes in all sizes, all colors, and all shapes" (p. 1). The concept has been labeled many different things, including "management by results," "management by goals and results," and "individual goal-setting," to name a few (Raia, 1974).

Although no research about MBO in nursing has been located, numerous references to MBO appear in the nursing literature; some describe the concept, and some suggest specific application to nursing practice or management.

Ganong and Ganong (1975) describe NMBO and NBO.

> NMBO is Nursing Management by Objectives. It is MBO applied by nurse managers as part of their management responsibilities for personnel, facilities, patient care, and budgetary planning within their own segments of the nursing department.

Other nursing management functions such as program development, nursing audit, career planning, and handling grievances and complaints can also use NMBO.

Nursing by objectives (NBO) is "a results-oriented technique using mutually-established patient care objectives, an implementation schedule, and evaluation of results and patient progress" (Ganong & Ganong, 1975, p. 73). It focuses on one nurse and one patient working together for management of that patient's care.

Rutkowski (1987) discusses the use of the MBO method as the most common method for implementing a performance appraisal system that provides for employee motivation and improved productivity, has employee appeal, involves employees in setting performance standards, and assists them in resource utilization and time management.

> The MBO method is well suited for decentralized settings and for nurses who require little supervision since it is objective and participatory. Users feel that it elevates morale and encourages nurses to be more productive (Rutkowski, 1987, p. 247).

Rowland and Rowland (1980) also present MBO as an effective system for performance appraisal of nursing staff, as do Beyers and Phillips (1979), who also point out that, although MBO might be difficult to implement at times, evidence shows that this method is superior to traditional appraisal systems.

Kirk (1981) presents MBO as an effective means of planning for the nurse manager and recommends the use of an MBO planning tool that organizes the activity, addresses not only the objectives but also the expected results, identifies additional resources and a target date for completion, and assigns responsibility for completion of the action(s).

Hollee and Batchley (1982) discuss the advantage of using MBO as a system to avoid ineffective planning as a nurse manager. Marquis and Huston (1987) state that each nurse manager should keep a list of objectives on top of her or his desk and refer to it periodically in order to steer a straighter course, should encourage subordinates to do likewise, and should formally and informally review their progress with them.

Nurse managers and staff nurses are responsible for management functions whether they be management of the organization, the department, the unit, a group of patients, or one patient. Management by objectives is a concept, used appropriately, that can assist the nurse to get the job done.

REFERENCES

Beyers, M., & Phillips, C. (1979). *Nursing management for patient care* (2nd ed.). Boston: Little, Brown, & Co.

Carroll, S.J., Jr., & Tosi, H.L., Jr. (1973). *Management by objectives: applications and research.* New York: Macmillan.

Drucker, P.F. (1954). *The practice of management.* New York: Harper & Row.

Ganong, J., & Ganong, W. (1975). *Help with management by objectives.* Chapel Hill, NC: W.L. Ganong Co.

Holle, M.L., & Batchley, M.E. (1982). *Introduction to leadership and management in nursing.* Belmont, CA: Wadsworth.

Ivancevich, J.M. (1972). A longitudinal assessment of management by objectives. *Administrative Science Quarterly, 17,* 126-138.

Ivancevich, J.M., Donnelly, J.H., & Lyon, H.L. (1970). A study of the impact of management by objectives on perceived need satisfaction. *Personnel Psychology, 23,* 139-151.

Kirchhoff, B.A. (1975). A diagnostic tool for management by objectives. *Personnel Psychology, 28,* 351-364.

Kirk, R. (1981). *Nursing management tools.* Boston: Little, Brown, & Co.

McGregor, D. (1957). An uneasy look at performance appraisal. *Harvard Business Review, 35,* 89-94.

Mali, P. (1975). *How to manage by objectives: A short course for managers.* New York: Wiley.

Marquis, B.L., & Huston, C.J. (1987). *Management decision making for nurses.* Philadelphia: Lippincott.

Meyer, H.H., Kay, E., & French, J.R.P. (1965). Split roles in performance appraisal. *Harvard Business Review, 43,* 123-129.

Miner, J.B. (1980). *Theories of organization behavior.* Hinsdale, IL: Dryden.

Odiorne, G.S. (1979). *MBO II: A system of managerial leadership for the 80s.* Belmont, CA: Fearson Pittman.

Preston, S.J. (1968). J. Stone's management by objectives. *Personnel* (London), *1,* 22-25.

Raia, A.P. (1974). *Management by objectives.* Glenview, IL: Scott, Foresman.

Rowland, H.S., & Rowland, B.L. (1980). *Nursing administration handbook.* Germantown, MD: Aspen.

Rutkowski, B. (1987). *Managing for productivity in nursing.* Rockville, MD: Aspen.

Wickens, J.D. (1968). Management by objectives: An appraisal. *Journal of Management Studies, 5,* 365-379.

Chapter 31 *

Goal Congruence Theory
Chris Argyris

Ann Marriner-Tomey
Janet Chorpenning

❙❙   CASE STUDY

After 2 months in the position of head nurse for the evening shift on a surgical progressive unit, Susan Jones was dealing with several major issues. Generally, the 24-bed unit was 95% occupied, the patients' care required management of various treatment modalities, patients needed major assistance with care, and typically the staffing pattern for the evening shift included one RN, one LPN, and two nursing assistants. Staff believed that the work was difficult, that no one really cared about them, and that they were owed "sick" time. Consequently, they took time off as frequently as they could. Susan frequently had to use float nurses without enough time to give them orientation. Reports were somewhat incomplete and affected continuity of care. Float nurses asked a lot of questions, did not know the procedures, seemed hesitant to act, and sometimes felt that they were more bother than worth.

The nursing model was designed for team nursing. The staffing availability caused Susan much concern about the quality of care, as she was constantly confronted by staff discontent about workload as well as frequent patient or family concern about the lack of timely delivery of care.

Susan wondered what she could do to make a difference. She approached management to express concern about the level of care required, quality of care, and monetary issues and to request additional staffing.

❘❘❘

GOAL CONGRUENCE THEORY

Chris Argyris was influenced by E. Wright Bakke, with whom he worked at Yale University, when he developed goal congruence theory. Although Argyris has published prolifically, goal congruence theory is presented in three primary sources: *Personality and Organization* (Argyris, 1957), *Integrating the Individual and the Organization* (Argyris, 1964), and "Personality and Organization Theory Revisited" in *Administrative Science Quarterly* (Argyris, 1973).

Argyris discussed the healthy adult personality in *Personality and Organization.* He labeled the multidimensional process of striving to meet objectives as *internal maintenance* and adaptation to the external environment as *self-actualization* (p. 49). He described the developmental trends from immature infants to mature adults as movement from a state of passivity to a state of increasing activity, from a state of dependence upon others to a state of relative independence, from being able to behave in only a few ways to being capable of behaving in many different ways, from erratic, casual, shallow, quickly dropped interests to deeper interests, from a short time perspective to a longer time perspective, from being in a subordinate position to an equal or superordinate position, and from lack of awareness to awareness of and control over self (p. 50). Various forces within organizations and individuals themselves inhibit the process of moving along those dimensions.

Argyris also presented the classical management theory principles of formal organization, including task specialization, chain of command, unity of direction, and span of control (pp. 58-66). He indicated that a basic incongruity between the needs of a mature personality and the requirements of formal organizations results in frustration, conflict, failure, and a short time perspective (pp. 66-75). He identified individual and group adaptations, such as leaving the organization, climbing the organizational ladder, using defense mechanisms, lowering work standards and becoming apathetic, placing more value on material rewards and depreciating human and nonmaterial rewards, and teaching children not to expect satisfaction on the job (pp. 76-122). Managers are likely to conclude that employees are lazy, uninterested, apathetic, money-crazy, and creators of errors and waste. Consequently, management often becomes more directive and imposes more controls, resulting in more undesired behavior (pp. 123-162).

Argyris concluded *Personality and Organization* with the following propositions:

I. There is a lack of congruency between the needs of healthy individuals and the demands of the formal organization.
II. The resultants of this disturbance are frustration, failure, short time perspective, and conflict.
III. Under certain conditions the degree of frustration, failure, short time perspective, and conflict will tend to increase.
IV. The nature of the formal principles of organization causes the subordinate, at any given level, to experience competition, rivalry, inter-subordinate hostility, and to develop a focus toward the parts rather than the whole.
V. The employee adaptive behavior maintains self-integration and impedes integration with the formal organization.
VI. The adaptive behavior of the employees as a cumulative effect, feedbacks into the organization, and reinforces itself.
VII. Certain management reactions tend to increase the antagonisms underlying the adaptive behavior.
VIII. Other management actions can decrease the degree of incongruency between the individual and formal organization.
IX. Job or role enlargement and employee-centered leadership will not tend to work to the extent that the adaptive behavior (propositions III, IV, V, and VI) has become imbedded in the organizational culture and the self-concept of the individuals.
X. The difficulties involved in proposition IX may be minimized by the use of reality-oriented leadership. (p. 233-237)

Argyris modified his theory, dropped the infant-adult comparison, and focused on psychological energy in *Integrating the Individual and the Organization* (1964). He indicated that the higher the self-esteem, the greater the potential psychological energy a person has available. A climate of trust enhances the opportunity for psychological success, which creates the proper state of mind for psychological energy (pp. 29–31). He replaced "healthy individuals" with "individuals aspiring for psychological success" and noted that not everyone wants psychological success. Placing a person who does not desire psychological success where it is required is incongruent, as is placing someone who aspires to psychological success in a pyramidal organization. The incongruity between the organizational form and the individual's needs causes disturbance that leads to unintended consequences such as passivity or aggression, thus diverting energy from the organizational goals.Argyris addresses organizational pseudo-effectiveness as a state where no discomfort is reported but ineffectiveness exists. He analyzed it as

1. The unintended activities with their protective defenses and the resulting employee attitudes toward being productive lead to a situation in which (a) increasing increments of energy will be used nonproductively, (b) the potential energy input will decrease, and (c) the probability of resolving these problems is decreased. . . .
2. Participants will tend to experience feelings of uncomfortableness that are beyond their control to correct.
3. In order to protect the unintended activities, the participants at all levels feed up to the top information that makes the organization look (to the top) more effective than it actually is. This will lead to organizational pseudo-effectiveness. (pp. 132-133)

Argyris reported his findings about hosts (people who are receptive to ineffectiveness) and carriers (people who carry ineffectiveness around and infect others) as identified by their self-actualization in the organization scores.

1. The lower the self-actualizing score a person has, the greater are the chances that he will be a carrier of the "illness" low morale, and the greater are the chances of his infecting others.
2. Every carrier of "low morale" is also a "host" for further infection of "low morale." Subsequent infection from others will tend to have a "spiraling" or "snowballing" effect that is noticeable in an individual as his morale becomes increasingly lower.
3. The degree of infection with "low morale" is not only dependent on the number of carriers carrying this disease, but it is also a function of the number of "hosts" available within the environment of the carriers. This number, in turn, is a function of a complex set of variables in the milieu of the department in which the carriers and hosts exist.
4. Another variable that influences the chances of infection is the existence of natural boundaries in the environment to prevent a carrier from coming into contact with a host.
5. Categorizing people in terms of high, medium, and low self-actualizing scores, we find that a low-score individual tends to be a carrier of ineffectiveness. The host tends to be a medium-score individual. Apparently the high-score individual is perceived by the carrier as being immune to infection (p. 143).

Argyris defined "organizational effectiveness as a system manifesting increasing outputs with constant or decreasing inputs or constant outputs with decreasing inputs" (p. 146). Inputs include psychological energy. Consequently, effectiveness is increased by increasing the amount of psychological energy available to work.

Argyris proposed that incongruities between individual and organizational needs can be overcome by modifying pyramidal organizations to provide opportunities for psychological success. He presented a mix model and six hypotheses for integrating organizational and individual goals (pp. 146-191). Then organizational structures of the new system were presented, and the conditions for use of various structures were discussed. The pyramid may be used when time is important; decisions are routine; distribution of power, reward, controls, work specialization, or the centralization of information are not affected; a large number of scattered people are involved; and individuals do not desire psychological success. Overlapping groups are useful when the decision is not routine and does not affect the distribution of power, time is important, and change cannot be delegated to everyone involved. Power according to functional contribution may be used for new product development, when solutions to problems involve more than one department, and for long-range policy planning. Power according to inevitable organizational responsibilities is appropriate when decisions affect control or define the rules for use of the structures (pp. 197–211). Argyris concluded that leaders need to develop competence in several leadership styles, internalize their philosophy of leadership, and shift styles with personal security as the situation indicates (p. 216).

In "Personality and Organization Theory Revisited," Argyris (1973) reduced the infant-adult dimensions from seven to four, discussed interaction of personality and organization, and presented research designed to test the theory, results that were predictable by the theory, and results that could be explained by the theory.

CASE ANALYSIS

After reviewing Argyris's work, Susan decided she wanted to help build her staff's self-esteem so they would have more psychological energy to work toward the organizational goals. She changed the modality of care to a modular or modified primary nursing. The RN was responsible for about half of the patients and the LPN the rest. One aide was assigned to work with each. The RN and LPN served as role models to the aides as they worked together to move and ambulate patients. They gave explicit directions to the aides as they delegated passing water and trays and helping patients eat and ambulate. They explained why the delegated duties were important and gave positive reinforcement for jobs well done. Susan tried to assign the same personnel to the same patients as much as possible to facilitate continuity of care. She requested that some float aides be oriented to her unit and that those aides be the ones pulled to her unit as much as possible. Susan noted that the quality of care started improving and that absenteeism decreased.

RESEARCH

Few studies have directly tested Argyris's theory. He conducted some studies during the 1950s and early 1960s and identified a number of studies, the results of which could be explained by goal congruence theory. Then his focus changed to organizational change.

Employees of various departments in a bank were interviewed to assess the degree of goal congruence (Argyris, 1954). When the degree to which employees actualize themselves and the degree to which the organization expressed itself were both high, as in three departments, the departments were assessed to be effective. When both indexes were low, as in one department, the department had more apparent conflict and less organizational commitment.

Two manufacturing plants were used to study self-actualization (Argyris, 1957, 1959, 1960a, 1960b). High scores characterized the more effective plants. The self-actualization data supported a number of theory-based predictions. Foremen emphasized promotion and pay, and employees felt more pressure in the less effective plant; employees were more prounion, less friendly, and less concerned with quality in the less effective plant. However, concurrent findings do not establish cause and effect, and the coding reliability was about 70% agreement.

Argyris noted several studies that support goal congruence hypotheses in reviews of the literature (1964, 1973). However, most of the studies have not been published in easily obtained professional literature, and they cannot be evaluated from Argyris's description of them.

Bonjean and Vance (1968) developed a questionnaire to measure self-actualization that correlated .61 and .72 with Argyris's index in two separate samples. High and low self-actualized personnel did not differ regarding lack of interest in the job, restriction of output, or aggression toward co-workers. The low self-actualized subjects reported more errors in their work, more anger with supervisors, less job satisfaction, and more thoughts about earning money and seeking other work.

Pennings' (1976) findings generally supported the theory when he used 40 offices of a brokerage firm to test hypotheses by relating measures of organizational autonomy and participation to various criterion indexes. However, he found a significantly higher level of anxiety under participative conditions.

Dewar and Werbel (1979) found that high levels of formalization and routinization of technology were related to reduced job satisfaction but that neither showed any relationship to the amount of conflict. Conflict was related to directive leadership, but whether conflict elicited the directive leadership or directive leadership elicited the conflict was not clear.

Goal congruency theory predicts that the tendency to oppose bureaucratic procedures increases at each lower organizational level, but Rossel (1971) found negative attitudes most pronounced just below top management. They were less at the top and at first-level supervision levels. These attitudes were apparently related to opportunities for promotion.

Burke and Weir (1978) found that in mutually helping operations individuals seek help from each other as well as help each other more. This help is more personal than work related and consequently has questionable effects on quantity or quality of production.

No testing of goal congruence theory or Argyris's work was located in the nursing literature.

REFERENCES

Argyris, C. (1954). *Organization of a bank: A study of the nature of organization and the fusion process.* New Haven, CT: Labor and Management Center, Yale University.

Argyris, C. (1957). *Personality and organization.* New York: Harper & Row.

Argyris, C. (1959). Understanding human behavior in organizations: One viewpoint. In M. Haire (Ed.), *Modern organization theory.* New York: Wiley.

Argyris, C. (1960a). *Understanding organizational behavior.* Homewood, IL: Dorsey.

Argyris, C. (1960b). Organizational effectiveness under stress. *Harvard Business Review, 38*(3), 137-146.

Argyris, C. (1964). *Integrating the individual and the organization.* New York: Wiley.

Argyris, C. (1973). Personality and organization theory revisited, *Administrative Science Quarterly, 18,* 141-167.

Bonjean, C.M., & Vance, G.G. (1968). A short form measure of self-actualization. *Journal of Applied Behavioral Science, 4,* 299-312.

Burke, R.J., & Weir, T. (1978). Organizational climate and informal helping process in work settings. *Journal of Management, 4*(2), 91-105.

Dewar, R., & Werbel, J. (1979). Universalistic and contingency predictions of employee satisfaction and conflict. *Administrative Science Quarterly, 24,* 426-448.

Pennings, J.M. (1976). Dimensions of organizational influence and their effectiveness correlates. *Administrative Science Quarterly, 21,* 688-699.

Rossel, R.D. (1971). Autonomy in bureaucracies. *Administrative Science Quarterly, 16,* 308-314.

Chapter 32

Behavior Modification
B.F. Skinner

Patricia Lynn Burgamy

▌▌ **CASE STUDY**

Betty Paton is a newly appointed head nurse on a busy medical-surgical floor in a community hospital. Although administration is committed to having an all-professional staff, the current nursing shortage has rendered this goal impossible. Only six registered nurses are available to cover all three shifts, with the bulk of the direct patient care administered by practical nurses and nurse's aides. Consequently, Betty has a great interest in establishing and maintaining good working relationships with these nurses. Her observations have led her to believe that the registered nurses are basically capable, caring professionals, but she has observed some disturbing trends that she feels must be addressed. Chronic absenteeism has become a problem and seems to be increasing. In addition, several employees are frequently late and take longer than the allotted time during coffee and meal breaks. This type of behavior has led to an increased workload for all that has further decreased morale because everyone is already overworked due to the staff shortage. The previous head nurse reinforced these poor working habits not only by failing to address the problem but also by engaging in these same behaviors herself on occasion. Betty feels that the problem necessitates immediate action, but she is unsure of how to approach the situation because she has not yet established any relationships with her staff.

│ │

BEHAVIOR MODIFICATION THEORY

Organizational behavior modification has its origin in the work of B.F. Skinner and his principles of operant conditioning. Skinner (1953) believes that human behavior can be predicted by identifying and analyzing its causes. Once the causes are analyzed, behavior can be controlled if the causes can be manipulated. Skinner (1972) postulates that all human problems involve human behavior and therefore cannot be solved by physical or biological technology alone. He contends that what is needed is a technology of behavior. A scientific analysis from which such a technology might be drawn would shift responsibility and achievement to the environment rather than to the individual.

The purpose of behavior modification is to create desirable new behavioral patterns in place of behavior considered undesirable (Luthans, 1973a). Organizational behavior modification assumes that observable behavior is the unit of analysis. An individual's beliefs, attitudes, or values are not of any direct concern. Observable behaviors such as absenteeism, tardiness, or task completion are analyzed in relation to the organization's goals.

A systematic evaluation of an intervention's impact on performance is essential to determine where effort should be expended. Behaviors are not targeted for change unless a direct relationship exists between the behaviors and the performance of the organization. For example, any unusual work habits would not be of concern unless they adversely affected the organization's goals (Luthans, Maciag, & Rosenkrantz, 1983).

Four intervention strategies are used to bring about desired behavior change. The first and most powerful is positive reinforcement. A positive reinforcer is any stimulus that strengthens the probability of a certain response. Behavior that leads to a positive consequence is usually repeated, whereas behavior that leads to negative consequences is not (Hamner, 1974).

Negative reinforcement is like positive reinforcement in that it increases the frequency of some desired behavior. However, its reinforcement property comes from the termination or withdrawal of some condition. An example would be an employee who works harder to avoid the nagging of the supervisor. It is frequently confused with punishment, but the difference is that negative reinforcement increases the frequency of a behavior and punishment does not (Luthans & Kreitner, 1975).

Punishment strategies are designed to decrease the frequency of a behavior. Punishment has been perhaps the most widely used strategy, although it is not the most effective. It must be systematically applied and also be a direct consequence of the undesired behavior to have the appropriate results. Luthans (1973b) states that punishment must be personal and individualized. In other words, what is punishing for one person is not for another. A manager must assess the response frequency of the undesired behavior to ascertain the effectiveness of the punishment.

Although punishment is capable of changing behavior, behaviorists stress the undesirable side effects that can occur. Punishment may lead to anxiety and temporary rather than permanent behavior change. Also, punishment may lead to hostile feelings between manager and employee because the employee does not distinguish between the punishment and the punisher.

Extinction is a very potent strategy in spite of the fact that nothing is done. Behaviors must be reinforced to recur; if no reinforcement is available, the behavior decreases in frequency and eventually disappears. The behaviors are then replaced by new responses that are reinforced (Luthans & Kreitner, 1975).

These strategies may be used individually or in various combinations. Extinction and positive reinforcement are used together, as are punishment and positive reinforcement, and punishment and negative reinforcement.

The success of the behavior modification program depends on the timing of the contingent consequences. The rewards or reinforcers are administered systematically through one of several predetermined reinforcement schedules. Although certain rewards may already be familiar to most managers, the significant difference here is the systematic application of the reinforcers (Luthans & White, 1972).

A continuous reinforcement schedule exists when reinforcement follows every desired response. It is effective at maintaining behavior as long as the reinforcer can always occur, but the response is usually stopped as soon as the contingent reinforcement ceases. It may be appropriate initially for weak or low-frequency responses, but reinforcing every desired response is simply not practical.

An intermittent reinforcement strategy actually promotes stronger behavior that is less subject to extinction. This strategy may take one of four forms. A fixed-ratio strategy occurs when a fixed number of responses must be emitted before any reinforcement occurs. This schedule tends to produce a high rate of response that is steady. A variable-ratio schedule exists when a random or varying number of desired responses must occur before reinforcement is offered. This schedule also produces a high rate of response that is resistant to extinction. A fixed-interval schedule exists when the first response after a given period of time is reinforced. This schedule usually produces an uneven response pattern. Response may be slow immediately following reinforcement or very vigorous immediately preceding it. A good example of this type of schedule is the weekly or monthly paycheck. The variable-interval schedule occurs when the first response after a varying or random period of time is reinforced. It usually produces a vigorous, consistent response pattern that is highly resistant to extinction (Luthans & Kreitner, 1975).

Most behaviors are expected to become self-reinforcing after a sufficient period of time; that is, satisfaction is found in the completion of the task itself rather than in the reward or reinforcer (Luthans & Kreitner, 1975).

Hamner and Organ (1978) have formulated rules for using these operant conditioning techniques. Although they may appear simple, research indicates that they are often violated.

Rule 1: Do not reward all people the same. Many managers seem to believe that the only fair system is to treat all employees in a certain job classification in the same manner, but most employees want differentiation so that they can recognize their importance to the organization. If all rewards are the same, the behavior of high-performance workers is being extinguished because it is being ignored and poor-performance workers are being reinforced because they are receiving the same rewards as the others. In other words, no one has any incentive to excel.

Rule 2: Failure to respond has reinforcing consequences. Some managers may be uncomfortable differentiating between workers and therefore may choose not to respond, but this behavior, in itself, has reinforcing properties and can modify behavior. Performance consequences of inaction as well as action must be considered.

Rule 3: Be sure to tell a person what he or she can do to receive reinforcement. A manager increases the individual freedom of employees by clarifying the contingencies of reinforcement. The employee then has a standard by which to measure her or his performance.

Rule 4: Be sure to tell a person what he or she is doing wrong. If a manager fails to specify why reinforcement is being withheld, the employee may associate the action with some past undesirable response rather than the undesired response the manager is trying to extinguish. The manager may be extinguishing good performance while not affecting the undesired behavior.

Rule 5: Do not punish in front of others. Punishment should be sufficient only to extinguish the undesired behavior. When administered in front of peers, it also serves to ridicule an employee and may have negative side effects.

Rule 6: Make the consequences equal to the behavior. Be fair by making sure rewards are offered appropriately. Employees should be advised when their performance is not satisfactory. An overrewarded employee may feel guilty, and an underrewarded employee may feel resentful.

The principles of operant conditioning have been used in mental hospitals and schools with success, but the organizational manager must be able to apply the same intervention strategies and reinforcement schedules in achieving the desired goals within the organization. Luthans and Kreitner (1975) have developed an organizational behavior modification problem-solving model called behavioral contingency management with five major steps.

Step 1: Identify performance-related behavioral events. Organizational activity consists of behavioral events, performance, and organizational consequences. Organizational behavior modification deals primarily with behavioral events that are classified as either desirable, undesirable, or irrelevant. Desirable behaviors lead to the accomplishment of the organization's goals. They must be strengthened and maintained. Undesirable behaviors detract from the organization's goals. They must be weakened and extinguished when possible. Irrelevant behaviors do not affect organizational objectives.

A manager desiring to use the behavioral contingency model must first reduce the behaviors in question to observable, countable events. A behavior such as thinking could not be considered because it is not quantifiable, but correctly completing questions on an exam could be measured. This step is necessary to establish acceptable measures of performance.

Identifying only performance-related behavior ensures that effort is not expended in modifying behavior that has no bearing on the organization's objectives. For example, an employee may have an irritating habit such as complaining. If this habit has no bearing on job performance, the manager should concentrate on other, more salient behaviors.

Performance-related behavior may be identified by considering its organizational consequences. Would production be increased if the behavior in question ceased? To illustrate this point, attendance may be a more critical behavior for certain employees because production may cease when they are not present.

Certain nonbehavioral performance problems may exist in organizations. Such things as lack of individual ability, outdated equipment, or unfair output standards may be responsible for unmet goals. The behavioral contingency management model cannot cure these types of difficulties.

Step 2: Measure the frequency of response. Once performance-related behavioral events are identified, steps should be taken to measure the strengths of these behaviors before any attempt is made to change them. A manager may find that certain behaviors are more or less damaging than previously thought. A variety of methods for recording the frequencies may be utilized, but care should be taken to ensure that the data collected are accurate.

Employees may have questions about the data collection. Managers should always be straightforward about their efforts; however, the Hawthorne effect may cause some distortion of reality. Recording activities should be as unobtrusive as possible to minimize this effect.

Step 3: Identify existing contingencies through functional analysis. A functional analysis communicates to the manager where the responding is occurring and what the consequences are. It is usually completed during the data-collecting period and determines what is reinforcing undesirable behaviors. Once these reinforcers are identified, they can be either removed or replaced. The analysis is also important in establishing the antecedents of the behavior.

Step 4: Intervention strategies. This step actually consists of four substeps: developing intervention strategies, applying them, measuring their impact on response frequency, and maintaining desirable outcomes. Managers must consider such variables as organizational structure, decision-making processes, communication, and the nature of the task involved. Appropriate intervention strategies are selected after the variables have been appraised. The results of the intervention are then carefully monitored and charted. Schedules of reinforcement are applied to maintain desirable behaviors.

Step 5: Evaluate. Behavioral contingency management is geared to bottom-line performance improvement. Subjective statements or opinions should not be regarded. If objective evaluation determines that the intervention strategy is not affecting the targeted individual or group, other interventions may be attempted.

Desirable behaviors that have never occurred cannot be positively reinforced and subsequently strengthened. Miner (1980) summarizes two learning methods—shaping and modeling—that address this situation.

Shaping involves defining the target behaviors, reducing them to a measurable sequence of steps that the individual is capable of meeting, selecting positive reinforcers, allowing antecedent conditioning to foster desired behavior, making all reinforcement contingent on increasingly close approximations to the desired behavior, and reinforcing the target behavior on a continuous and then variable basis.

Modeling is a type of learning that is somewhat inconsistent with a strict behavior modification approach. Internal constructs such as memory and imagination must be used to understand the technique. Modeling entails identifying the target behavior, selecting the model and the medium to be used, structuring a favorable learning environment, modeling the target behavior and supporting it with such activities as role playing while demonstrating the positive consequences of the modeling behavior, reinforcing all progress, and reinforcing the target behavior on a continuous and then variable basis.

The concept of self-control is also considered in behavior modification. However, self-control is seen only as manipulation of the environment by an individual to determine her or his own behavior (Miner, 1980). Luthans and Davis (1979) have postulated that with behavioral self-management, individuals can manipulate stimuli and rewards to change their own behavior in desired ways. They believe that behavioral self-management may be the first step in increasing managerial effectiveness.

Any analysis of operant conditioning as it relates to human resource management must include a discussion of money as a reinforcer. Schneier (1974) states that money is the most frequently used reinforcer in the workplace. He further elaborates that money is both a conditioned reinforcer and a discriminative stimulus. It is considered a conditioned reinforcer because it is necessary to acquire such primary reinforcers as food and shelter. It is a discriminative stimulus in that it serves as a cue to the individual that he or she will receive more money upon completion of work.

Although money is the most frequently used reward in organizations, it is not always a positive reinforcer. Luthans and Kreitner (1975) suggest that the changing environment may be rendering money a less powerful reinforcing tool. Social attitudes have diminished the significance of money earned through work. Also, money received as salary is frequently not contingent on performance. If, however, the receipt of money or some equivalent prize is really contingent on a specific desired behavior, it then becomes a positive reinforcer. A piecerate incentive program in which a designated amount of pay is received for a designated amount of work is the most contingent.

An appropriate concluding topic of discussion is the ethical controversy surrounding behavior modification. Nord (1969) states that modern Americans, particularly those of the managerial class, consider themselves self-actualizing individuals rather than animals manipulated by their environment. Significant numbers of managers feel that manipulating people to accomplish one's own objectives is unethical. What must be considered is the fact that people are constantly manipulating others and being manipulated themselves through reinforcing actions. This manipulation most often occurs without any awareness on the part of either person, but it nevertheless exists. Behavior modification techniques are distinctive only in that behavior is influenced in a systematic manner (Stolz et al., 1975). The behavioral approach to management makes the individual behavior of both leader and subordinate, as well as their interactive behavior, the focus of analysis (Luthans & Davis, 1979). Luthans and Kreitner (1975) feel that organizational behavior modification is no more or less manipulative than any other approach to human resource management. If manipulation does exist, it is manipulation of the environment rather than of the individual.

CASE ANALYSIS

The head nurse in the case presented faces some interesting challenges. How does she motivate her employees to improve their performance without alienating them? As a new manager, if she approaches the situation with a strict, punishing attitude, she may never be able to establish the kind of cooperative environment she desires.

The principles of organizational behavior modification are particularly useful in dealing with the types of behaviors that this head nurse must address. The chronic absenteeism and tardiness are observable, countable behaviors that directly influence the goal of the organization to provide quality health care. Implementation of a behavioral contingency management plan as outlined above may provide the necessary solution to the problem.

The target behaviors of absenteeism and tardiness have already been identified, so the next step is gathering the baseline data. Data collection provides the basis for detecting trends and problem areas (McDonald & Shaver, 1981). The head nurse may find that the problem is not as significant as she suspected. If, however, these behaviors are indeed found problematic, a functional analysis of the situation should follow.

The antecedents and consequences of the behaviors should be identified. Does the excessive workload cause the nurses to fail to perform at an optimal level or are other personal factors involved? What reinforcers have existed in the past to strengthen the undesirable behaviors? A complete analysis should help to identify all behavioral contingencies.

Intervention strategies are planned after the functional analysis is complete. A vast number of reinforcers could be used, but the nurse may find that she is limited to some degree by budgetary concerns. For example, lotteries, cash bonuses, and time off work have been used successfully in some organizations, but the resources may or may not be present to implement such a program.

A combination of praise, recognition, and feedback may be all that is necessary to reinforce desirable behavior. Studies have found that recognition is the strongest means to improve morale and augment motivation (Edwards & Powers, 1982). The head nurse may praise each employee for being on time and attending work regularly. Clear expectations about attendance and punctuality should be established, and employees should receive feedback on how well they are doing (Roach, 1984).

After the appropriate intervention strategy has been chosen and applied, more data should be gathered to determine the frequency of desired and undesired responses. Making this information accessible to all employees may be pertinent. The nurse manager can then assess the effectiveness of the intervention strategy. If the intervention strategy has been successful, care should be taken to maintain the desired behavior through a suitable reinforcement schedule. If the intervention has not been effective, alternative strategies should be developed and implemented.

Behavioral contingency management may allow the head nurse in this situation to improve performance on her unit and establish positive working relationships with her employees without resorting to punishment and its negative sequelae. Nord (1969) believed that the gains from behavioral modification may well be limited only by a manager's creativity and resources.

RESEARCH

Studies investigating the efficacy of operant conditioning in the organizational setting have not been numerous, especially in recent years, but several should be noted.

The Emery Air Freight positive reinforcement program was perhaps the most widely known and demonstrated how effective behavior modification can be in the organizational arena. Feeney (1973), Vice President of System Performance, stated that Emery was selective in its application of positive reinforcement by using it only where it was most needed and where the potential for improvement was the greatest. An appropriate example was in the manner in which small shipments were packed. By encouraging employees to increase their use of containers from 45% to 95% of all shipments, Emery realized an annual savings of $650,000.

A performance audit was done to find the areas where the largest potential profit existed and to convince managers with these quantitative data that they had room for improvement. Emery never used money as a positive reinforcer but found instead that praise and recognition expressed in quantitative terms were most effective. Feeney encouraged managers to praise their employees at least twice a week during the beginning of the program and to continue the positive reinforcement on a descending scale of frequency.

Positive reinforcement was fully implemented in sales, operations, and containerized shipments. Benefits were sustained during the 3-year study period, and the savings amounted to more than $3 million in 3 years. Emery's past experience had shown that continuous feedback must be administered daily or performance rapidly deteriorated.

Hamner and Hamner (1976) surveyed ten companies and found that positive reinforcement offered considerable rewards. The companies claiming to be implementing and using positive reinforcement programs were Emery Air Freight, Michigan Bell Maintenance Services, Connecticut General Life Insurance Company, General Electric, Standard Oil of Ohio, Weyerhaeuser, City of Detroit, B.F. Goodrich Chemical Company, and ACDC Electronics. Managers were questioned on their successes and failures as well as whether they considered positive reinforcement a legitimate management technique.

Most companies reported significant benefits from the program, including increased productivity and job satisfaction, increased profit, decreased absenteeism and tardiness, and fewer customer complaints. Hamner and Hamner conclude that positive reinforcement is a powerful tool when the reinforcers are sufficiently powerful, when the reinforcers are strictly contingent on performance, and when a reliable training procedure is established for inducing the desired responses.

Komaki, Waddell, and Pearce (1977) applied behavior modification techniques to improve performance in a neighborhood grocery store and a downtown game room. In the grocery store study, time off with pay, feedback, and self-recording were introduced as reinforcers, and desired tasks were clarified. The mean performance level of the three behaviors improved from 53%, 35%, and 57% to 86%, 87%, and 86%, respectively. The game room study involved goal clarification and a contingent pay system. Performance in this study increased from baseline means of 62% and 63% to 93% and 97%, respectively. These results certainly seem to indicate further potential for the program.

The problem of absenteeism was addressed in one major study by Pedalino and Gamboa (1974). A behavior modification plan was implemented at a manufacturing facility employing 215 hourly workers. Employees in four adjoining plants were studied as comparison groups. A lottery incentive system was designed and implemented with great success. Absenteeism in the experimental group decreased significantly following the intervention but did not decrease in the comparison groups.

Otteman and Luthans (1975) conducted a study to evaluate the effectiveness of an organizational behavior modification program in an industrial setting. Their findings indicate that the production rates of supervisors trained in behavioral contingency management increased significantly over the supervisors who had not received the training. The organizational behavior modification aproach was found to be more effective than other conventional human resource techniques. Although they grant that their results may prove to be only temporary, the fact that the training sessions were spread out over 10 weeks and the performance data was collected for 3 months after completion of the training might indicate that the program has some permanency.

Wexley and Nemeroff (1975) evaluated the effectiveness of positive reinforcement and goal setting as a method of managerial development. Two managerial training programs were studied. One program utilized role playing, delayed appraisal sessions, and assigned goal setting; the other program utilized these techniques as well as immediate reinforcement through telecoaching. Data were collected 60 days after completion of training. The results indicated that the experimental group was more effective in improving the integration skills of managers and reducing absenteeism among their subordinates.

Kim and Hamner (1976) investigated the effects of performance feedback and goal setting on productivity and satisfaction in a large telephone company. Their results indicate that goal setting alone can enhance performance but that adding performance feedback can greatly augment performance. These results give further credence to behavior modification principles.

The role of modeling has been the subject of research among behaviorists. Weiss (1977) studied lower-level supervisors and their superiors and concluded that modeling is indeed a mechanism for the socialization of organizational behaviors.

Moses and Ritchie (1976) developed a behavior modeling program at Amerian Telephone & Telegraph and concluded that the process is effective. They state that modeling is a powerful type of learning that provides appropriate examples for staff interaction. Their training procedures provide a method of systematically internalizing management principles.

Sorcher (1971) has commented on a behavior modification approach to supervisor training. He believes this approach can provide a supervisor with more adaptive ways to deal with subordinates. The process he suggests for exploring and learning these new behaviors is role playing. During role playing, a supervisor's more adaptive behavior is positively reinforced by peers and the instructor and therefore strengthened.

Organizational behavior modification has critics as well as proponents. Locke (1977) contends that behavior modification techniques commonly used in organizations are neither behavioristic nor new. He states that the behavior modification model is not a valid tool for the manager because the facts of human behavior do not correspond to it. All behavior is not controlled by reinforcements because people also learn by imitation and self-instruction. The behaviorist position does not acknowledge the impact of an individual's values or knowledge on behavior. He also states that reinforcers do not condition behaviors automatically but rather affect action through the individual's mental content and processes. According to Locke, the very fact that we can think proves the behaviorist view to be false.

Mawhinney (1975) has examined problems of interpretation, application, and evaluation of operant concepts and found that problems exist in the extant literature. For example, in the Pedalino and Gamboa study (1974) cited previously, absenteeism was significantly reduced before anyone received a lottery prize. Thus, something other than the prize must have reinforced the punctual behavior of the employees. Mawhinney believes that current methods of data collection leave much to be desired and must be improved before a body of scientific fact about operant conditioning can be generated.

In spite of these criticisms, Mitchell (1976) points out some similarities between certain cognitive approaches and a Skinnerian philosophy that are frequently overlooked. For example, equity, expectancy, and exchange theories all emphasize outcomes and rewards. Consequently, the effect of reinforcement on cognition and behavior can be recognized without accepting that all operant behavior is completely caused by environmental contingencies.

A review of the nursing literature reveals that the principles of organizational behavior modification have not been researched to any significant degree in relation to nursing management. Sullivan and Decker (1985) have developed a behavior modeling training technique that has been used in industry to train management personnel. It has recently been adapted to teach management skills to nurses and is currently being utilized in Barnes Hospital in St. Louis and in the baccalaureate nursing program at the University of Missouri. However, this is the only application documented in the current literature. Behavior modification techniques are being implemented at the bedside, and research is ongoing in the area. Nurse managers are in a key position to implement some of these principles in their organizations to determine what benefit the approach may have to the field of nursing. Perhaps Skinner (1974, p. 251) was correct when he stated, "In the behavioristic view, man can now control his own destiny because he knows what must be done and how to do it."

REFERENCES

Davis, T.R.V., & Luthans, F. (1979). Leadership reexamined: A behavioral approach. *Academy of Management Review, 4,* 237-248.

Edwards, M., & Powers, R. (1982). Turning staff frustration to satisfaction. *Nursing Management, 13,* 51-52.

Feeney, E.J. (1973). At Emery Air Freight: Positive reinforcement boosts performance. *Organizational Dynamics, 1,* 41-50.

Hamner, W.C. (1974). Reinforcement theory and contingency management in organizational settings. In H.L. Tosi & W.C. Hamner (Eds.), *Organizational behavior management: A contingency approach.* Chicago: St. Clair Press.

Hamner, W.C., & Hamner, E.P. (1976). Behavior modification on the bottom line. *Organizational Dynamics, 4,* 3-21.

Hamner, W.C., & Organ, D.W. (1978). *Organizational behavior: An applied psychological approach.* Dallas: Business Publications.

Kim, J.S., & Hamner, W.C. (1976). Effect of performance feedback and goal setting on productivity and satisfaction in an organizational setting. *Journal of Applied Psychology, 61,* 48-57.

Komaki, J., Waddell, W.M., & Pearce, M.G. (1977). The applied behavior analysis approach and individual employees: Improving performance in two small businesses. *Organizational Behavior and Human Performance, 19,* 337-352.

Locke, E.A. (1977). The myths of behavior modification in organizations. *Academy of Management Review, 2,* 401-402.

Luthans, F. (1973a). *Organizational behavior.* New York: McGraw-Hill.

Luthans, F. (1973b). The role of punishment in organizational behavior modification. *Public Personnel Management, 2,* 156-161.

Luthans, F., & Davis, T.R.V. (1979). Behavioral self-management—the missing link in managerial effectiveness. *Organizational Dynamics,* 42-60.

Luthans, F., & Kreitner, R. (1975). *Organizational behavior modification.* Glenview, IL: Scott, Foresman.

Luthans, F., Maciag, W.S., & Rosenkrantz, S.A. (1983). O.B. Mod.: Meeting the productivity challenge with human resource management. *Personnel,* 28-36.

Luthans, F., & White D.D. (1972). Behavior modification: Application to manpower management. In F. Luthans (Ed.), *Contemporary readings in organizational behavior.* New York: McGraw-Hill.

Mawhinney, T.C. (1975). Operant terms and concepts in the description of individual work behavior: Some problems of interpretation, application, and evaluation. *Journal of Applied Psychology, 60,* 704-712.

McDonald, M.J., & Shaver, A.V. (1981). An absenteeism control program. *Journal of Nursing Administration, 11,* 13-18.

Miner, J.B. (1980). *Theories of organizational behavior.* Hinsdale, IL: Dryden.

Mitchell, T.R. (1976). Cognitions and Skinner: Some questions about behavioral determinism. *Organization and Administrative Sciences, 6,* 63-72.

Moses, J.L., & Ritchie, R.J. (1976). Supervisory relationships training: A behavioral evaluation of a behavior modeling program. *Personnel Psychology, 29,* 337-343.

Nord, W.R. (1969). Beyond the teaching machine: The neglected area of operant conditioning in the theory and practice of management. *Organizational Behavior and Human Performance, 4,* 375-401.

Ottemann, R., & Luthans, F. (1975). An experimental analysis of the effectiveness of an organizational behavior modification program in industry. *Academy of Management Proceedings,* 140-142.

Pedalino, E., & Gamboa, V.U. (1974). Behavior modification and absenteeism: Intervention in one industrial setting. *Journal of Applied Psychology, 59,* 694-698.

Roach, K.L. (1984). Production builds on mutual respect. *Nursing Management, 15,* 54-56.

Schneier, C.E. (1974). Behavior modification in management: A review and critique. *Academy of Management Journal, 17,* 528-545.

Skinner, B.F. (1953). *Science and human behavior.* New York: Free Press.

Skinner, B.F. (1972). *Beyond freedom and dignity.* New York: Alfred A. Knopf.

Skinner, B.F. (1974). *About behaviorism.* New York: Alfred A. Knopf.

Sorcher, M. (1971). A behavior modification approach to supervisor training. *Professional Psychology, 2,* 401-402.

Stolz, S.B., Wienckowski, L.A., & Brown, B.S. (1975). Behavior modification: A perspective on critical issues. *American Psychologist, 30,* 1027-1048.

Sullivan, E.J., & Decker, P.J. (1985). Using behavior modeling to teach management skills. *Nursing and Health Care, 6*(1), 41-45.

Weiss, H.M. (1977). Subordinate imitation of supervisor behavior: The role of modeling in organizational socialization. *Organizational Behavior and Human Performance, 19,* 89-105.

Wexley, K.N., & Nemeroff, W.F. (1975). Effectiveness of positive reinforcement and goal setting as methods of management development. *Journal of Applied Psychology, 1975,* 446-450.

Chapter 33

Social Learning Theory: Modeling
Albert Bandura

Sylvia L. Bond

▌▌ CASE STUDY

The nursing administrator looked up to see the chief of surgery standing in her doorway. His usual friendly smile was replaced by an angry scowl as he approached her desk and gave an account of what had just happened to him.

Dr. Johnson had been making patient rounds alone up on 5-East. Although aware the floor was busier than usual, he held out hope that a nurse would soon accompany him. As he gave discharge instructions to his last patient, he added another mental note to talk to her husband.

While finishing his charting at the nurses' station, he asked the charge nurse if the lab results on Mr. James were available. The charge nurse did not respond. Thinking she did not hear him, he repeated the question in a louder voice. She replied, "Can't you see I'm busy? If they're not on the chart, they're not in!" Stunned by the sharpness in her voice, Dr. Johnson said, "Look, I know you are busy, but it seems to me I'm not asking too much of you. It is your job." Mrs. Abbott replied, "Yeah, then why don't you try doing it" and stalked off.

Having told the story, Dr. Johnson stated he had observed the rudeness of this nurse before and that others had similar complaints about her behavior. He stated he would like to exercise his influence to rid the hospital of someone with such a bad attitude. To give credence to what he was saying, he reminded the nursing administrator that he was not a habitual complainer. The nursing administrator assured the physician she would investigate the matter and get back to him.

Mrs. Abbott was an exceptional clinician. She was well organized, she had an excellent attendance record, and her patients thought her to be competent and caring. Her lack of warmth and friendliness did not seem to diminish her positive rapport with them.

However, she was also noted for her abrupt manner. Other staff members would avoid her on some of her worse days, choosing to sidestep any would-be confrontation. She had been involved in several altercations in the past and had even been put on probation for inappropriate responses to peers on one occasion, but her behavior did not change. She was tolerated for all her other virtues.

Mrs. Abbott was asked to come down to the nursing administrator's office. When asked to relate what happened with Dr. Johnson, she became visibly angry and upset but explained that several things had gone wrong that morning, including the unanticipated death of a patient. Dr. Johnson's needs seemed minuscule compared to what was occurring on the unit. Furthermore, she believed Dr. Johnson was just being peevish because he was not getting the attention he felt was his due.

The nursing administrator asked Mrs. Abbott if she had observed this behavior before in Dr. Johnson. When the reply was negative, she tried to help the nurse explore reasons for this sudden change. During the discussion, the nursing administrator was never able to convince Mrs. Abbott that she, the nurse, had a role in provoking the incident, nor was she able to elicit alternative ways to handle the situation. Mrs. Abbott insisted her voice, manner, and expression were appropriate for the situation and that she was not the one that needed changing. Faced with this challenge, the nursing administrator considered her options.

| | | | | | | | | | | | | | | | | | | | | | | | | | | | | | | | | | | | | | | | | | | | | | | | | | | | | | | | | | | | | | | | | | |

SOCIAL LEARNING THEORY: MODELING

Bandura's social learning theory is based on the notion that human thought, affect, and behavior can be markedly influenced by observation (Bandura, 1977). The ability of humans to use symbols or coding to reflect experiences, to think through given situations, to communicate, to imitate, and to determine future action is central to his theory. In addition, the self-regulatory process people ordinarily engage in is a key component. It assumes a continuous process by which the reciprocal interaction that takes place between a person and an environment is a basis for decisions an individual makes to determine his or her own behavior.

Bandura concluded that learning could occur through vicarious reinforcement; that is, desired goals of behavior can be learned by watching those whom the observer admires and wants to emulate. The observer can learn more effectively if informed in advance of the consequences of engaging in a specific behavior rather than by waiting until the behavior is demonstrated and then receiving the reinforcer (Latham & Saari, 1979).

Modeling is viewed as a major source for learning behavior. Good or bad, children learn by observing their parents' behavior. The theory acknowledges that some behaviors are rooted in genetics, but in the main, behavior is learned.

Observational learning is conceptualized into four major processes:

1. *Attentional processes.* Several variables influence which modeling behaviors will be observed and imitated and which will be ignored. They are related to incentive conditions, to observer characteristics, and to the modeling itself. The modeled performance should be a descriptive demonstration of the correct behaviors that enables the observer to relate to the desired results. A person's motivation to perform a behavior is determined by (1) the results that the behavior is expected to produce and (2) the values placed on these results (Porras & Anderson, 1981).

2. *Retention processes.* For observers to profit from the behavior of models when they are no longer present to provide direction, the response patterns must be represented in memory in symbolic form (Bandura, 1977). The human being's ability to code information enables her or him to memorize the learning points demonstrated. Rehearsal operations have been shown to stabilize effectively and strengthen acquired responses (Bandura, 1969). The highest level of observational learning is achieved when the modeled behavior is first coded symbolically in the mind and then rehearsed.

3. *Motor reproduction processes.* This component is the rehearsal of the behaviors. The observer reenacts the modeled performance and, with each demonstration, makes corrective adjustments until the behavior meets the goal. In everyday learning, most people achieve a close approximation of the desired behavior by refining it through informative feedback with each performance and from focused demonstrations of segments that have been only partially learned (Bandura, 1977).
4. *Motivational processes.* People are more likely to adopt modeled behavior if it results in outcomes they value than if it has unrewarding or punishing effects (Bandura, 1977). The self-regulatory process is the influence at this stage.

Through these means the individual selects the behavior he or she wishes to mimic and discards at will those that are undesirable. Failure of the observer to imitate the desired behavior is attributable to the following causes:

1. Not observing the relevant activities
2. Inadequately coding modeled events for memory representation
3. Failing to retain what was learned
4. Physical ability to perform
5. Experiencing insufficient incentives (Bandura, 1977)

According to social learning theory, behavior is learned by processing key points while observing the desired behavior in a model. The observer combines and sequences the events to produce the new behavior and then rehearses it until it is the correct response.

CASE ANALYSIS

The nursing administrator asked Mrs. Abbott if she was interested in maintaining her role as a charge nurse. When the reply was an incredulous "yes," the nursing administrator explained this would not be possible unless her behavior radically changed.

Mrs. Abbott was told that although she had an engaging smile, she seldom used it. Further, she tended to carry over her home problems to the work setting, which may have accounted for some of the abrupt behavior. The nursing administrator made it clear that this behavior would no longer be acceptable and asked Mrs. Abbott if she would be interested in some suggestions. Mrs. Abbott asked if she had a choice. The reply was no, not if she wanted to remain in her position, whereupon Mrs. Abbott stated that she did not understand what she was doing that caused so many negative outcomes in her relationships.

The nurse manager began by demonstrating alternative responses when under pressure. She then compared these desired behaviors with what Mrs. Abbott exhibited during the incident. She role played the entire situation and stressed key points on which Mrs. Abbott was to focus. She then asked the nurse to go home and practice the new approach in front of a large mirror. She encouraged her to smile as appropriate during her rehearsal. Mrs. Abbott was instructed to return for an assessment in 3 days to determine if the new learned technique would be satisfactory. If so, she would be expected to retain these behaviors and also to teach others by example.

The social learning theory can easily be applied to this case study because it is a good example of vicarious learning. The negative reinforcement threat of losing her job created strong motivation for Mrs. Abbott to attend to the nursing administrator's approach. The assumption is that reinforcement and punishment can play important roles in the acquisition and performance of modeled behavior (Kanfer & Goldstein, 1986). The nursing administrator's role and obvious interest in Mrs. Abbott's welfare had the effect of causing Mrs. Abbott to participate in the process.

The nursing administrator was able to define the correct behaviors while reinforcing the good behaviors Mrs. Abbott already possessed, such as smiling. By so doing, she used methods that helped Mrs. Abbott retain the key elements pointed out to her. Mrs. Abbott was able to process and retain the information appropriately because she was committed to patterning her own behavior into a desired goal.

Mrs. Abbott gained insight while imitating and self-correcting her performance in front of the mirror. Her cognitive response was to think through the value of the altered behaviors and to perform them willingly.

When Mrs. Abbott returned to the nursing administrator's office, she was prepared to demonstrate her newfound skills. As she related her experience, she evidently felt positive about herself. The nursing administrator was able to praise her performance and her willingness to try harder. This reinforcement added to the positive outcomes of these behaviors and has served to help Mrs. Abbott continue in her role.

In this instance, modeling clearly transmitted and promoted a new style of behavior for an individual. This technique can easily be adapted to groups of individuals. It is especially effective in the supervisory role because the desired behavior could then be imitated by subordinates. Its informal, nonauthoritarian learning atmosphere is conducive to active participation, a prerequisite for problem solving (Sullivan & Decker, 1984).

RESEARCH

The social learning theory has been applied in a number of industrial settings. Extrapolators of Bandura's work have found good evidence that modeling is an important technique used by managers to develop their own leadership style. Weiss (1977) was able to show significant correlations between subordinates' perceptions of their supervisor's success and competence and the degree of supervisor-subordinate behavior similarity.

Goldstein and Sorcher (1974) explained the potential value of behavioral modeling procedures for first-line supervisory training. Their study was conducted at General Electric to facilitate the retention of disadvantaged employees. Different films were shown to the supervisor and employee groups emphasizing and rewarding desired behaviors for each group. The study showed the modeling training to have a significant impact on turnover rates.

Moses and Ritchie (1976) conducted similar studies at American Telephone & Telegraph. They developed a program called Supervisory Relationships Training to help frontline supervisors relate more effectively to their subordinates. The training program helps the supervisor confront issues that are unique to managing a work force composed of women and minorities. They have clearly demonstrated the modeling technique works.

Latham and Saari (1979) produced a study at the University of Washington designed to improve supervisors' interpersonal skills in dealing with their employees. They randomly assigned 40 first-line supervisors to a control group or to a behavioral modeling training program. Over a sustained period of time, the training group was found to be significantly better in supervisory methods than the control group. Moreover, when the control group was given the same training, their performance was equal to the first group.

Porras and Anderson (1981) created a management development program based on social learning theory at a large manufacturing operation. The object of the program was to increase interpersonal problem-solving skills for their first-line managers. The program included seven weekly workshops lasting 6 hours each and was based on learning and motivational procedures taken from the social learning theory. They concluded that supervisory behavior changed significantly and that behavior modeling is very useful in dealing with the many human relations problems faced by managers.

The nursing literature contains many articles related to modeling. An exceptional article, written by Clarke (1983), describes an audiovisual modeling program for adolescent parents. It depicts how nurses can facilitate adolescent parenting by providing opportunities for young mothers to observe and practice appropriate behavior to promote their infants' growth and development. The premise is that if adolescent parents improve their decision-making skills, they will become a much better resource to solve their children's health care maintenance problems.

Sullivan and Decker (1984) apply the social learning theory components to a nursing education and service setting. The techniques they outline are used in Barnes Hospital in St. Louis and the baccalaureate nursing program for registered nurses at the University of Missouri. They report modeling is particularly useful in an undergraduate course in leadership and management. Administrators state that nursing management practice improved as a result of the use of this technique.

Budgen (1987) applies the modeling process to program development in nursing. Use of this methodology guides program planning and design by creating a series of diagrams accompanied by a paragraph highlighting key points. The result is a visual representation of the program that defines how the program components relate to produce desired outcomes. Those who use this technique have acquired a tool as well as a program that can be used in practice or educational settings.

Through the use of predictive modeling, Hinshaw and Associates (1983) studied the impact of a perioperative teaching program on multiple patient outcomes. In addition, the influence of such a program on the nursing staff was examined. The assumption was that patients' postoperative outcomes would be influenced positively by receiving cognitive, sensory, and participative orientation to the surgical experience. Results showed the experimental patients evidenced higher satisfaction with their care and tended to have less postoperative vomiting. However, they also tended to recover more slowly and to cope less well than the control group. This complex study also showed the nurses seemed to derive a significantly greater amount of satisfaction with the care they gave to the experimental group.

Erickson, Tomlin, and Swain (1983) have used several theories as a basis for their theory of modeling and role modeling. They believe the art of modeling is the development of a mirror image of the situation from the client's perspective. Their initial study provided evidence that psychosocial factors are significantly related to physical health problems. Several doctoral students at the University of Michigan School of Nursing are pursuing various research questions based on this theory.

Modeling has been effective in leadership training outside the field of nursing. Now is the time to test the theory in nursing management.

REFERENCES

Bandura, A. (1969). *Principles of behavior modification.* New York: Holt, Rinehart and Winston.

Bandura, A. (1977). *Social learning theory.* Englewood Cliffs, NJ: Prentice-Hall.

Budgen, C.M. (1987). Modeling: A method for program development. *Journal of Nursing Administration, 17*(12), 19-25.

Clarke, B.A. (1983). Improving adolescent parenting through participant modeling and self-evaluation. *Nursing Clinics of North America, 8,* 303-311.

Erickson, H.C., Tomlin, E.M., & Swain, M.A.P. (1983). *Modeling and role-modeling: A theory and paradigm for nursing.* Englewood Cliffs, NJ: Prentice-Hall.

Goldstein, A.P. & Sorcher, M. (1974). *Changing supervisor behavior.* New York: Pergamon Press.

Hinshaw, A.S., Gerber, R.M., Atwood, J.R., & Allen, J.R. (1983). The use of predictive modeling to test nursing practice outcomes. *Nursing Research, 32*(1), 35-41.

Kanfer, F.H., & Goldstein, A.P. (1986). *Helping people change.* New York: Pergamon Press.

Latham, G.P., & Saari, L.M. (1979). Application of social-learning theory to training supervisors through behavioral modeling. *Journal of Applied Psychology, 64,* 239-246.

Moses, J.L., & Ritchie, R.J. (1976). Supervisory relationships training: A behavioral evaluation of a behavior modeling program. *Personnel Psychology, 29,* 337-343.

Porras, J.I., & Anderson, B. (1981). Improving managerial effectiveness through modeling-based training. *Organizational Dynamics, 9,* 60-77.

Sullivan, E.J., & Decker, P.J. (1984). Using behavior modeling to teach management skills. *Nursing & Health Care, 6*(1), 41-45.

Weiss, H.M. (1977). Subordinate imitation of supervisor behavior: The role of modeling in organizational socialization. *Organizational Behavior and Human Performance, 19*(1), 89-105.

PART V

EVALUATE

Chapter 34

Budget as Control

Lorraine B. Anderson

▮▮ CASE STUDY

Liz Kramer sits in her windowless 6 × 8-foot office and gazes despondently at the latest monthly budget variance report. She is thinking about how hard she has worked at controlling costs on the unit and how hard she has worked at enlisting all the staff to think cost control as they work. Use of purchased nursing services is down, and the staff is doing a good job of reporting supplies used so patient accounts can be charged. But it all seems so futile; the unit is in the red again!

Liz has been unit manager on 6 West, the renal transplant unit at West State University Hospital, for more than 3 years. She feels competent in her management of the day-to-day operations of the unit. Her skills in managing the human resources component of the job have developed more slowly than she anticipated they might, but she now feels at ease with that part of the job. In fact, her interactions with staff are now a very gratifying part of her work. Then there is the frustrating experience of dealing with the budget!

As a new unit manager, Liz has seen the budgeting responsibility as a special mark of advancement and has taken great pride in her participation in the process. Liz blamed her early failures to achieve a positive balance in the monthly variance reports of revenues and expenses on her lack of familiarity with the complicated process of budgeting. The unit's reported performance, however, has not improved over time.

The annual budgeting process is underway again, and the budget manual for this planning period is on Liz's desk. She plans to stay late this evening to begin the unpleasant task of budget preparation. West State University Hospital uses what Preston (1987) labeled a combination approach budget review procedure. Certain objectives are established at the corporate level and passed down through departments to the individual units. Using the assigned objectives, unit managers develop their operating objectives and forward them back through the hierarchy for approval or rejection. The work involves using provided formulas to make calculations and then completing the assigned forms. The directions for these processes are clear and easy to follow.

For Liz, dealing with the payroll segment has made previous budget-preparation experiences painful. Wages and salaries have been regularly increased in line with the economic situation and supply-and-demand conditions in her community, but each year budgeted staff seems to be the focus for cost cutting and cost control. The specifics of that focus on budgeted staff have differed from year to year. One year the edict was "No expansion of full-time equivalents (FTEs)." In the case of the renal transplant unit, this rule meant no increase in FTEs in spite of an increase in patient days. Another year all units were required to cut half an FTE. Because at the time Liz was recruiting for one FTE, this requirement had not entailed losing someone from the unit. It did, however, mean that if the unit had a generally sustained increase in patient days or acuity during the year and more regular staff were needed, getting approval would involve submitting a new position request and justification. With this history in mind, Liz sits down to begin the budgeting task, the part of her job that has over time become so distasteful to her. Figure 34-1 presents a list of the categories and line items included in this year's budget and the direct, indirect, and overall totals Liz will review.

Obviously, for Liz, staff development did not fill the gaps regarding the budgeting process that remained after formal education. Given the present diversity of focus in master's programs in nursing administration (Stark, 1987), the master's program in which Liz is presently enrolled is unlikely to fill her needs for knowledge and skills in financial management. The irregular picture of fiscal management practice among present nurse executive managers suggests that Liz is unlikely to find (and she has not yet found) an appropriate role model from whom to learn the ropes and the skills she needs. If Liz's past academic preparations did not prepare her for budgeting responsibilities, if the organization is not expected to prepare her, if the number of role models available is very limited, and if education in graduate nursing programs will not prepare her to deal effectively with the budgeting responsibilities of her job, what recourse has she, besides either suffering gradual erosion of her professional self-esteem or leaving nursing management?

| | | | | | | | | | | | | | | | | | | | | | | | | | | | | | | | | | | | | | | | | | | | | | | | | | | | | | | | | | | | | | | | | | |

THEORY

A budget is a plan for the use of money. Budgeting is the process of making decisions about the use of money and implementing those decisions. Most of the nursing literature about budgets and budgeting is focused on application (Hoffman, 1984; Rowland & Rowland, 1985; Sheridan Bronstein, & Walker, 1984; Stevens, 1985; Vanderzee & Glusko, 1984). When theory is included in nursing texts and articles about budgeting, it is usually economic theory (e.g., Strasen, 1987).

Does economic theory explain or predict the budgeting process? Mansfield (1983) has defined and differentiated the two major branches of economic theory as microeconomics, which "deals with the economic behavior of individual units like consumers, firms, and resource owners," and macroeconomics, which "deals with the behavior of economic aggregates like national output, the price level, and the level of unemployment" (p. 3). Although economic theory does provide one very necessary base of understanding to people involved in developing budgets for nursing organizations (Greenfield, 1988; McGivern, 1988), it does not provide explanations or predictions about how or why the operating budgets for individual nursing units are developed and implemented. This gap in the explanation of budgeting suggests that economic theory provides an essential but not sufficient theoretical framework for understanding budgeting.

DIRECT EXPENSES	INDIRECT COSTS

Payroll
    Administrative staff
    Salaries
    Wages—regular time
    Wages—overtime

Nursing Administration
Occupational Therapy
Social Services
Intern/Resident Staff
Medical Records
Nutrition and Dietetics
Engineering and Maintenance

Employee Benefits
    Fringe benefits
    Social Security
    Retirement

Accounting
Patient Referral and Utilization
Credit and Collections
Administration, General
Volunteer Services

Supplies and Expenses
    Central stores supplies
    Publications
    Telephone and telegraph
    Office supplies
    Purchased services, nursing
    Repairs, maintenance
    Durable supplies
    Medical/surgical supplies
    Supplies and expenses, general

Depreciation
Interest Expense
Hospital Epidemiology

TOTAL DIRECT EXPENSES

$ 405,297

TOTAL INDIRECT COSTS

$ 378,415

TOTAL EXPENSE BUDGET

$ 783,312

FIGURE 34-1 Budget categories and line items; direct, indirect, and overall totals for the past year.

The general management sciences literature about budgeting is, like the nursing literature, primarily focused on application. However, a segment of the general management literature addresses theory relevant to budgeting. Behavioral theories have been used to explain some of the what, how, and why of the budgeting process (Chandra, 1987; Chenhall & Brownell, 1988; Hirst, 1987; Mia, 1987). The content of these reports and analyses suggests that budgeting, seemingly a quintessentially quantitative process, is a psychosocial process as well.

Comprehensive theories and models of management usually suggest some combination of functions that include at least planning, organizing, directing, and controlling. If budgeting is specifically included in a theoretical framework or model, it is usually included as a part of the planning function (e.g., Mackenzie, 1969). It has been suggested, however, that the ultimate purpose of a budget is control.

The role of the accounting and budgeting system is to provide information that helps managers in *controlling* [italics added] subordinates by pinpointing inadequate and unsatisfactory performance (Chandra, 1987, p. 839).

Programming, budgeting, and controlling processes (PBCP) represent the three major phases of a formal management *control* [italics added] system (Vraciu, 1980, p. 117).

The *control* [italics added] of spending is accomplished through the budget.... Managers are usually evaluated based on their financial performance and budget adherence. It is the factor that allows the budget to actualize the control of the spending function (Strasen, 1987, p. 124).

A budget is the quantitative representation of a set of decisions about how an organization's money will be used to achieve the organization's goals. In that sense, it is an explicit, objective directive, and compliance is easily monitored. Because all human and material resources in organizations are ultimately money dependent, the control exerted by the budget extends to the smallest functional units of organizations. With this understanding, it becomes apparent people who have final decision power over an organization's budget control the direction of the organization.

In 1958, Tannenbaum and Schmidt presented a model of the decision-making authority dimension of leader behavior. In that model the decision-making authority dimension was presented simply as a balance between the amount of authority the boss exercised and the amount of freedom subordinates had. The model presented these two concepts—authority exercised by the boss and freedom of subordinates—on a continuum with boss-centered leadership at one end and subordinate-centered leadership at the other end. Seven points along the continuum described different balances between the extremes. Making decisions is an integral part of the budgeting process.

In a 1973 *Harvard Business Review* classic, Tannenbaum and Schmidt revised and expanded their 1958 model (Figure 34-2). In the revised model, boss-centered leadership became manager power and influence, and subordinate-centered leadership became nonmanager power and influence. Points along the continuum are defined in terms of how much freedom the manager has rather than in terms of how much authority the leader must yield in decision-making situations. Tannenbaum and Schmidt (1973) noted that these changes reflected societal changes that had occurred during the intervening 15 years. Additions to the model integrated concepts from open-system theory (Tannenbaum & Schmidt, 1973). In the 1973 model concentric bands representing the internal (organization) environment and the external (societal) environment encircle the continuum of behavior. Tannenbaum and Schmidt (1973) stressed the interdependency among elements of the model and emphasized two changes in the dynamics of the decision-making process. First, they gave a great deal more attention to what they called "the realities of power" (p. 168) on both sides. Second, they emphasized the concept of continual change occurring in an open system. Tannenbaum and Schmidt's 1973 model provides an excellent conceptual framework for analyzing the case of Liz Kramer, unit manager on 6 West.

CASE ANALYSIS

At this time Liz obviously believes that the only power she has in this situation is the power to withdraw. She can choose to leave. Liz had anticipated that participation in the budgeting process would be a satisfying growth experience. She would make decisions about the use of unit resources. If those decisions were good decisions, unit staff would be enabled to achieve

---

FIGURE 34-2 Continuum of manager-nonmanager behavior. *Reprinted by permission of the* Harvard Business Review. *An exhibit from "How to Choose a Leadership Pattern" by Robert Tannenbaum and Warren H. Schmidt (May/June 1973). Copyright © 1973 by the President and Fellows of Harvard College; all rights reserved.*

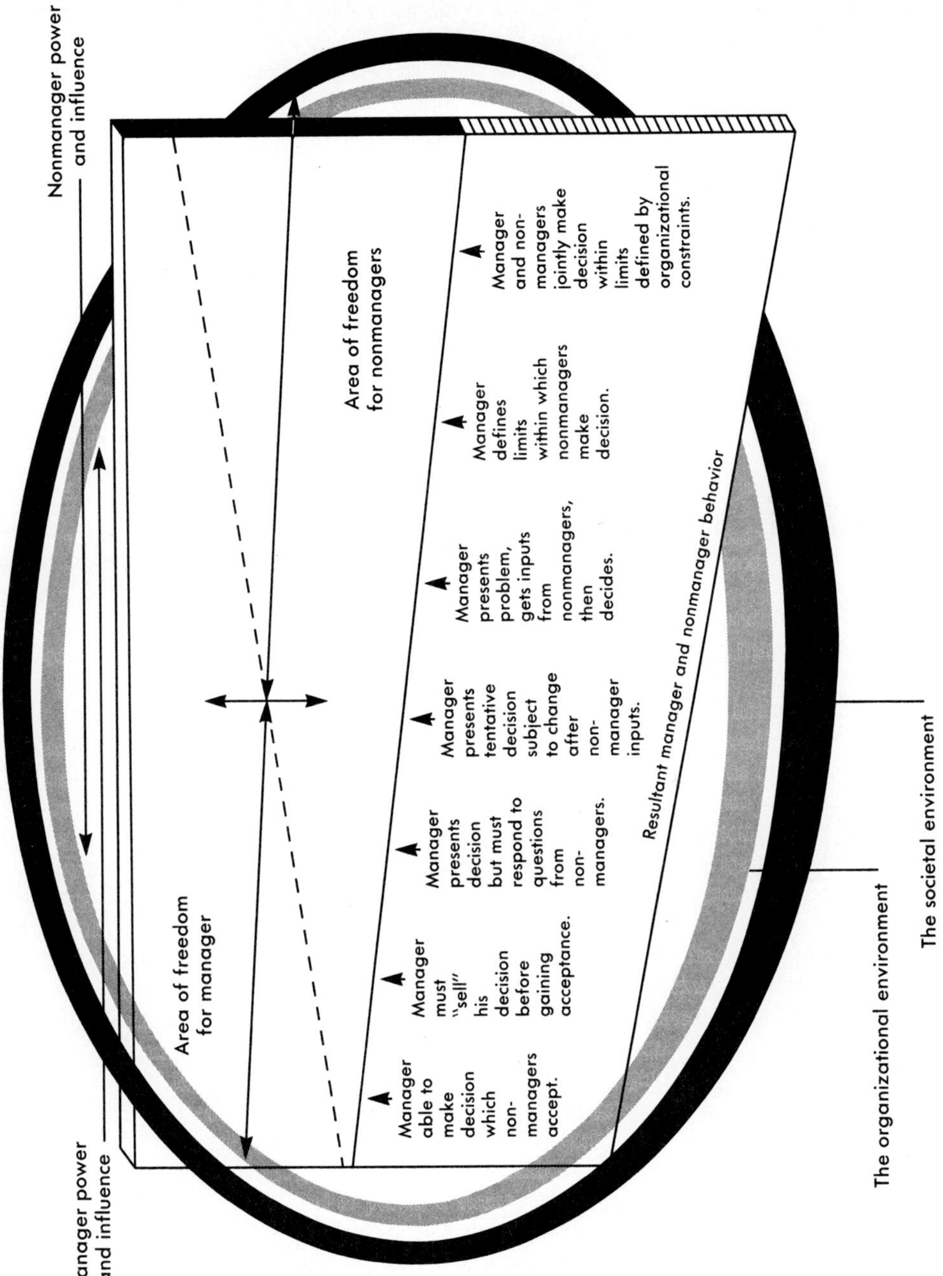

FIGURE 34-2   For legend, see opposite page.

nursing unit goals for patient care, and Liz would be enabled to realize her professional goal to be an effective manager. What went wrong?

Chandra (1987) noted two types of budgets: imposed and participative. These two budget types might be visualized as being at opposite ends of a continuum, much as manager power and influence and nonmanager power and influence appear in Tannenbaum and Schmidt's continuum of manager-nonmanager behavior in decision making. If imposed and participative do represent the two ends of a continuum, then when participation is present in budgeting the nature and extent of that participation must be determined. Although some first-line managers may find themselves included early on in the beginning phases of planning, others find themselves included only in the budget preparation and control phases of the budgeting process. By the time the budgeting process has reached the budget-preparation phase, options are necessarily limited. The control phase involves monitoring adherence to the budget and making adjustments as possible to maintain adherence.

Decentralization of budget preparation responsibilities to nursing units promotes among unit managers a sense of ownership of the budget. Decentralization of the monitoring accountability to nursing units also enhances organizational control. The hospital's nursing unit managers operate at a major intersection of hospital resources and patients. Promoting a sense of ownership of the budget among first-line managers would certainly be considered a prudent management tactic. However, precisely this ownership of the budget and the attendant accountability for its successful implementation has brought Liz to the point of making a major career decision to leave nursing, or at least to leave nursing management.

In spite of her diligent attention to staffing, scheduling, and assuring that supplies used for patients are charged to patient accounts, Liz has been, more often than not, "in the red." A second look at the list of expense categories included in Liz's budget suggests that the budget violates an important management principle, the principle of controllability. Chandra (1987) suggested that when budgeted and actual results are reported to a manager the report should contain information about only those budget items that the manager can control. If the lists of items in Figure 34-1 are reviewed with the principle of controllability in mind, obviously Liz is being held accountable for many items over which she has little or no control. For example, if food service costs or engineering and maintenance costs are poorly controlled, a part of the cost overrun is charged to 6 West, as part of indirect costs. The formulas used to calculate indirect cost assignments are sometimes reasonable and logical, sometimes not. For example, on given days several patients on a unit may receive no meal trays during a 24-hour period. Nevertheless, if the formula for calculating the nutrition and dietetics indirect cost assignments to nursing units is

Patient days $\times$ 3 (standard cost per meal)

then the unit could could easily be charged several thousand dollars each month for something that was never delivered!

Liz's performance is thus regularly evaluated on the basis of the performance of other organizational components over which she has no control. How might such an inappropriate assignment of accountabilities occur? Birkofer, Wasch, and Kramer (1987) observed that reporting requirements to external parties often influence internal budgeting practices and reduce the usefulness of the various reports. Given the array of indirect costs that are by a variety of formulas prorated to units, determining the actual financial status of a unit becomes virtually impossible. As Birkofer, Wasch, and Kramer noted, "The quality of the original budget determines the quality of the review of variances that can be performed" (1987, p. 635).

Covaleski and Dirsmith (1984) reported that executive nurse managers were very concerned about the nature of their involvement in the budgeting process, as "budgeting systems were being increasingly imposed on them by hospital administrators" (p. 8) and suggested that nurse managers must become more active in their own behalf. They suggested that nurse managers initiate communications with hospital administrators, administration staff, and financial staff about the budget and the budgeting process during planning and implementation.

Harrison and Roth's (1987) findings support those of Covaleski and Dirsmith (1984). Harrison and Roth concluded, following their survey of 206 chief nurse executives, that: "Although chief nurse executives were highly involved in most decision areas pertaining to nursing operations, formulation/control of the nursing budget and implementation of reward systems for nursing were areas of moderate involvement" (p. 74).

However, the literature shows some disagreement about the nature and extent of the involvement of nurse managers in budgeting processes. On the basis of 416 returns from a national survey by Witt Associates, Inc., Andrica (1988) presented a vastly different picture: "The financial responsibilities of the nurse executives were extensive. They controlled an average operating budget of $22 million, with a range from $5 million to $333 million" (p. 112). (Note that this report is based on a 26% return.) The differences in findings across situations may in part be explained by the recency of involvement of nurse executives in the budgeting process. As lately as 1978, Goertzen reported that for some nursing directors "it was a new experience to be asked by the hospital administrator or controller to develop a budget for the nursing department" (p. 62).

The variety of opinions expressed in the literature suggests that the nurse executive's role in budgeting varies significantly across institutions. Obviously many nurse managers — even chief nurse executives — feel uneasy or unprepared to engage the budgeting process in their organizations (Covaleski & Dirsmith, 1984). Liz, too, felt ill prepared to understand and participate in the budgeting process at West State University Hospital.

Preparation for nursing practice takes place both in academic settings and on the job. On-the-job preparation occurs in group and one-on-one staff development encounters and through role-modeling exposures. Nurse writers have recently expressed concern about the lack of, or poor quality of, the financial management component of formal educational programs in nursing. Poteet and Goddard (1989) concluded that "the legacy of nursing education at the undergraduate and graduate levels has produced almost three decades of nurses with little or no theoretical basis for sound financial management" (p. 100). Poteet and Goddard noted further that with the end of what they termed "the golden years of health care financing" (p. 700) nurses in management positions at all levels have found themselves ill prepared for financial management. Simms's (1989) review of the history of nursing administration content in nursing education programs illustrates that educators have often resisted and rejected the inclusion of nursing management content in nursing curriculums. Other recent reviews have focused on the management knowledge and skills components of undergraduate (Norton, 1989), master's (Carroll, 1989), and doctoral (Singleton, 1989) programs in nursing. All three reviews suggest that preparation in financial management is still far short of adequate.

Stark (1987) also recently prepared a content overview of master's programs in nursing. Among nursing administration programs, she found a great diversity in focus and content. Stark noted disagreement as to what is an appropriate focus for aspiring nurse managers — clinical content or business management content. At least in part, the problem seems to be that the content nurse managers need is about two degrees' worth!

Staff development is often used to bridge gaps between formal preparation and the workplace, but most staff development is designed to focus on the specifics of applications in a particular workplace. Staff development programs are based on an assumption that employees come to their positions with basic preparation for these positions completed. Is this assumption valid in regard to nurse managers' preparation for financial management? Based on the content reviews of Carroll (1989), Norton (1989), Singleton (1989), and Stark (1987), the answer may be no.

Liz and other aspiring managers like her must assert their need for appropriate preparation in financial management. At least three avenues for assertion are available. First, these nurses should communicate to the leaders of academic programs that they are seeking courses in financial management, and that, if these courses are not made available within nursing programs, then they will look elsewhere for the preparation they need. Second, aspiring nurse managers can look for immediately available noncredit academic courses that address their needs. Third, in addition to seeking formal learning programs in financial management, these nurses should look for jobs in organizations that have nurse executives who are full partners in the fiscal management of their organizations. They should look also for top-level nurse managers who express a willingness and intent to mentor new nurse managers and to facilitate their development in the vital skills of financial management. Sonberg and Vestal (1983) stressed the importance of mentoring down the nursing management lines.

Covaleski & Dirsmith (1984) observed that the control philosophy adopted by an organization should reflect its external environment. Standardization can be effective in stable environments; shifting, unstable environments call for flexibility and adaptability. In the introduction to his recent book, *Thriving on Chaos* (1987), Peters declared that chaos is the present state of things, and flexibility is paramount to success. He exhorts top management to achieve flexibility by empowering people: "Involve everyone in everything" (p. 285), "Delegate" (p. 451), and finally "Decentralize information, authority and strategic planning" (p. 505). In terms of Tannenbaum and Schmidt's model, Peters seems to be suggesting that the balance of power in decision making must approach a fifty-fifty balance, with manager-nonmanager (top managers–other managers) interwoven or interlaced to form a strong, flexible, resilient organization that can survive the buffeting of a chaotic external environment.

If nurse managers should be involved as completely and integrally in everything as Peters has suggested, they would be involved in decision making during all phases of management, from planning (including financial planning) through implementation and evaluation. As Harrison and Roth (1987) remind readers, to function effectively nurse managers must have several sorts of power, and one of these is expert power. Nurse managers must bring to the work setting a variety of knowledges, competencies, and skills, with one of the most important of these being fiscal management skills. Liz presents one very simple example of what happens when nurse managers do not bring to the job the knowledge, competence, and skills — the expert power — to perform the job responsibilities effectively. When nurses fall short in this respect, they cannot assume their full potential in the organization.

RESEARCH

In education and practice, nurse managers make use of literature from a variety of other disciplines. A review of current nonnursing research dealing with aspects of financial management is therefore worthwhile. Mia (1987) examined the nature of the relationship between participation in budgetary decision making and attitude toward the job in relation to locus of control and task difficulty. Mia's findings have implications for manager selection and placement. Chenhall and Brownell (1988) also studied an aspect of participative budgeting, the process by which participation in budgeting affects the performance and job satisfaction of managers. On the basis of study results Chenhall and Brownell developed a model in which role ambiguity acts as an intervening variable between participation and job satisfaction and job performance. Both studies should be of interest to nurse managers.

Nearly 15 years ago Lindeman (1975) surveyed a panel of more that 300 nurse and nonnurse experts about research priorities for nursing. Among the top 15 research focuses judged to have value for the profession, two related directly to financial management: "Determine valid, reliable methods for establishing nursing staffing patterns that adequately reflect patient needs and cost containment" (p. 440), and "Determine the different effects on patient welfare of care provided by nursing personnel having different educational preparation" (p. 440). Clinicians and administrators ranked these topics between 6 and 11, but educators and researchers ranked them between 16 and 32.

The report of a recent survey to delineate administration research priorities noted that the high-priority questions identified in the survey reflected the "intense, price-sensitive, economic environment" (Henry et al., 1987, p. 314). The report also noted that in the field relatively few investigators were focusing on nursing management concerns and suggested that efforts were needed to define better how nursing and management knowledge are integrated in order to determine the best ways to go about researching these concerns.

In a 1987 article, Hinshaw and Smeltzer proposed as one characteristic of a researchable problem that it should "represent long-term practices and/or policies for which accurate information or data will be necessary for decision-making" (p. 21). Financial management concerns in nursing services certainly meet that criterion. However, Hinshaw and Smeltzer also noted that studies easily involve one, two, or more years of work. This amount of time may be difficult to sustain in balance with the relentless daily press for immediate answers to problems. Tuttle (1988) also noted that although health services research, which she described as "the study of the organization, economics, financing, and delivery of health services" (p. 48), had the potential to help service organizations create sound master strategies, the immediate opportunity costs were often viewed as prohibitive in the light of meeting day-to-day pressures.

Among the research program focuses established for the National Center for Nursing Research in the National Institutes of Health is one on the delivery of nursing services, including a focus on nursing systems, notably assessment of the costs of providing care under different systems. Moreover, even when financial management concerns do not comprise the chief intent of a research focus, financial management concerns are, or should be, embedded in the fabric of every study. Health services literature shows an increasing emphasis on the central significance of having accurate, appropriate financial information on which to base a variety of organization and service component decisions (Dowd, 1988; Huckabay, 1988; Jones, 1988). Market feasibility studies, for example, depend on such information. Nurses must either (1) take the initiative in obtaining financial information, analyzing it in quality of nursing and financial terms, and entering the planning and decision-making arena; or (2) become the collectors of information for use by planners and decision makers who lack knowledge about nursing and are prepared to bring only financial management knowledge and skills to bear on decisions about nursing services (Covaleski & Dirsmith, 1984).

Dowd (1988) recommended a framework for making planning decisions about health services. Of the five critical decision factors Dowd recommended, two have directly to do with financial matters. The framework included five critical factors in any health services decision: compatibility with purpose, community service, profitability, feasibility, and quality of service. If nurses want to be part of the decision-making processes, so that the budget will be based on decisions in which nurses have fully participated, then they must prepare themselves to be conversant and prepared to deal with financial management subjects and activities. Concluding a recent review of approaches to cost accounting under the prospective payment system,

Huckabay maintained that "understanding the cost and revenues that nursing produces for each diagnosis can lead to increased control over practice" (1988, p. 80). Jacox (1987) recommended that nursing research should go beyond determining costs and revenues for present services and that nurses should take the lead in determining the costs of doing work in different ways.

Earlier in this chapter, attention was given to preparing nurses to deal with financial management concerns and tasks. What about nursing research? Are nurses demonstrating initiative in the research areas suggested as relevant to financial management? A review of recent research suggests that nurses are actively researching costs of nursing services (Halloran, 1983; Wolf et al., 1986) and the methods for determining costs (Richards, Hexum, & Anderson, 1987; Rosenbaum, Willert, Kelly, Grey, & McDonald, 1988). Staffing methodology directly concerns both cost and quality (Kinley & Cronenwett, 1987; Misener, Frelin, & Twist, 1987). Several recent articles have presented overviews of research in costing of services, methods of costing, and staffing methodology (Edwardson & Giovanneti, 1987; Halloran & Vermeersch, 1987; McCloskey, Gardner, & Johnson, 1987). However, none of the nursing research reviewed examined budgeting processes directly or examined behavioral aspects of budgeting.

The role of research is generally agreed to be one of bringing rigorous and systematic study to bear on a problem or area of concern (Burns & Grove, 1987). The greatly increased emphasis on cost control in health care services suggests that all aspects of financial management warrant research attention.

REFERENCES

Andrica, D.C. (1988). Changing profiles of nurse executives. *Nursing Economics, 6*(3), 112-115.

Birkofer, J.R., Wasch, R.S., & Kramer, C.C. (1987). Budgeting in nonprofit organizations. In H.W.A. Sweeny & R. Rachlin (Eds.), *Handbook of budgeting* (2nd ed.). New York: Wiley.

Burns, N., & Grove, S.K. (1987). *The practice of nursing research: Conduct, critique and utilization.* Philadelphia: W.B. Saunders.

Carroll, T.L. (1989). Administration and organization content in master's programs in nursing. In B. Henry, C. Arndt, M.D. Vincenti, & A. Marriner-Tomey (Eds.), *Dimensions of Nursing Administration.* Boston: Blackwell.

Chandra, G. (1987). The behavioral aspects of budgeting. In H.W.A. Sweeny & R. Rachlin (Eds.), *Handbook of budgeting* (2nd ed.). New York: Wiley.

Chenhall, R.H., & Brownell, P. (1988). The effect of participative budgeting on job satisfaction and performance: Role ambiguity as an intervening variable. *Accounting Organizations and Society, 13,* 225-233.

Covaleski, M., & Dirsmith, M. (1984). Building texts for nursing services through budgeting negotiation skills. *Nursing Administration Quarterly, 8*(2), 1-11.

Dowd, R.P. (1988). Participative decision making is strategic management of resources. *Nursing Administration Quarterly, 13*(1), 11-18.

Edwardson, S.R., & Giovanneti, P.E. (1987). A review of cost-accounting methods for nursing services. *Nursing Economics, 5*(3), 107-117.

Goertzen, I. (1978). Regulation of hospital rates and its implications for nursing. *Nursing Administration Quarterly, 3*(1), 59-65.

Greenfield, J. (1988). Budget-driven era demands new lesson plan. *Nursing & Health Care, 9*(3), 133-135.

Halloran, E., & Vermeersch, P.E.H. (1987). Variability in nurse staffing research. *Journal of Nursing Administration, 17*(2), 26-32.

Halloran, E.J. (1983). RN staffing: more care—less cost. *Nursing Management, 14*(9), 18-22.

Harrison, J.K., & Roth, P.A. (1987). Empowering nursing in multihospital systems. *Nursing Economics, 5*(2), 70-76.

Henry, B., Moody, L., Pendergast, J.F., O'Donnell, J., Hutchinson, S.A., & Scully, G. (1987). Delineation of nursing administration research priorities. *Nursing Research, 36*(5), 309-314.

Hinshaw, A., & Smeltzer, C. (1987). Research challenges and programs for practice settings. *Journal of Nursing Administration, 17*(7, 8), 20-26.

Hirst, M.K. (1987). The effects of setting budget goals and task uncertainty on performance: A theoretical analysis. *The Accounting Review, 62*(4), 774-784.

Hoffman, F.M. (1984). *Financial management for nurse managers.* Norwalk, CT: Appleton-Century-Crofts.

Huckabay, L.M.O. (1988). Allocation of resources and identification of issues in determining the cost of nursing services. *Nursing Administration Quarterly, 13*(1), 72-82.

Jacox, A.K. (1987). Determing the cost and value of nursing. *Nursing Administration Quarterly, 12*(1), 7-12.

Jones, K.R. (1988). Strategic planning in hospitals: Applications to nursing administration. *Nursing Administration Quarterly, 13*(1), 1-10.

Kinley, J., & Cronenwett, L.R. (1987). Multiple shift patient classification: Is it necessary? *Journal of Nursing Administration, 17*(2), 22-25.

Lindeman, C. (1975). Delphi survey of priorities in clinical nursing research. *Nursing Research, 24,* 434-441.

Mackenzie, R.A. (1969, November-December). The management process in 3D. *Harvard Business Review,* 80-87.

Mansfield, E. (1983). *Principles of microeconomics* (4th ed.). New York: W.W. Norton.

McCloskey, J.C., Gardner, D.L., & Johnson, M.R. (1987). Costing out nursing services: An annotated bibliography. *Nursing Economics, 5,* 245-253.

McGivern, D.O. (1988). Teaching nurses the language of the marketplace. *Nursing & Health Care, 9*(3), 127-130.

Mia, L. (1987). Participation in budgetary decision making, task difficulty, losses of control and employee behavior: An empirical study. *Decision Sciences, 18,* 547-561.

Misener, T.R., Frelin, A.J., & Twist, P.A. (1987). Sampling nursing time pinpoints staffing needs. *Nursing & Health Care, 8,* 233-237.

Norton, B. (1989). Organization and administrative content in baccalaureate nursing programs. In B. Henry, C. Arndt, M.D. Vincenti, & A. Marriner-Tomey (Eds.), *Dimensions of nursing administration.* Boston: Blackwell.

Peters, T. (1987). *Thriving on chaos.* New York: Alfred A. Knopf.

Poteet, G.W., & Goddard, N.L. (1989). Issues in financial management. In B. Henry, C. Arndt, M.D. Vincenti, & A. Marriner-Tomey (Eds.), *Dimensions of Nursing Administration.* Boston: Blackwell.

Preston, J.G. (1987). The budget manual. In H.W.A. Sweeny & R. Rachlin (Eds.), *Handbook of budgeting* (2nd ed.). New York: Wiley.

Richards, M., Hexum, J., & Anderson, R. (1987). Patient care demands by DRG: A pilot study. *Nursing Economics, 5*(3), 125-129.

Rosenbaum, H.L., Willert, T.M., Kelly, E.A., Grey, J.F., & McDonald, B.R. (1988). Costing out nursing services based on acuity. *Journal of Nursing Administration, 18*(7, 8), 10-15.

Rowland, H.S., & Rowland, B.L. (Eds.). (1985). *Nursing administration handbook* (2nd ed.). Rockville, MD: Aspen.

Sheridan, D., Bronstein, J., & Walker, D. (1984). *The new nurse manager.* Rockville, MD: Aspen.

Simms, L. (1989). The evolution of education for nursing administration. In B. Henry, C. Arndt, M.D. Vincenti, & A. Marriner-Tomey (Eds.), *Dimensions of Nursing Administration.* Boston: Blackwell.

Singleton, E.K. (1989). Organization and administration content in doctoral nursing programs. In B. Henry, C. Arndt, M.D. Vincenti, & A. Marriner-Tomey (Eds.), *Dimensions of Nursing Administration.* Boston: Blackwell.

Sonberg, V., & Vestal, K.W. (1983). Nursing as a business. *Nursing Clinics of North America, 18,* 491-498.

Stark, P.L. (1987). The master's-prepared nurse in the marketplace: What do master's-prepared nurses do? What should they do? In P.L. Stark (Ed.), *Issues in graduate nursing education* (NLN Pub. No. 18-21, 96). New York: National League for Nursing.

Stevens, B.J. (1985). *The nurse as executive.* Rockville, MD: Aspen.

Strasen, L. (1987). *Key business skills for nurse managers.* Philadelphia: Lippincott.

Tannenbaum, R., & Schmidt, W.H. (1958, March-April). How to choose a leadership pattern. *Harvard Business Review,* 95-101.

Tannenbaum, R., & Schmidt, W.H. (1973, May-June). How to choose a leadership pattern. *Harvard Business Review,* 162-168, 173, 175, 178-180.

Tuttle, W.C. (1988). The evolving role of health care organizations in research. *Hospital & Health Services Administration, 33*(1), 47-56.

Vanderzee, H., & Glusko, G. (1984). DRG: Variable pricing, and budgeting for nursing services. *Journal of Nursing Administration, 14*(5), 11-14.

Vraciu, R.A. (1980). Programming, budgeting, and control in health care organizations: The state of the art. In G.E. Birbes & R.A. Vraciu (Eds.), *Managing the finances of health care organizations.* Ann Arbor, MI: Health Administration Press.

Wolf, G., Lesic, L.K., & Leak, A.G. (1986). Primary nursing. The impact on nursing costs within DRG's. *Journal of Nursing Administration, 16*(3).

Chapter 35

Analyzing Performance Problems
Robert F. Mager and Peter Pipe

Jo Anne Clanton
Marilyn Sue Doub

❚❙   CASE STUDY

John Andrews was a 28-year-old nurse transferred to the intensive care unit after various jobs throughout the hospital. His reputation as lackadaisical with an attitude problem preceded his transfer. Upon transfer, John infrequently tried to interact with the staff. He came to work, accepted his assignment, and started his day with usually less than a "hello." He always took his breaks alone and ate his meals off the unit. No matter what type of day he had, he always managed to leave work on time, often leaving extra work for the next shift.

The transfer itself was a dramatic change for John. He had worked as a staff nurse on a general ward where most activities were considered routine. He could take his time and complete his job at his own speed. The intensive care unit, however, was a high-stress environment of constantly changing situations and patients. The work demanded intense prioritizing and organizational skills.

The majority of the intensive care nurses were assertive, outstanding performers. They were committed to their patients and thrived on challenges. Frequently, many of the nurses put in numerous hours of overtime helping the next shift.

John's patient care was less than average. Because he never seemed to get around to the daily basic care of hygiene, his patients always appeared in disarray. They were not shaved, and their hair was never combed. His bedside area was continuously cluttered with all sorts of paraphernalia.

In addition to what appeared to be slovenly work, he often missed critical changes in patients. The subtle details seemed unimportant to him. Many of the nurses recognized his inattentiveness and often complained that he would not ask for help when he got in over his head. John's passive attitude accentuated his nonacceptance by the other nurses. Many resented working with him, for they felt he did not carry his load and certainly was not capable of caring for the more critical patients.

Not only was John's performance less than desirable but he also started arriving late for work several times a week. Although his tardiness was only 3 to 5 minutes, this factor created another source of animosity among his co-workers. They felt as though they could not count on John even for report.

❘❘❘

MAGER AND PIPES: ANALYZING PERFORMANCE PROBLEMS

In applying Mager and Pipe's theory of analyzing performance problems, first the problem must be understood in detail before a workable solution can be found. The nature of the performance discrepancy—the difference between what is desired and what exists—must be identified. If the discrepancy does not affect the end result, the solution might be to ignore the discrepancy. If the consequence is important, however, action should be taken to eliminate it.

Once the discrepancy is identified as important, the cause must be determined. The cause may be a skill deficiency. A skill that the individual has not learned to perform will require some type of formal training; refresher training methods will be needed for a skill that the individual used to do but does not do often. If the skill is used frequently, feedback may assist in providing a better level of performance.

Sometimes a simpler solution may be obtained without formal training. The job could be changed to meet the individual's skills by using job aids such as checklists, memoranda, or instructions. On-the-job training may be a better route than formal training. "See one, do one" is easier than sitting in a classroom hearing about how to do one.

An individual may try to do his or her best, but that best does not meet standards. The individual just cannot develop the skills necessary to perform. In this case, termination or transfer is the answer.

When the discrepancy is not a skill deficiency, modification of conditions associated with performance or consequences should be explored. Mager and Pipe suggest trying to change something in the environment so that effort will be more attractive, less repulsive, or less difficult (Mager & Pipe, 1970). Four general questions to assess nonperformance are: (1) Is it punishing to perform as desired? (2) Is it rewarding to perform other than as desired? (3) Does it matter if performance is as desired? (4) Are these obstacles to performing as desired? (Mager, 1970, p. 48). Managers should stop punishing desirable performance, such as giving good workers additional work without additional rewards. Reward desirable behavior, let workers know their efforts are noticed, and remove obstacles to good performance.

CASE ANALYSIS

John's performance problem could not be ignored, so intervention was necessary. His actual performance was less than desired, constituting a performance discrepancy. Prior to the interview, the head nurse decided that John's performance was not a skill deficiency, for he had the ability to perform. He had been taught the skills and had had the opportunity to practice them. She realized that she would have to modify the conditions associated with John's performance before improvement could be obtained.

The head nurse considered the possibility that John might feel that desired performance would lead to unfavorable consequences. Perhaps John was late some mornings so that he would avoid being assigned the most difficult patient. If he arrived early, he would have to have some interaction with the staff. Did he think that if he gave better patient care he would receive more difficult assignments?

The head nurse needed to find out how John perceived his performance. If difficult assignments were the issue, she could reassure him that he could have input into his assignments. By doing this, she could do as Mager and Pipe suggest and remove the punishment.

The head nurse decided to explore Mager's second question regarding performance. Was performing other than as desired rewarding for John? The result of his performance led to decreased responsibility. Did he think because of this he did not have to work as hard? Supposedly, John had had a performance problem in the past. Was this his way of getting attention? As a result of his present performance, he was usually assigned the least difficult patient and always left work on time. If his assignments were less, did that mean he just had to worry less? If he did not accept responsibility and make decisions, he would not have to worry about getting into trouble.

If John was anxious about his responsibility and decisions, she could encourage him to utilize the senior nurses when faced with difficult issues. Therefore, he would not have to feel totally responsible for uncertain situations. No matter what shift would be involved, resource personnel were always on the unit.

The head nurse then wondered if John's performance mattered to him. What consequence — favorable or unfavorable — did his performance have? Was he getting any satisfaction — personal or professional — from his work? She could call his attention to how his performance mattered, such as a patient who got relief from pain because of his action. She could pass patient compliments on to him.

Something could definitely be done to make consequences for John's performance. The head nurse could give him a low performance evaluation, which would certainly affect chances of promotion and in turn hinder salary increases. She could notice when he did something desirable and thank him. If his performance improved, she could reward him by approving the evening shift he had requested. A positive consequence of a personal value could produce a more desirable performance.

In order to give his performance a fair analysis, the head nurse considered Mager's fourth cause — obstacles. What was preventing John from performing? Maybe he was not sure what was expected of him. Did he feel inferior with a group of aggressive, mostly female nurses? Did he lack the authority to master his role as a critical care nurse? Possibly he felt that he did not have enough time to give care to all of this patients. Did the unit have too much sensory overload?

Obstacles were certainly prevalent in the unit. John had not overcome the obstacle of acceptance by his peers. He was not a team player. Moreover, the unit itself provided many obstacles. Patients, physicians, and procedures were constantly changing. Solutions could definitely be explored in counseling sessions.

The head nurse decided to use Norman R.F. Maier's model for problem solving as her interview technique with John. Maier's Appraisal Interviewing Model appears in Chapter 36. The main objective for the interview was John's development in the intensive care unit. By using the problem-solving method, the head nurse and John could learn and communicate with the hope that discussing John's problems would lead to improved performance. The head nurse realized that she had to accept John as he was, for a personality cannot be changed. Some kinds of behavior John had control over, and some he did not. She also knew that she must understand and try to see the job as John saw it.

When the head nurse called John in, she explained that the purposes of the session were to see how John felt about his job, the progress he had made, and where they were going. Because John did not believe he was being judged in this meeting, he felt less threatened.

The interview generated several clarifications of John's problems. When John expressed his fears of the unit and the anxiety associated with coming to work, a direct line of communication started. The issues John brought up were pertinent. He stated that he disliked coming to work, for everything was chaotic and always changing. He felt that in only a few hours, he would be behind in his work. He was frustrated because he had no control over the many changing situations.

Different alternatives were discussed, and they agreed on some changes. Patient assignments had been changed daily. A plan was initiated whereby John would keep the same assignment for 3 to 5 days to allow him to feel comfortable with the routine of specific patients. Because he was always behind, he would write a plan of care at the beginning of each shift to help him organize his time more efficiently. Intrinsic motivation was instilled by removing the fear of constantly changing patients. Having more input in his assignments gave John more control over his environment.

Because of his lack of experience with the new equipment, John was overwhelmed with the technology. Therefore, he requested a critical care course. A more detailed understanding of the changing technology would certainly give him more confidence.

Some of John's problems, such as staff interaction and tardiness, were not discussed at this time. The head nurse knew that results of positive staff interaction would not be immediate, but she hoped that as John became more confident a change would take place. She also hoped that his punctuality would improve as his anxieties lessened.

The objective of this technique was the development of better future performance. John was included in all decision making for improved performance. All John's fears and concerns would not disappear overnight, but this stage was a starting point. A future session was scheduled in 6 weeks to review and determine progress.

RESEARCH

Mager and Pipe's model to analyze performance appraisals as part of needs assessment has been used and found to enhance training programs. Mager's *Preparing Instructional Objectives* (1962) has been used to develop staff and patient educational programs. A search of the Social Citation Index revealed 40 citations of Mager in nursing journals, two of which appeared in *Journal of Nursing Administration*, "The Hospitalwide Education Department," by P.J. King (1978), and "Evaluating the Quality of Patient-Care through Retrospective Chart Review," by S. Watson and M. Mayers (1976).

Mager and Pipe's model to analyze performance appraisals was used by R.B. MacAfree (1982) in "Using Performance Appraisal to Enhance Training Programs" and by Bowman, Wolkenheim, Beck, O'Donnell, and Schneider, in "Needs Assessment: An Information Processing Model" (1985). MacAfree felt that in a comprehensive needs assessment, individual performance measures needed to be reviewed through auditing performance appraisals of a random sample of staff and analyzing the results with the Mager and Pipe model (MacAfree, 1982). Bowman and co-workers (1985) found that not all performance problems are corrected through education. Some may, in fact, be attributable to supervision, procedures, or other obstacles to performance. They used Mager and Pipe's model for analyzing performance problems at Milwaukee Children's Hospital. Mager's *Preparing Instructional Objectives* (1962) was used to develop "A Model for Employee Development" (Huntsman, 1987; instructional goals for educating outpatients at a Veterans Administration clinic (Berger & Wesley, 1986); and a modular curriculum for community health nursing at the State University of New York (Weitzel & Robinson, 1986). Byrnes (1986) wrote an article on "Bridging the Gap Between Humanism and Behaviorism in Nursing Education" in which she referred to Mager's *Preparing Instructional Objectives* (1962).

REFERENCES

Berger, M.S., & Wesley, W. (1986). Can we educate outpatients effectively? Certainly. *Nursing Management, 17*(12), 34-37.

Bowman, B., Wolkenheim, B., Beck, M.L., O'Donnell, D., & Schneider, K. (1985). Needs assessment: An information processing model. *The Journal of Continuing Education in Nursing, 16,* 200-204.

Byrnes, K.A. (1986). Bridging the gap between humanism and behaviorism in nursing education. *Journal of Nursing Education, 25,* 304-305.

Huntsman, A.J. (1987). A model for employee development. *Nursing Management, 18,* 51-54.

King, P.J. (1978). The hospitalwide education department. *Journal of Nursing Administration, 8*(14), 13-19.

MacAfree, R.B. (1982). Using performance appraisal to enhance training programs. *Personnel Administrator,* *29*(11), 31.

Mager, R.F. (1962). *Preparing instructional objectives.* Palo Alto, CA: Fearon Publishers.

Mager, R.F., & Pipe, P. (1970). *Analyzing performance problems or "You really outa wanna."* Belmont, CA: Fearon Publishers.

Watson, S., and Mayers, M. (1976). Evaluating the quality of patient-care through retrospective chart review. *Journal of Nursing Administration, 6*(3), 17-21.

Weitzel, A.R., & Robinson, M.E. (1986). Modular curriculum development in community health nursing. *Public Health Nursing, 3,* 257-263.

Chapter 36

Maier's Appraisal Interviewing Model
Norman R.F. Maier

Marilyn Sue Doub
Jo Anne Clanton

❚❚ CASE STUDY

Jane Smith was a 30-year-old nursing assistant who had been trained on the job. During her 6 years of employment in the long-term care facility, she had proven herself to be caring and dependable. She had completed training as a qualified medication aide and functioned in this capacity whenever requested. Although she was unable to work double shifts, she would come into work on her days off. However, she no longer was willing to take call. She organized her work well, gave high-quality resident care, participated in care planning, and completed her work on time. She was equally good at rehabilitation, maintenance, and terminal care. She could get her residents to eat and often trained them to feed themselves as they progressed from puree diets to mechanical soft diets. Her firmness, effective in the rehabilitation of some elderly residents, resulted in uncooperative behavior from other residents with domineering personalities. She never avoided the difficult or terminal resident. She could do the work of three new employees without appearing to hurry. She was thorough at training new employees but obviously disliked that job.

The manager could not understand why Jane frequently passed up call lights and refused to help other nursing assistants with lifting. She insisted on lifting heavy residents by herself instead of getting help. She was overweight, limped around on arthritic heels, often did not acknowledge instructions, by stating that she had a hearing loss, and showed little enthusiasm for her work. Her lack of enthusiasm and sluggish behavior irritated her co-workers. She was frequently observed engaged in long personal conversations with co-workers during resident care time. Two days in a row she was observed talking to a co-worker for 20 minutes before three o'clock rounds. Both days she worked about 30 minutes overtime and clocked out late. She took a good half hour to chart and frequently extended her break time. She rarely offered to help other employees finish their assignment. When asked to stay over and help the next shift when they were short of staff, she would refuse. However, if her ride was not on time, she would find work to do and clock out late in order to obtain the overtime. Because of this behavior, the nurse manager arranged an interview with Jane to discuss her behavior.

MAIER'S APPRAISAL INTERVIEW MODEL

Norman R.F. Maier's appraisal interview model includes three different interviewing techniques: tell and sell, tell and listen, and problem solving. The technique or combination of techniques used depends on the situation, the goal of the interview, and the skills of the manager.

Tell and Sell

The objectives of the tell-and-sell method are to communicate the evaluation of the employee's work performance and to persuade the employee to improve. The evaluation needs to be accurate and fair, resulting from objective observations and not from hearsay. The supervisor is expected to let the employee know how he or she is doing, gain the employee's acceptance of the evaluation, and have the employee agree to follow a plan for improvement. These objectives can be achieved if the employee wants to correct the faults, accepts the judgment of the superior, and has the ability to change.

The tell-and-sell method has its greatest potential when the superior is respected because of position, knowledge, and experience, and the employee is inexperienced and insecure and wants advice and assurance from an authority figure.

Harmful effects may result from the tell-and-sell method when the appraisal is perceived to be unfair, the interview becomes personal, and face-saving problems develop that affect the day-to-day relationship between the superior and the subordinate. Another risk occurs, particularly where appraisals include middle and top management, when subordinates accept the judgment of the superior and try to please her or him, thus suppressing their own initiative and potential. The tell-and-sell method is bound to encourage this kind of reaction with employees who are not assertive. The employee may continue to function at a minimal level but feel anger and frustration, which result in stress-related physical conditions, depression, and/or burnout. Because the tell-and-sell interview is a form of downward communication that makes no provision for upward communication, it perpetuates existing values. When used with experienced, educated, highly motivated individuals who are used to acting autonomously, the tell-and-sell method may result in resignations (Maier, 1976).

Tell and Listen

The values promoted by the tell-and-listen interview include trust, tolerance, and respect for the dignity of the individual. The purpose of the tell-and-listen interview is to evaluate the employee and establish two-way communications that enable the supervisor to understand the subordinate's viewpoint. Understanding then should result in increased respect, trust, and motivation for the employee. The interviewer covers the strong and weak points of a subordinate's job performance, avoids interruption, and puts off controversy for later consideration. The second part of the interview is spent encouraging the employee to express his or her feelings. It is assumed that verbal expression or release of frustrated feelings tends to reduce or remove them. It is also assumed that individuals have a right to their feelings and a need to express them. The interviewer must be mature and accept the interviewees' defensive reactions. The necessary skills include active listening, effective use of pauses, reflection of feelings, and summarizing of feelings. Motivation can result if the interview results in solving some job problems, clarifying misunderstandings between supervisor and subordinates, or solving a personal problem (Maier, 1976).

Problem-Solving Method

Maier's problem-solving method of interviewing takes the interviewer out of the role of judge and into the role of helper. It offers four ways to improve the performance of subordinates: (1) changing the subordinates' behavior, (2) changing the job duties or the job procedure, (3) changing jobs, and (4) changing the pattern of supervision (Maier, 1976).

CASE ANALYSIS

Previous evaluations with Jane Smith using the tell-and-sell method did not result in a change of behavior. Jane appeared easygoing, uncritical, and unimaginative, and she accepted authoritarian leadership. She would verbally agree with her evaluation and then continue to do the work "her way." Jane could not resign, she cared for her patients and her family, and she continued to function at a minimal level, determined to survive.

The supervisor considered using the tell-and-listen method and listed the following goals: understanding Jane's feelings, attitudes, and behavior; utilizing Jane's skills in orienting new employees; developing Jane's image as a role model, and developing Jane's awareness that some residents found security in her firmness and other residents felt she was rude. What started out as a tell-and-listen interview ended up as a problem-solving interview. By combining the tell-and-listen and problem-solving interviewing methods, the supervisor became both employee minded and production minded.

During the tell-and-listen part of the interview, Jane expressed the following feelings: She felt that the more work she did, the more she was asked to do. Many times she passed up call lights and refused to help other employees because if she did she ended up doing not only her work but also much of theirs. Having organized and worked all of the assignments, she knew when other employees needed help and assisted them but refused to help co-workers who "just goofed off, got behind, and then tried to use me to catch up." She was reluctant to help orient and train new nursing assistants because "they don't always stay and I feel like I'm wasting my time. Training a person is double duty. I have the assignment to do plus showing the new person everything. If the employee doesn't work out, I feel like I'm to blame." Jane felt entitled to extra breaks and easy overtime at her convenience because she had not been compensated for training new employees or shown appreciation for her flexibility and quality care.

Jane had many stresses at home. Her husband and daughter had chronic health problems that resulted in expensive doctor bills. She was frequently the only source of income. Both fatigue and transportation were problems. She worked hard at home as well as on the job. Any suggestions by more enthusiastic aides overwhelmed her, and her response was, "Don't tell the boss or she will make me do it too." She had to pace herself to survive.

Jane's ability to organize her work and maintain quality care had resulted in more work for her. She had been delegated the job of a clinical nurse instructor without any training, support, recognition, or financial reimbursement.

Listening to Jane enabled the supervisor to understand her behavior and established the two-way communications needed to focus on the problem of how to orient and train nursing assistants in the 3 days allowed by corporate management. At this time classroom training was not required for nursing assistants, but the regulations were specific as to what was to be covered during orientation.

During the problem-solving portion of the interview, the supervisor and Jane set goals for each orientation day, selected residents, and decided who would do what. Instead of the supervisor delegating her duties to Jane, they shared them and made the best use of the skills of both. Continued use of the combination of the tell-and-listen and problem-solving models resulted in the supervisor learning more about the residents and staff and Jane learning more about nursing and teaching. New employees learned more, stayed longer, and became better nursing assistants. As Jane and the supervisor developed their communication, teaching, and problem-solving skills, they developed procedures for handling problem residents. Their respect and tolerance for each other increased. Jane felt good about herself, improved as a role model, and realized that she had to set an example for the others to follow. The supervisor, a perfectionist, learned to accept the limits of reality and pace herself. A support system developed by the use of the tell-and-listen and problem-solving interviewing styles during the orientation period. The tell-and-sell method was infrequently used, even for disciplinary action.

RESEARCH

Norman R.F. Maier is the author of more than 200 research publications, a management training film, and 14 books, including the classic *Supervisory and Executive Development* (1957), which has been revised and published by University Associates as *The Role-Play Technique* (1975). He has also done research on increasing the creative potential of management groups. Comparisons of the six taped simulated interviews that were included in his book and the Tape-Assisted Learning Program show the following interrelationships among objectives, methods, and skills: (1) the tell-and-sell method yielded more words than the other two methods and took more time; (2) the tell-and-listen interviews showed about fifty-fifty participation; and (3) the subordinate does most of the talking in the problem-solving interviews. The interviewers recorded in this book often failed to achieve their objective of improving the subordinate's job performance with the tell-and-sell and tell-and-listen methods. If the objectives of the interview are (1) let the employee know where he or she stands, (2) warn the employee, (3) evaluate the employee for promotion or transfer, (4) provide a record of job performance, (5) obtain a record of ratings by various supervisors, and (6) supply higher management with an inventory of talent available, the tell-and-sell or tell-and-listen method could be used. The tell-and-listen method recognizes the importance of the employee's feelings and the need to express and clarify them. Once the emotional obstacles are recognized and expressed, behavior changes follow (Maier, 1976). "Listening may be in conflict with the objective of informing the employee where he stands, but if it results in the employee gaining insight into his own problems, both acceptance and communication of the appraisal may be achieved" (p. 146). The problem-solving approach seems most natural in a setting in which power does not play a part in the interaction and in which two people respect each other and search together for a better way to do the job. Using the problem-solving approach to focus on the task does facilitate change (Maier, 1976).

Since the publication in 1958 of *The Appraisal Interview: Objectives, Methods, and Skills,* real-life studies of the appraisal interview support the conclusions reached in Maier's simulation experiments (Burke & Wilcox, 1969; Kay, Meyer, & French, 1965; Meyer & Walker, 1961; Meyer & Kay, 1964.) They show the ineffectiveness of persuasion approaches by revealing the hostility generated and the failure to make changes in behavior (Maier, 1976).

A review of the Social Science Citation Index showed frequent reference to Maier's work in psychology and business journals. In the nursing literature, however, Maier was cited only briefly in two articles appearing in the *Journal of Nursing Administration:* "Using Management Literature to Enhance New Leadership Roles" (Calkin, 1980) and "Managerial Decision-Making" (Lamonica & Finch, 1977). His *Frustration: The Study of Behavior without a Goal* was used as a reference for "How to Deal with Overt Aggression" (Fernandez, 1959, 1986).

REFERENCES

Burke, R.J., & Wilcox, D.S. (1969). Characteristics of effective employee performance review and development interviews. *Personnel Psychology, 22,* 291-305.
Calkin, J.D. (1980). Using management literature to enhance new leadership roles. *Journal of Nursing Administration, 10*(4), 24-29.

Fernandez, T.M. (1959, 1986). How to deal with overt aggression. *American Journal of Nursing, 59,* 658-660; *Issues in Mental Health Nursing, 8,* 79-83.

LaMonica, E., & Finch, F.E. (1977). Managerial decision-making. *Journal of Nursing Administration, 7*(5), 20-ff.

Kay, E., Meyer, H.H., & French, J.R.P. (1965). Effect of threat in a performance appraisal interview. *Journal of Applied Psychology, 69,* 311-317.

Maier, N.R.F. (1958). *The appraisal interview: Objectives, methods, and skills.* La Jolla, CA: University Associates.

Maier, N.R.F. (1975). *The role-play technique* (Rev. ed.). La Jolla, CA: University Associates.

Maier, N.R.F. (1976). *The appraisal interview: Three basic approaches,* La Jolla, CA: University Associates.

Maier, N.R.F., Solen, R.A., & Maier, A.A. (1957). *Supervisory and executive development,* New York Science Edition. La Jolla, CA: University Associates.

Meyer, H.H., & Kay, E. (1964). A comparison of a work planning program with the annual performance appraisal approach. *Behavior Research Services Report No. ESR 17,* General Electric Company.

Meyer, H.H., & Walker, W.B. (1961). A study of factors relating to the effectiveness of a performance appraisal program. *Personnel Psychology, 14,* 291-298.

Chapter 37

Role Theories

Mary C. Harrell
Lou Ellen Sears

|| CASE STUDY

Nancy Brown, RN, had performed the role of charge nurse on the skilled unit of a health care facility for 6 months. She worked day shift with every other weekend off. Her duties included making assignments for licensed practical nurse team leaders and nurse's aides and supervising the care of all 45 residents on her unit. She was responsible for all paperwork, communicating with physicians, and admitting, discharging, and transferring residents.

Nancy was known to be very efficient, cheerful, and pleasant. The staff respected her and the unit functioned well. Therefore, when the assistant director of nursing (ADON) was promoted to director of nursing at another facility, Nancy was offered the position of ADON, a salaried weekday position with responsibility for teaching and supervising nurse's aides. The ADON's duties also include planning in-service training, participating in evaluations of employees, and functioning as the director of nursing in her absence. Because of this, the two work closely together and alternate call every other week and weekend. Nancy cheerfully accepted and was eager to assume her new duties.

After only 2 months in the new position, Nancy tearfully asked to be relieved of the duties and placed back into the position of charge nurse on the skilled unit. She explained that her two teenagers participated in many activities and she feared she would not have the time to be involved. Another concern was that her husband attended school at night, which placed an added burden on her at home. She could not deal with the strain of being on call, which might necessitate coming into the facility during the night or on a weekend. Even though she had not had to come in, she felt the added strain of that possibility when she was on call and therefore was unable to sleep. Also, the phone ringing at night disturbed her family.

Nancy returned to the charge nurse position, which she enjoyed. She felt confident in her abilities as a charge nurse.

||||||||||||||||||||||||||||||||||||||||||||||||||||||||||||||||||

ROLE THEORY

Role theory provides a framework to examine and discuss many social issues. It explains roles by presuming that persons are members of a social position and hold expectations of their own behavior and that of other persons. Hardy and Conway (1988) explain that the development of role theory began in the 1930s when publication of several early social theoreticians formally created the basic knowledge area. Marino, a psychiatrist from Germany, pioneered psychodrama, the use of groups and role playing in psychiatric treatment. He introduced the idea of role playing as a method for learning to play a role more effectively. He also linked types of role behavior to different sets of expectations. George Herbert Mead, a social philosopher, had a significant impact on his associates and students at the University of Chicago. His main interest was in mind, self, and understanding human nature in terms of group and society. Mead is considered the originator of symbolic interaction. The concept of role began to be the focus of study in 1920 when Park, Mead's colleague at the University of Chicago, identified the concept that roles are linked to structural positions. Within these positions, the self is ultimately linked to playing multiple roles. Lenton further conceptualized the social organization and the individual's place within it—a status distinction. These approaches dominated the work in the sociological literature during the 1950s and 1960s and significantly influenced the applied social health sciences. Biddle (1986) reviewed the current state of role theory, noted ideas basic to it, examined these ideas from several perspectives of social thought, and reviewed empirical research for key issues in the theory. Disagreement over the actual definition of *role* has hampered progress toward a universally accepted theory. These differences are focused more in terminology than in actual substance.

The various perspectives of role theory include functional, symbolic interactionist, structural, organizational, and cognitive. Biddle (1986) summarizes the focus of each:

1. *Functional.* This approach focuses on the characteristic behavior of persons who occupy a social position within a stable social system. Roles are conceived as the shared, normative expectations that prescribe and explain these behaviors.
2. *Symbolic interactionist.* This perspective stresses the role of individual actors, the evolution of roles through social interaction, and various cognitive concepts through which social actors understand and interpret their own and others' conduct. Roles are thought to reflect norms, attitudes, contextual demands, negotiation, and the evolving definition of the situation as understood by the actors.
3. *Structural.* In this approach the attention is focused on *social structures,* conceived as stable organizations of sets of persons (*social positions* or *statuses*) who share the same patterned behaviors *(roles)* that are directed toward other sets of persons in the structure.
4. *Organizational.* This version of role theory focuses on social systems that are preplanned, task oriented, and hierarchical. Multiple sources for norms exist, and therefore individuals are subject to role conflict, which often leads to role strain. The core of this theoretical approach concerns variables that affect the actors' choice of strategies for coping with the situation.
5. *Cognitive role theory.* This approach deals with the relationship between role expectations and behavior. The various subfields include discusson of role playing, group norms, and the roles of leader and follower, anticipating role expectations, and role taking. Unlike most theorists, Biddle assumes that role expectations can occur in at least three modes of thought: norms, preferences, and beliefs.

The concepts of role theory are numerous and include:

1. *Consensus.* There is agreement among expectations that are held by various persons (Biddle, 1986).
2. *Conformity.* There is compliance in some pattern for behavior. Studies here investigate the relationship between expectation and behavior (Biddle, 1986).
3. *Role conflict.* Two or more incompatible expectations for the behavior of a person appear concurrently (Biddle, 1986).
4. *Role taking.* The suggestion here is that the adequate development of self and

participation in social interaction require that a person "take the role of the other" (Biddle, 1986).

5. *Role competence.* A person in an interdependent or exchange relationship that is ongoing in time is able to carry out lines of action that are task and interpersonally effective (Hardy & Conway, 1988).

6. *Role transition.* The process of personal change makes it possible to move from one position to another.

Role theory is concerned with a triad of concepts: patterned and characteristic social behavior, parts or identities that are assumed by social participants, and scripts or expectations for behavior that are understood by all and adhered to by performers. Most versions of role theory presume that expectations are major generators of roles, that expectations are learned through experience and that persons are aware of expectations they hold. This discussion focuses on role stress and strain and the conflicts that result from assuming new roles.

Individual participants in society function in a number of roles at the same time. Goode (1960) described a theory of role strain defined as "the felt difficulty in fulfilling role obligations." This approach countered the widely accepted theoretical view that explained the continuity of social roles and thus the maintenance of society as being due to two major variables: the normative consensual commitment of the individuals of the society and the integration among the norms held by these individuals. Some persons cannot conform and thus are unable to meet the expectations of themselves or others. The cause may be insufficient resources, lack of time, lack of energy, or other factors. The result of this unmet expectation is role strain. According to Goode (1960), sources of role strain include (1) even when role demands are not onerous, difficult, or displeasing, they are required at particular times and places; (2) all individuals take part in many role relationships and each may have different obligations; (3) each role relationship typically demands several activities or responses; and (4) many role relationships are "role sets," that is, the individual engages, by virtue of one of his or her positions, in several role relationships with different individuals. A person, therefore, is likely to face varying, distracting, and sometimes conflicting expectations. According to Goode's theory, meeting all demands to the satisfaction of all those who comprise an individual's role network is not possible. Therefore, having difficulty in meeting given role demands is normal. The problem becomes how to make the whole system manageable or how to allocate energies and skills so as to reduce role strain to some bearable proportion.

Hardy and Conway (1988) describe a role stress typology based on a role stress–role strain framework. Definitions pertinent to the discussion include the following:

1. *Role occupant.* A person who holds a position within the social structure
2. *Status set.* The complex of distinct positions held by an individual
3. *Role expectations* (obligations, demands). Position-specific norms that identify the attitudes, behaviors, and cognitions required and anticipated for a role occupant
4. *Role performance* (role behavior or role enactment). Behavior or action relevant to a specific position
5. *Role identity.* An individual's interpretation of role expectations
6. *Focal position.* The position under consideration or study
7. *Role partner* (counter role occupancy). A person who, while occupying an interdependent position with the occupant of the focal position, holds expectations for the focal occupant
8. *Role set.* Constellation of relationships with the role partners of a particular position; all of an actor's role partners

9. *Role stress.* External to a role occupant, a social structural condition in which role obligations are vague, irritating, difficult, conflicting, or impossible to meet; a characteristic of the social system, not of a person in the system
10. *Role strain.* A subjective state of emotional arousal in response to the external conditions of role stress

Hardy and Conway (1988) identified major difficulties that lead to role stress for a role occupant.

1. *Role ambiguity.* Vagueness, lack of clarity of role expectations
2. *Role conflict.* Incompatible role expectations
3. *Role incongruity.* Self-identity and subjective values grossly incompatible with role expectations (role transition and poor self-role fit)
4. *Role overload.* Too much expected in the time available
5. *Role underload.* Minimal role expectations that underutilize the role occupant's abilities.
6. Role overqualification. Motivation, skills, and knowledge far greater than those required
7. *Role underqualification* (role incompetence). Lack of the necessary resources (commitment, skill, knowledge)

The changing state of health care in this society contributes to role strain for those who are health care providers. Hardy and Conway (1988) outline conditions that contribute to role stress in health care. The first is socialization deficit. Most preparation to assume a role in health care is focused in the basic education process. As experience is gained, an individual may be promoted into a new position, staff nurse to assistant head nurse, for example. Often the transition into the new role is difficult and accompanied by feelings of uncertainty, overload, and unclear expectations. Providing programs that would facilitate modification and expansion of existing attitudes, knowledge, values, and behaviors that are appropriate for the new role would assist the transition for the role occupant.

Another source of role stress is the ambiguity that naturally occurs as new roles are established. Health care facilities are changing as a result of technological advances and specialization. New roles and the expertise needed to meet the demands require an ongoing process of clarification and evaluation in order to provide the necessary service. During this process, role ambiguity is very evident. Changes in the organization and delivery of health care — outpatient centers, a focus on wellness, and greater involvement of the consumer in health care, including interest in increasing self-care activities rather than seeking medical care — have also had an impact on those who occupy health provider roles.

Economic controls have certainly placed health care providers and those who receive care in changing positions. Traditional expectations by the client and the provider have been modified. The resulting behaviors of nurses and physicians, for example, may leave the client dissatisfied and unhappy if the client expects responses and approaches that are no longer feasible because of financial cutbacks. The advances in technology, particularly in information systems, require participants in the health care field to adapt to new methods of communication and data storage and retrieval. This change requires willingness on the part of those who occupy specialized roles — intensive care unit nurses, for example — to acquire new values, skills, and knowledge.

Role conflict and role overload for women have been areas for research since the 1960s. These stressors are major obstacles for women in the single-parent or dual-career family. Some of the stress can also be attributed to the forced choices a woman must make between coordinating household and family activities and being goal directed at work. Hardy and Conway (1988) address the career commitment of women in nursing and conclude that the career choice is not given priority over marriage and family. The effects of role overload are significant in that the role occupant is unable to carry out all the obligations in the time available.

Goode (1960) described two main sets of techniques for reducing role strain: those that determine whether or when an individual will enter or leave a role and those that deal with the actual role bargain. Role bargaining is defined as a process of negotiation, involving two or more actors, on acceptable role behaviors to be enacted by the parties involved. Hardy and Conway (1988) point to "A promising new direction in the social sciences . . . the examination of social behavior in terms of transactions or exchanges." In role relationships or social exchanges, the role occupants are aware of the resources (skill, experience, education) they contribute, the costs (role strain, frustration, anxiety) they bear in the transaction, and the reward (approval, feeling of self-worth, monetary gains) they gain from the transaction. In determining whether to enter or leave a role, an individual must consider the implications. Some positions such as age, race, and gender cannot be discarded. Others such as parent and wage earner carry obligations that are more difficult to abandon. Positions that represent considerable commitment are difficult to eliminate. The negotiation process is often necessary when transactions with role partners occur. Two negotiation techniques, role taking and role making, have been described in symbolic interaction theory. Role taking may be viewed as synonymous with empathy, the ability to place oneself in another's position. Role making deals with one's own role prescriptions and emphasizes the positive process of creating and modifying one's own role. These processes require communication and interaction with role partners. During periods of role stress, oftentimes communication diminishes and the level of role stress increases.

The ability to role bargain and negotiate can be influenced by certain conditions. The presence and affects of others greatly influence a bargaining action. An actor's self-esteem and need for approval dictate the position he or she maintains on a certain issue. A neutral party can often reduce conflict in a bargaining situation. Open communication is vital for perception and resolution of role stress. The rank and power of the individual who is bargaining influence the interactions, as does that person's behavioral disposition.

CASE ANALYSIS

Nancy Brown functioned comfortably as the charge nurse on a skilled care unit. She had integrated the role of nurse leader on a shift basis with her roles as wife and mother. The unit functioned well, and the staff respected her. Therefore, role stress for Nancy was apparently minimal in this position. Role expectations were clear; she performed at a level acceptable to her and to the staff on the nursing unit (role set). We can assume that expectations of the roles of wife and mother were also met at levels acceptable to her and to the members of her family (role set).

The role of assistant director of nursing affected Nancy in a variety of ways. Role strain became increasingly evident over a 2-month period. Nancy began to worry about the possibility of being called in during off time. She recognized that being on call was an expectation of the role but experienced definite role conflict when she anticipated having to go to work in the evening or on weekends. Nancy also experienced role overload. She could not determine a method of meeting the expectations she held of herself as a mother while also meeting the expectations of an assistant director of nursing. Obviously, Nancy's priority roles were as wife and mother. Therefore, she chose to deal with role strain by returning to a role that met her needs of self-esteem in her career while allowing her the time to meet the expectations she held of herself as a mother. Nancy demonstrated role-bargaining techniques with the director of nursing in negotiating to return to her previous position. Nancy's goal was to reduce the strain she was feeling with her new role.

Nancy may have benefited from a better understanding of the transition process. If the expectations were unclear and confusing, some frank discussions with the administrators may have provided the opportunity to negotiate role expectations. Nancy did not have the benefit of a mentor or coach who would help her identify coping strategies and networking skills to deal with the stress associated with a position of this type.

Knowledge of role theory and the associated concepts can help to ease the stressful conflicts between expectations and feasibility at many levels. Nurse managers play a pivotal role in making this happen.

RESEARCH

Ward (1986) points out that difficulty in fulfilling role obligations is a frequently observed phenomenon in health care for both recipients and providers. The nursing profession is 96% female. The literature suggests the benefits of occupying multiple roles outweighs the strains (Froberg, Gjerdingen, & Preston, 1986). Women are expected to devote themselves to their families to the exclusion of other major roles. Stress results from having to make forced choices between the options of coordinating household activities and being goal directed at work (Hardy & Conway, 1988). Meisenholder (1986) studied the influence of five variables of self-esteem: perceived reflected appraisals of husband, employment, occupational prestige, husband's preference for wife's work role, and woman's preference for her work role. The results show that the perceived reflected appraisal of the husband was a strong predictor of self-esteem for all women but was three times more influential for homemakers than for employed women. Child care is a concern for today's working women. Rodman, Pratto, and Nelson (1985) studied child care arrangements and children's functioning. Forty-eight self-care children were compared with 48 matched children in adult care to investigate whether the self-care (latchkey) arrangement has negative consequences for children. On several measures of social and psychological functioning, no significant differences were found between the two matched samples. The authors suggest further research in this area.

In addition to concerns about children at home, the concept of role transition deserves some attention. In role transition, the self and self-perceptions are incompatible with the expectations associated with a new role (Hardy & Conway, 1988). Benner (1984) describes levels of competence for new practitioners of nursing: novice, advanced beginner, competent, proficient, and expert. Kramer (1974) described *reality shock,* defined as the specific, shocklike reactions to a work situation of new workers who have spent several years preparing for the work, thought they were going to be prepared, and suddenly find they are not. Preceptor programs and transition programs exist for new graduates, but the effectiveness of these programs is not clear (Schempp & Rompre, 1986).

The transition into a nurse manager's role is accompanied by unclear expectations, fear of the unknown, and feelings of loneliness (Rice, 1988). Minimizing the stress that nurses experience after a promotion requires understanding the dynamics of fledgling managers. Darling and McGrath (1983) interviewed nurses over a 3-year period about their experiences of moving up in management. Their four areas of concern were unawareness of the transition process, unclear role descriptions and expectations, unmet needs, and unplanned programs of follow-up. The authors then described actions that nursing administrators could have taken to ease the transition process. Building an awareness of the transition process is a vital consideration that facilitates receptive attitudes toward coaching and mentoring by supervisors of the new managers. Clarifying roles and expectations must occur not only in the form of job descriptions but also in frank discussions between the administrators and potential managers. The mismatches that often occur result in a high cost to the individuals involved and also to the institution (Kotter, 1973). Another component is attending to the needs of new managers, which can be accomplished by a mentoring or coaching process. The new manager is guided in the skills of networking, empowering strategies, and problem solving. Orientation programs need to be formalized. Dunne, Ehrlich, and Mitchell (1988) describe an orientation curriculum plan with a framework for advanced management enhancements that addresses this need.

What of managers who have been in a position for a period of time? The role transition phase may be over, but role stress remains and may become the important issue. Scalzi (1988) conducted a survey of nurse executives and identified four major role stress factors: (1) overload, defined as conflicting and/or too many expectations, along with a large span of control; (2) quality of care concerns that include the competence of nurses and physicians and general quality-of-care issues related to cultural differences; (3) role ambiguity or lack of clear job expectations, policies, and guidelines; and (4) role conflict associated with working within and between groups that have different orientations and/or priorities, such as hospital administrators and practicing nurses at the bedside. The participants in the study identified positive and negative coping strategies. Awareness of these strategies in the context of role stress may allow the nurse executive to concentrate on the more productive strategies.

REFERENCES

Barnett, R.C., & Baruch, G.K. (1985). Women's involvement in multiple roles and psychological stress. *Journal of Personality and Social Psychology, 49,* 135.

Benner, P. (1984). *From novice to expert.* Reading, MA: Addison-Wesley.

Biddle, B.J. (1986). Recent developments in role theory. *Annual Review of Sociology, 12,* 67-92.

Darling, L.W., & McGrath, L.G. (1983a). The causes and costs of promotion trauma. *Journal of Nursing Administration, 13*(4), 29-33.

Darling, L.W., & McGrath, L.G. (1983b). Minimizing promotion trauma. *Journal of Nursing Administration, 13*(9), 14-19.

Dunne, R.S., Ehrlich, S.A., & Mitchell, B.S. (1988). A management development program for middle level nurse managers. *Journal of Nursing Administration, 18*(5), 11-16.

Froberg, D., Gjerdingen, D., & Preston, M. (1986). Multiple roles and women's mental and physical health: What have we learned? *Women and Health, 11*(2), 79-96.

Goode, W.J. (1960). A theory of role strain. *American Sociological Review, 25,* 483-496.

Hardy, M.E., & Conway, M.E. (1988). *Role theory: Perspectives for health professionals.* Norwalk, CT: Appleton & Lange.

Kelly, J. (1982). Role theory as a model for human interaction: Its implications for nursing education. *The Australian Nurses Journal, 12*(1), 42-43, 51.

Kotter, J.P. (1973). The psychological contract: Managing the joining-up process. *California Management Review, 15*(3), 91-99.

Kramer M. (1974). *Reality shock: Why nurses leave nursing.* St. Louis: C.V. Mosby.

Marriner-Tomey, A. (1988). *Guide to nursing management.* St. Louis: C.V. Mosby.

Meisenholder, J. (1986). Self-esteem in women: The influence of employment and perception of husband's appraisal. *Image, 18,* 8-14.

Rheiner, N.W. (1982). Role theory: Framework for change. *Nursing Management, 13*(3), 20-22.

Rice, J.M. (1988). Transition from staff nurse to head nurse: A personal experience. Notes from the field. *Nursing Management, 19*(4), 102.

Rodman, H., Pratto, D., & Nelson, R. (1985). Child care arrangements and children's functioning: A comparison of self-care and adult-care children. *Developmental Psychology, 21,* 413-418.

Sarbin, T., & Allen, V.L. (1968). Role Theory. In G. Linzey & E. Aronson (Eds.), *The handbook of social psychology.* Reading, MA: Addison-Wesley.

Scalzi, C. (1988). Role stress and coping strategies of nurse executives. *Journal of Nursing Administration, 18*(3), 34-38.

Schempp, C.M., & Rompre, R.M. (1986, Fall). Transition programs for new graduates. How effective are they? *Journal of Nursing Staff Development,* 150-155.

Ward, C.R. (1986). The meaning of role strain. *Advances in Nursing Science, 8*(2), 39-49.

Chapter 38

Conflict Mode Model
K.W. Thomas and R.H. Kilmann

David Eugene Hunt

David Eugene Hunt

❘❘   CASE STUDY

Sarah Goodamin has been the vice president of nursing in a rural hospital for the past 10 years. A change in reimbursement from prepayment to a prospective payment system has forced management to seek new avenues of maintaining hospital revenue and to focus on increasing market shares. The major purpose of such activity has been to stabilize the institution's financial viability during a period of transition from a noncompetitive to a competitive era. Secondary to the reimbursement changes, Sarah had identified an increase in patient acuity on all nursing units. There were fewer admissions; however, those patients admitted were requiring an increased number of patient care hours. By analyzing monthly and quarterly data, Sarah had identified the need to employ an additional 25 registered nurses. The need to employ additional registered nurses was confirmed by the numerous complaints received weekly by the nursing staff. To complicate the situation, Sarah was reminded almost daily of the nursing shortage by means of newspaper and journal articles. Although Sarah had previously considered such situations challenging, the pressure from hospital administration to increase productivity and efficiency while the employees complained of being overworked and stressed had left this vice president of nursing in a very perplexing situation.

More recently, Sarah "sensed" a better feeling in regard to staff satisfaction based on the fact that she was experiencing fewer employee complaints. During this same time frame, patient beds were running on the average of 90% capacity, and the units were continuing with high patient acuities. That approximately 12 of the 25 vacant registered positions had been filled has added to her "sense" of overall improvement in staff satisfaction. To Sarah the entire system appeared to be functioning smoothly; revenue was up because of the high percentage of filled beds, and complaints from the staff had decreased.

Then, one morning while she was entering the hospital to begin her day's work, she noticed an individual passing out information to all interested nursing employees. Curious, she asked the individual for a copy. Reading the first sentence was like having a bolt of lightning pierce her body. The staff was in active pursuit of recruiting a union to represent them during future deliberations between the nurses and management. Sarah could not believe what was occurring. She paused and, with feelings of failure surrounding her, reflected back momentarily on the changes that had occurred. Staffing had improved, and employee complaints had decreased. Why was this happening? Frustration, fear, anger, and discontent were just a few of the emotions she felt. She had a grave sense of failure yet at the same moment realized that management had little time to organize and respond. Sarah recalled a continuing education program about labor and employment law she attended a few years ago.

After meeting and consulting with hospital administration in relation to the employees' organization attempts, legal representation for the hospital was notified and counter proceedings were put into motion immediately. While reviewing her notes from the continuing education program, she vividly remembered one point. When employees ask about a union, encourage them "not to sign the card." Sarah also promptly reviewed the restraints placed on management while the employees are in process of organizing. Management *cannot* (1) interfere with the employees' organizing activities, (2) discriminate against an employee for participating in union activities, (3) dominate a union by gaining influence by paying union expenses or providing union leaders with special benefits, (4) refuse to bargain in good faith, or (5) turn their heads to unfair practices committed by a supervisor (Potter, 1984). Sarah also reviewed management's rights as protected by the National Labor Relations Board (NLRB). Management *can* (1) inform employees of the disadvantages of belonging to a union, (2) inform employees of their right to refuse to sign union authorization cards, and (3) encourage employees to participate in the union election (Potter, 1984).

Sarah now feels that she has failed as a vice president of nursing in this hospital and is seeking advice and direction in dealing with this immediate problem. Part of the problem, she feels, is associated with the lack of communication between the nursing staff and herself over the previous year.

| | | | | | | | | | | | | | | | | | | | | | | | | | | | | | | | | | | | | | | | | | | | | | | | | | | | | | | | | | | | | | |

CONFLICT THEORY

Katz and Lawyer (1985) describe *conflict* as "an expressed struggle in which two or more interdependent parties are experiencing strong emotion resulting from a perceived difference in needs or values." They identified four criteria apparent in a conflict situation (p. 93):

1. At least two parties are involved.
2. Mutually exclusive needs or mutually exclusive values either exist or are perceived to exist.
3. Interaction is characterized by strong emotion and behavior designed to defeat, reduce, or suppress the opponent.
4. Parties face each other with mutually opposing actions as they attempt to gain a forward position of power relative to each other.

Dipolarization exists in conflict. Positive conflict can be constructive, provide prestige to the winner, offer personal gain, and be an incentive for creativity (Blake & Mouton, 1964; Marriner, 1982). Negative conflict can be destructive if permitted to continue without intervention from management. Conflict of this nature should warn management that an organizational imbalance exists and stimulate efforts to investigate new solutions through problem solving, clarification of objectives, and determining group boundaries (Marriner, 1982). Over the past two decades, social science researchers have worked diligently to develop an increased understanding of conflict and, ultimately, a classification system to identify interpersonal modes of handling conflict. Blake and Mouton (1964) suggested that the functionality or dysfunctionality of a given conflict situation is extensively influenced by the manner in which individuals approach and manage disagreement. Thomas (1971) was concerned that Blake and Mouton had focused on the individual's attempts to deal with interpersonal conflict as individual predispositions or styles, that Blake and Mouton's studies were unclear as to what extent the occurrence of these modes was determined by situational factors, and that the amount of information available in the literature in relation to dealing with interpersonal conflict was limited. Thomas was also interested in whether the effect of one individual's use of conflict-handling modes would influence the mode of another during a disagreement.

After identifying these concerns, in "Conflict-Handling Modes in Interdepartmental Relations" (1971), Thomas identified that candor was generally viewed as being associated with positive sentiments, perceived cooperation, efficient decision making, and related supervisors' ratings of respondents' promotability by managers and coordinates (members of other departments with whom the managers negotiated). In contrast, Thomas identified that coordinates associated forcing and avoiding with negative sentiments, noncooperation, and inefficient decision making, yet the respondents' forcing and avoiding were not significantly related to promotability. Accommodation was viewed positively by coordinates but was negatively related to promotability. Compromise was viewed neutrally by both coordinates and supervisors. Thomas also concluded that a manager's interdepartmental conflict-handling behavior was directly influenced by four variables: (1) the manager's personal characteristics, (2) factors stemming from the manager's membership in the department, (3) technology, and (4) the manager's coordinates behavior. The strongest influence identified upon conflict-handling behavior was conflict of interest between departments. Thomas concluded that conflict of interest was associated with competitive conflict-handling behavior, negative sentiments, and inefficient decision making. A final component discussed in this study was the effects of social desirability. Thomas did not feel that the tool used accurately identified the influence of social desirability. He was also concerned that the relationships between responses to different items were subject to the halo effect. Both were considered weak components of the study, requiring further attention in future studies.

In the mid-1970s, Kilmann joined Thomas to assist in the development of a forced-choice measure of conflict-handling behavior, known today as the Thomas and Kilmann Conflict MODE Instrument (Thomas & Kilmann, 1974); MODE is an acronym for the management-of-differences exercise, which includes 30 forced-choice questions that attempt to control for social desirability. Prior to developing the new tool, Thomas reinterpreted Blake and Mouton's (1964) scheme for classifying interpersonal conflict-handling behavior. The new conflict-handling modes were identified as competing, collaborating, compromising, avoiding, and accommodating. Thomas and Kilmann (1974) defined each of the five conflict-handling modes.

1. *Competing* is a power-oriented mode whereby an individual uses the appropriate power strategy to win his or her own position. Competing might mean "standing up for what you feel is right" or simply trying to win.
2. *Accommodating* is the opposite of competing; the individual neglects her or his own concerns to satisfy the concerns of others. Accommodating involves giving in to another's wishes or point of view with some degree of self-sacrifice.
3. *Avoiding* involves sidestepping an issue for diplomatic reasons, postponing confrontation until a better time, or withdrawing from a threatening situation.
4. *Collaboration* is the opposite of avoiding; it involves working with another individual in an attempt to identify a solution and exploring insights to determine different viewpoints as related to a conflict situation for the purpose of creatively resolving the problem.
5. *Compromising* focuses on identifying a prompt, mutually acceptable solution that partially meets the needs of both parties. Although similar to collaboration, compromising focuses on seeking a quick middle-ground position and lacks the extensive exploration of individual insights.

Thomas (1976) and Ruble and Thomas (1976) identified two separate dimensions that exist in the new classification: cooperation and assertiveness. *Cooperation* was defined as the attempt to satisfy the other person's concerns; *assertiveness* was defined as the attempt to satisfy one's own concerns. Incorporation of the two dimensions with the five modes of handling conflict enhances the understanding and clarity when dealing with interpersonal conflict. Competing is both assertive and uncooperative, collaborating is assertive and cooperative, avoiding is unassertive and uncooperative, accommodating is unassertive and cooperative, and compromising is intermediate in both cooperativeness and assertiveness. The advantage of this classification scheme is that the five specific modes reflect independent dimensions of interpersonal conflict behavior. Blake and Mouton (1964), Lawrence and Lorsch (1967), and Hall (1969) had also developed tools similar to the Conflict MODE Instrument. Thomas and Kilmann (1973, 1975) examined the instruments and found all to be strongly susceptible to social desirability biases. They discovered that the scores on the Hall and Lawrence-Lorsch tools were nonipsative and that reliabilities were modest. Thomas and Kilmann also discovered that Blake and Mouton scores on competing and compromising were unstable, with all three instruments measuring somewhat different constructs.

Thomas and Kilmann felt that a more valid instrument needed to be developed to assess the five modes, especially relating to the profound social desirability factor identified in the three instruments examined, so that further research in the area of conflict management would not be severely limited.

CASE ANALYSIS

From the information provided in the case study, the predominant mode used by this vice president of nursing appears to be avoiding. Although avoiding in select situations may be a functional mode, in this situation it seems dysfunctional. The repeated use of avoidance escalated both the number and degree of conflicts Sarah had to resolve.

Although a few social science and management experts challenge the validity of Thomas and Kilmann's MODE instrument, certainly increased knowledge of the five conflict-handling modes can contribute positively to a manager's effectiveness in dealing with conflict (Woodtli, 1987).

What if Sarah were knowledgeable and proficient in utilizing the five conflict-handling modes? Would Sarah be faced with the current problem of unionization if her repertoire of management skills included understanding and proficient use of the five modes of handling conflict behaviors? The possibility exists that the staff may pursue union representation regardless of the mode or modes used by leaders in nursing. However, the chance of unionization is greatly reduced if managers actively listen to nursing staff complaints. Sarah could have greatly reduced the chance of unionization if she had collaborated with her staff instead of avoiding them in this particular situation. By avoiding the issues presented by the staff, Sarah exhibited both unassertive and uncooperative behaviors in response to the employees' needs. Sarah could have been more effective by utilizing collaboration when dealing with employee issues, whereby both assertive and cooperative behaviors would have been exhibited and subsequently perceived by the staff. The staff most likely perceived Sarah's use of avoidance as not really caring about their needs. An important issue for Sarah to conceptualize is the nurses' actual perceptions of her efforts in alleviating the problems repeatedly identified. Probably the most effective way Sarah could have obtained this vital information would have been through employee meetings that allowed individual nurses to have a voice in resolving the continued problems. Such an approach in dealing with disgruntled staff members could have potentially saved this vice president of nursing a great deal of grief and misery, possibly even her job.

RESEARCH

Kilmann and Thomas (1977) presented the MODE instrument and the initial validity results. Development of the instrument specifically focused on eliminating biases identified in previous tools. The authors sought to achieve substantive validity, structural validity, and external validity in the development of the instrument.

Kilmann and Thomas (1977) identified and confirmed one aspect of the MODE's external validity by identifying meaningful correlations with a few instruments used in measuring personality. Only one of the personality instruments will be discussed.

Meyers-Briggs Type Personality Indicator

Thomas and Kilmann (1975) identified that Jungian functions associated with judging, such as thinking versus feeling, and the type of enactment, such as introverted versus extroverted, were significantly related to an individual's conflict-handling behavior. More specifically, the authors identified the following statistical correlations. Sensation-intuition significantly correlated with accommodating on the MODE instrument with $r = .27$ $(p < .05)$. Individuals scoring higher on feeling showed a significant tendency to be relatively less taking than giving with $r = -.38$ $(p < .001)$. The strongest and most consistent correlations noted were with the integrative dimension of conflict behavior, suggesting that individuals higher on extroversion are more likely to strive for integrative solutions, with $r = .29$ $(p < .01)$ (Thomas & Kilmann, 1975). Extroversion was also correlated wth assertiveness, with $r = .28$ $(p < .05)$. In contrast, extroversion correlated negatively with avoiding, with $r = .20$ $(p < .10)$.

Three Other Instruments Used in Measuring Conflict

Blake and Mouton's instrument on conflict entails five statements. Each one of the statements describes one of the five modes used in handling conflict.

The Lawrence-Lorsch instrument contains 25 proverbs that describe the five different modes of handling conflict. In this particular instrument, subjects rate the proverbs according to how closely they describe the behavior of individuals within their organization.

Hall's instrument consists of 12 groups of five statements. Preceding each group is a statement addressing conflict phenomena and a question for the subject to answer about himself or herself. The subject is then required to rate each of the five statements from 1 (completely uncharacteristic) to 10 (completely characteristic). According to Thomas and Kilmann (1978), for the different instruments to be compared on test-retest reliability and internal consistency, changes had to be made in the instruction component of both the Blake and Mouton and Lawrence-Lorsch instruments. An identified weakness of the results focused on the potential effects of making such changes. Thomas and Kilmann suggested further investigation in this area.

Criticisms of the MODE

The MODE is presently considered to be the preferred instrument to identify conflict-handling behaviors. Boris Kabanoff (1987), an affiliate of the Australian School of Management, doubts the utility of this instrument in predicting conflict behavior. Kabanoff identified that the MODE has been utilized in only a few research settings. Kilmann and Thomas (1977) recommended that the instrument should be tested in different research settings to identify further the tool's validity. Kabanoff has identified an interesting point. An in-depth investigation of the literature indicates that repeated testing of the instrument has in fact *not* occurred in the research setting. In Kabanoff's (1987) study, conducted to identify the MODE's lack of predictive validity, 63 students enrolled in a first-year organization behavior course were given the MODE instrument and also four other instruments measuring personality characteristics: Machiavellianism, locus of control, and expressed needs for control and inclusion. Twelve to 15 months after the initial testing, class members were sent a letter and questionnaire asking them to rate their peers on their observed use of one of the five conflict styles: competing, collaborating, compromising, avoiding, and accommodating. Based on previous experience with the MODE instrument, Kabanoff emphasized that instructions on the MODE focused on identifying behavioral characteristics when taking the test. In an attempt to neutralize the titles, Kabanoff decided to change the names to: "let's do it my way" (competing), "split the difference" (compromising), "better let the situation cool down before we act" (avoiding), "maybe we can work this one out" (collaboration), and "I see your point of view" (accommodating). He believed the students would be ideal subjects because they had been in previous classes and had worked in numerous settings together. Ratings were obtained by developing a questionnaire listing all student names and five columns for rating each classmate's likelihood of using each of the five conflict-handling modes. The choices were "fairly likely," "somewhat likely," "neither likely or unlikely," "somewhat unlikely," "fairly unlikely," and "don't know." After compiling the data from 54 of the 77 questionnaires, data were analyzed using the Spearman-Brown correction formula to determine the interrater reliabilities of the five modes of handling conflict. The results were as follows: competing (.82), collaborating (.50), compromising (.59), avoiding (.72), and accommodating (.78). From the results, Kabanoff (1987) stated that the "notion of measuring general styles of conflict behavior is inherently invalid." For example, competing in one context may not be perceived as competing in another. Kabanoff suggested that in applied settings individuals taking the MODE may learn more about their conflict intensions even if the actual behavior is not described. To the contrary, problems occur when the MODE is presented as a "behavior-diagnostic" tool. Kabanoff (1987) suggested that individuals have difficulty differentiating between intentions and behavior and summarized his study by contending that "subject to further research, there are reasons to doubt the utility of the MODE instrument as a means of predicting conflict behavior," yet he contended that the MODE can and should be used as a learning tool in identifying one's own conflict-handling strategies.

Nursing Research

One particular study identified in the literature was "Deans of Nursing: Perceived Sources of Conflict and Conflict-Handling Modes" (Woodtli, 1987). The three purposes for conducting the study were: (1) identification of potential sources of conflict between deans of nursing and faculty as perceived by deans; (2) identification of conflict-resolution modes used as perceived by deans; and (3) exploration of relationships among sources of conflict, modes of conflict resolution, and selected demographic data. This study surveyed deans from 257 NLN-accredited colleges of nursing where the bachelor of science degree in nursing was the only nursing degree offered. The researcher used 158 returns from 43 states. The instrument consisted of three sections, the first of which was six categories of demographic data. The first part of the second section asked the deans to select and rank in order three sources of conflict they perceived to be most disruptive from a provided list of 25 potential sources of conflict. The deans were then asked to respond to the Thomas and Kilmann MODE, keeping in mind the three chosen sources of potential conflict. The third section asked the deans to choose, from the list of 25 choices, three sources of conflict perceived to be least disruptive and again respond to the MODE. Statistical analysis included the use of chi square, analysis of variance, and Pearson product moment correlation. Modes of handling conflict used by deans in all situations were compromising, collaborating, avoiding, accommodating, and competing, in descending order based on frequency. The study concluded that:

1. Deans need to be aware of potential sources of conflict in conjunction with identification and utilization of the most effective modes of handling each source of conflict.
2. Deans must first be aware of their own conflict-handling styles before increasing their effectiveness in handling conflict situations with faculty.
3. There may be a need for additional preparation in the management of conflict at all levels of the educational process.
4. The management of conflict is associated with managerial effectiveness, suggesting the need for development and refinement of conflict-handling skills (Woodtli, 1987).

Marriner (1982) studied 182 nurses and found that their distributions of frequency favored essentially normal curves on each mode, and nurses used each mode with about the same frequency as a group of 339 managers in business and government organizations. The nurses analyzed previous conflict situations they had encountered and identified collaborating and compromising most frequently with successful conflict resolution, whereas avoiding and competing were used most frequently in unsuccessful conflict resolutions.

REFERENCES

Blake, R.R., & Mouton, J.S. (1964). *The managerial grid*. Houston: Gulf.

Hall, J. (1969). *Conflict management survey: A survey on one's characteristic reaction to and handling conflicts between himself and others*. Conroe, TX: Teleometrics International.

Kabanoff, B. (1987). Predictive validity of the MODE conflict instrument. *Journal of Applied Psychology, 72*, 160-163.

Katz, N.H., & Lawyer, J.W. (1985). *Communication and conflict resolution skills*. Dubuque: Kendall/Hunt.

Kilmann, R.H., & Thomas, K.W. (1975). Interpersonal conflict-handling behavior as reflections of Jungian personality dimensions. *Psychology Reports, 37*, 971-980.

Kilmann, R.H., & Thomas, K.W. (1977). Developing a forced-choice measure of conflict-handling behavior: The "MODE" instrument. *Educational and Psychological Measurement, 37*, 309-325.

Lawrence, P.R., & Lorsch, J.W. (1967). *Organization and environment: Managing differentiation and integration*. Boston: Harvard University, Graduate School of Business Administration.

Marriner, A. (1982). Managing conflict. *Nursing Management, 13*, 29-31.

Potter, D.O. (Ed.) (1984). *Practices: Legal risks, ethics, human relations, and career management*. Springhouse, PA: Springhouse.

Ruble, T.L., & Thomas, K.W. (1976). Support for a two-dimensional model of conflict. *Organizational Behavior and Human Performance, 16*, 143-155.

Thomas, K.W. (1971). *Conflict-handling modes in interdepartmental relations*. Unpublished doctoral dissertation, Purdue University.

Thomas, K.W. (1976). *Handbook of industrial and organizational psychology*. Chicago: Rand-McNally.

Thomas, K.W., & Kilmann, R.H. (1973). *Some properties of existing conflict behavior instruments*. Working Paper #73-11. Los Angeles: Human Systems Development Center, Graduate School of Management, University of California, Los Angeles.

Thomas, K.W., & Kilmann, R.H. (1974). The Thomas-Kilmann conflict mode instrument. Tuxedo Park, NY: Xicom.

Thomas, K.W., & Kilmann, R.H. (1975). The social desirability variable in organizational research: An alternative explanation for reported findings. *Academy of Management Journal, 18*, 741-752.

Thomas, K.W., & Kilmann, R.H. (1978). Comparison of four instruments measuring conflict behavior. *Psychology Reports, 42*, 1139-1145.

Woodtli, A.O. (1987). Deans of nursing: Perceived sources of conflict and conflict-handling modes. *Journal of Nursing Education, 26*, 272-277.

Chapter 39

Integrative Stress Theory
John M. Ivancevich and
Michael T. Matteson

Mary Lorraine Riegner

I I   CASE STUDY

The management of the five intensive care units (ICUs) in a large Midwest community hospital decided to implement the concept of all professional staffing. This concept meant the deletion of the licensed practical nurse (LPN) role within these designated areas. The two managers and five head nurses of the ICUs (the management team) met on several occasions to define the roles of the professional nurse. They decided that the professional nurse was needed to implement the holistic care of the ICU patient within these highly technical areas. Although several of the licensed practical nurses had developed good technical skills, the management team recognized that their scope of practice was very limited in the ICU setting. The LPN was not educationally prepared to meet the standards of the nursing process required of a professional nurse. Certain technical duties could not be performed by the LPN, which created extra work and stress for the professional nurse.

The proposal for a professional staff was presented to upper management, who endorsed this action unequivocally. The proposal was then presented to the professional staff nurses and the LPNs in separate meetings. The LPNs were informed at this time that they had 1 year to find other employment within the hospital. The effect and impact of what was proposed created profound reactions from both levels of nursing staff.

The next few weeks produced stress for the management team as well as for both levels of staff nurses. The decision of management was clearly understood by some of the staff; other staff members were emotional and perceived management as uncaring in deleting nursing positions for their co-workers. More important, they felt as though their relationships and camaraderie with their co-workers were threatened. Feelings of anger and frustration were present.

The level of stress in the management team was heightened also. Guilt feelings had to be worked through. Listening to the staff ventilate their feelings was unpleasant. The management team had anticipated feelings of distress from the group but not to the magnitude that it existed. Clearly, management interventions were needed.

THE INTEGRATIVE STRESS MODEL

Many of the various models of stress overlap in their approach to studying the concept of stress. Primarily these models use a medical-psychological approach or a behavioral approach. Neither approach alone encompasses an area of practical application for the manager within an organization.

Acting on the supposition that a model is needed that integrates the medical and behavioral approaches and that has practical applications that are more general than specific for managers in organizations, Ivancevich and Matteson (1980) proposed an integrative stress model. Their eight goals in support of the model (p. 31):

1. The model should improve managerial understanding of stress and work relationships.
2. The model should use terminology and concepts that make sense from a managerial perspective.
3. The model should appeal to managers in general and not a specific or a small group of managers.
4. The model should not be viewed as the complete or final solution to issues concerning stress and work.
5. The model should integrate medical and behavioral science variables that are relevant to managers.
6. The model should suggest courses of action that managers can take to counter stress in subordinates and in themselves.
7. The model should offer suggestions for testing and research on stress and work variables.
8. The model should incorporate individual, group, and organizational outcome variables.

The goals of the model are concise and applicable to the working environment. Ivancevich and Matteson have provided to management a workable tool that can be utilized as a guide.

According to Ivancevich and Matteson (1980), the integrative model has been adapted to utilize some of the concepts of the medical, behavioral, and behavioral medicine approaches to stress (p. 42). The model is composed of four main units: antecedents (stressors), stress (perceived), outcomes, and consequences (Figure 39-1). Introduced into the model is the moderator set of individual differences, which provides for cognitive-affective differences and demographic-behavioral differences (p. 45). These individual differences may affect the various relationships in the model, especially in the units of perceived stress and outcomes. None of the variables in the four units comprises an exhaustive list.

The antecedent stressors consist of intraorganizational and extraorganizational factors. Ivancevich and Matteson (1980) explain the relationship of these two factors by stating that "extra organizational life stress interacts with organizationally related job and career stress" (p. 45). The four subsets to intra organizational stress are physical environment (light, noise, etc.), individual level (work overload, role conflict, role ambiguity), group level (intragroup conflict, group dissatisfaction), and organization level (organizational climate, management styles). Extraorganizational stressors may include such variables as disruptive family relationships or economic problems. Extraorganizational stressors may interact with intraorganizational stressors to cause the individual to perceive stress within the job.

Unit two shows that the way stress is perceived is influenced by individual differences such as personality type, lack of control, and self-esteem. The third unit of the model consists of physiological and/or behavioral outcomes of stress. Physiological outcomes may be manifested as alterations in physiological processes, such as blood pressure changes. Behaviorally, the individual may exhibit signs of job dissatisfaction or poor job performance. The individual may have increased absenteeism or frequent job changes. Ivancevich and Matteson (1980) state that "these two relationships are extremely important to managers, since they can influence the development and maintenance of organizational conditions (e.g., job design, reward systems, leadership style) which minimize dysfunctional stressors (p. 45).

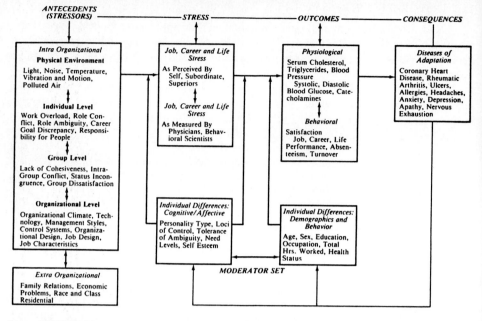

ANTECEDENTS
(STRESSORS) ———————————— STRESS ——————————— OUTCOMES ——————— CONSEQUENCES

Intra Organizational	Job, Career and Life Stress	Physiological	Diseases of Adaptation
Physical Environment	As Perceived By Self, Subordinate, Superiors	Serum Cholesterol, Triglycerides, Blood Pressure	Coronary Heart Disease, Rheumatic Arthritis, Ulcers, Allergies, Headaches, Anxiety, Depression, Apathy, Nervous Exhaustion

Intra Organizational

Physical Environment

Light, Noise, Temperature, Vibration and Motion, Polluted Air

Individual Level

Work Overload, Role Conflict, Role Ambiguity, Career Goal Discrepancy, Responsibility for People

Group Level

Lack of Cohesiveness, Intra-Group Conflict, Status Incongruence, Group Dissatisfaction

Organizational Level

Organizational Climate, Technology, Management Styles, Control Systems, Organizational Design, Job Design, Job Characteristics

Extra Organizational

Family Relations, Economic Problems, Race and Class Residential

Job, Career and Life Stress

As Perceived By Self, Subordinate, Superiors

Job, Career and Life Stress

As Measured By Physicians, Behavioral Scientists

Individual Differences: Cognitive/Affective

Personality Type, Loci of Control, Tolerance of Ambiguity, Need Levels, Self Esteem

Physiological

Serum Cholesterol, Triglycerides, Blood Pressure
Systolic, Diastolic Blood Glucose, Catecholamines

Behavioral

Satisfaction
Job, Career, Life Performance, Absenteeism, Turnover

Individual Differences: Demographics and Behavior

Age, Sex, Education, Occupation, Total Hrs. Worked, Health Status

Diseases of Adaptation

Coronary Heart Disease, Rheumatic Arthritis, Ulcers, Allergies, Headaches, Anxiety, Depression, Apathy, Nervous Exhaustion

MODERATOR SET

FIGURE 39-1 A model for organizational stress research. *From* Stress and work *by John M. Ivancevich & Michael T. Matteson. Copyright © 1980 by Scott, Foresman and Company. Reprinted by permission.*

The fourth unit, or consequence, is comprised of diseases of adaptation that result from the outcomes of stress. These include coronary heart disease, ulcers, headaches, anxiety, and depression.

The moderator set of individual differences has a direct bearing on perceived stress and outcomes and, in turn, the consequences. Such variables as personality type, age, sex, and education are individual differences that may affect the relationships of the last three units.

Ivancevich and Matteson approached the use of this model from an organizational and managerial perspective. The manager must understand that each individual is unique and different from every other individual. What one person perceives as stress may not be stressful to another individual.

CASE ANALYSIS

The case study can be analyzed from various elements of the integrative model of stress. At the individual level of antecedent stressors, the deletion of the job role of the LPNs caused a loss of group cohesiveness and increased group dissatisfaction, which are stressors from within the organization on the group level. The LPN role was deleted because of the professional education that was required to fulfill the requirements of the job as redesigned. Redesigning the job description created role conflict and role ambiguity. The organization had redesigned the job so that only professional nurses could work in the ICU.

Extraorganizational stressors interact with intraorganizational stressors to create job stresses. Several of the LPNs supplemented the family's income or were the sole financial support of the family. Losing their jobs was a financial threat to their security and well-being. The LPNs perceived this loss as real, even though they could seek employment in other areas of the hospital.

The second unit of the model is the job, career, and life stresses that are perceived by the individuals in the work situation or by their superiors. The management team acknowledged that stress did occur in the LPNs during the ensuing weeks. Job security was certainly threatened, even though employment was possible outside of the ICU setting. The loss of group or peer support was evident by the anger that was projected by the LPNs to the professional staff and the management staff. The moderator set of individual differences interacted strongly with the perceived stress of each individual.

The outcomes of the stress (unit three of the model) were demonstrated by the nurses' behavioral responses rather than by physiological responses. Behavioral changes were demonstrated by anger and outbursts of crying. Some of the LPNs were outwardly angry and verbalized their feelings. Other LPNs appeared withdrawn, as demonstrated by their nonverbal behavior and avoidance of management personnel. One LPN was absent for a short period of time.

The fourth unit of the model or the consequences (diseases of adaptation) to the stress are probably the most difficult to identify in this particular group of nurses. Physiological illnesses were not reported. Anxiety and depression were probably the most observable later outcomes. Interventions by the management staff included individual meetings with the LPNs, meetings with the hospital chaplain, who is proficient in guidance and counseling, and referral to the employee assistance program. Job threat was a very large issue, but the LPNs were assured of other positions within the hospital. Talking out the issues that had arisen proved beneficial.

During the following months, the LPNs eventually decided on courses of action that suited their individual needs, including other employment, retirement, or returning to school. Within the following year, each LPN found employment on other nursing units. Two of the LPNs were able to retire and did so, and one opted for an office job within the hospital. Two of the LPNs have earned associate degrees in nursing and have returned to the ICU to work.

The integrative model provides a framework that addresses stress and work relationships. All of the variables did not apply to this particular case study. However, the model provided the manager with a tool that helped to identify the causes of work-related stress. Ivancevich and Matteson (1980) state that "the goals [of their model] pay particular attention to providing managers with practical ideas and guidelines for understanding and coping with stress and work" (p. 41).

Other models of stress theory could be applied to the case study; however, these models focus more on the individual's response to stress. The perspectives of these models are not manager oriented, but managers can draw upon the information and apply the meanings in an organizational setting.

Lazarus and Folkman (1984) describe the cognitive theory of stress in terms of cognitive appraisal. Their definition of cognitive appraisal is that it is an "evaluative process of categorizing an encounter, and its various facets, with respect to its significance for well-being" (p. 31). Lazarus and Folkman claim that

> although personality factors such as needs, commitments, and preferred styles of attention influence perception, appraisals are generally correlated with reality; an appraisal of threat is inferred from what the person says. (p. 53)

They identify three types of appraisal: primary, secondary, and reappraisal:

Primary appraisal consists of the judgement that an encounter is irrelevant, benign-positive or stressful. Stressful appraisals can take forms: harm/loss, threat, and challenge. Secondary appraisal is a judgement concerning what might and can be done. Reappraisal refers to a change appraisal based on new information from the environment and/or the person. (p. 53)

This model of stress could be applied to the case study. The primary appraisal is that the LPNs experienced the harm/loss aspect (loss of job and financial security) and the threat aspect (loss of peer support and camaraderie and the perception that another job might not be available). The secondary appraisal evaluates what might be done in order to cope with a given situation. The management team met with the LPNs on several occasions to discuss options that they could make regarding their future. Although this process was long and tedious, some changes of attitude did occur from these meetings. They eventually accepted that this role change was meant to be. Reappraisal refers to a changed appraisal of the situation. Eventually the LPNs reevaluated their individual needs, and they made decisions based on these needs (returning to school, retirement, or searching for other employment).

Farmer, Monahan, and Hekeler (1984) describe the stress behavioral model. The sources of stress may occur from a combination of factors, such as the individuals themselves, families, friends, and the work environment. The effect of stress is what is felt by the individual in reacting to a stressful situation. These feelings are usually described in terms of depression or anxiety. An extension of these feelings range from feeling keyed up to feeling hopeless and frustrated. The effects of stress may be experienced on a physical or psychological level. Reactions to stress often cause the individual to behave in such a way that his or her feelings are expressed in specific actions, such as anger (Farmer et al., 1984, pp. 20-21). In the case study, the work environment was the source of stress. The loss of job created the stress, which manifested itself in behavioral changes. These changes were in the form of anger and frustration.

RESEARCH

Ivancevich and Matteson (1980) offer ten potential hypotheses for their model that might be suitable for testing with rigorous research designs. If this model has been tested by researchers, literature on the findings could not be located.

The relevant nursing research on stress from a manager or nurse administrator perspective is very limited. Much is written on various aspects of stress and burnout for staff nurses, however.

Several descriptive works and studies were reviewed but only a few had any practical application to the case study. Huckabay (1984) published an article on coping mechanisms for nurse administrators and supervisors. Nurse managers have very stressful jobs, and each individual manager reacts differently to stress. Huckabay infers that these nurse managers need to adopt behaviors to cope with job-related stress. Most of Huckabay's article cites the studies of Selye (1978), McClelland (1976), Kobasa, Hilker, & Middi (1979), Pines (1980), Antonovsky (1979), and Janis (1958) and summarizes the reactions to stress found in these studies. The following behaviors have been advocated: "Set realistic goals, practice altruistic egoism, adopt a set of attitudes that view change as a challenge, have a commitment to what one is doing, maintain control over the environment, develop a social support system, and acquire knowledge about what is producing the stress" (p. 19). Huckabay maintains that resilience to stress is an acquired behavior that should be learned by all nurse administrators.

Norbeck (1985) studied 164 female critical care nurses from eight hospitals to test the theoretical model of occupational stress developed by La Rocco, House, and French (1980). Norbeck measured the variables of perceived social support, perceived job stress (role conflict or excessive work load), job dissatisfaction, and psychological symptoms. She found that the model of occupational stress could be applied to the human service area. Norbeck's study found that unmarried nurses had more support from friends and less support from relatives than married nurses. According to Norbeck, her findings were consistent with the propositions of Litwak and Szelenyi (1969), who proposed that different subgroups of a network contribute different functions; that is, family networking provided support for long-term involvements, neighbors provided support for immediate tasks, and friends provided support for values that were similar (p. 226). Applying these results to the case study, the LPNs perceived a loss of this networking from their co-workers who had similar professional and work values.

Gentleman, Faulconer, and Goldman (1983), discuss managerial stress. They state that "one of the most common situations producing fear, stress, and anxiety for the nurse manager is change, which usually means some disruption of the environmental status quo and of professional relationships" (p. 31). They briefly allude to the fact that supervisory nurses may experience burnout because of the continuous pressures that they feel in trying to provide a support system to staff nurses who are in burnout. The management team in the case study also experienced stress while trying to act as a support system to both groups of staff nurses. Although the issue was not burnout, a major change in effect affected all the staff members. The job of acting as a support group to these nurses was made more difficult by their initial anger and frustration over the situation.

Huckabay and Jagla (1979) studied intensive care nurses to identify the origins of stress as the nurses perceived them. They found that the physical workload for the ICU nurse was rated as the most stressful event. Huckabay and Jagla contend that the nursing administrators have the responsibility to provide the ICU with qualified nurses in adequate numbers to reduce the workload. Nurses must be prepared educationally and should have some previous nursing experience. Huckabay and Jagla inferred that these two factors are more important than having an increased staffing ratio with unqualified nurses (p. 25). This study supports the view that the LPN is not educationally prepared to work in the ICU. The professional nurse had an increased workload in the ICU, as they had to do the technical jobs that the LPN was not allowed to do.

The integrative stress theory is applicable to nursing and provides the potential for considerable research.

REFERENCES

Antonovsky, A. (1979). *Health, stress, and coping.* San Francisco: Jossey Bass.

Farmer, R., Monahan, L., & Hekeler, R. (1984). *Stress management for human services.* Beverly Hills, CA: Sage.

Gentleman, C., Faulconer, D.R., & Goldman, V.B. (1983). Managerial stress. *Nursing Administration Quarterly, 7*(2), 1-34.

Huckabay, L. (1984). Stress and leadership: A coping mechanism. *Nursing Administration Quarterly, 8*(3), 17-20.

Huckabay, L., & Jagla, B. (1979). Nurses' stress factors in the intensive care unit. *Journal of Nursing Administration, 9,* 21-25.

Ivancevich, J., & Matteson, M. (1980). *Stress and work: A managerial perspective.* Glenview, IL: Scott, Foresman.

Janis, I. (1958). *Psychological stress.* New York: Wiley.

Kobasa, S.C., Hilker, R.R.J., & Middi, S.R. (1979). Stressful life events, personality and health: An inquiry into hardiness. *Journal of Personality and Social Psychology, 37*(1), 1-11.

La Rocco, J.M., House, J.W. & French, J.F.P. Jr. (1980). Social support, occupational stress, and health. *Journal of Health and Social Behavior, 21,* 202-218.

Lazarus, R., & Folkman, S. (1984). *Stress, appraisal, and coping.* New York: Springer.

Litwak, E., & Szelenyi, I. (1969). Primary group structures and their functions: Kin, neighbors, and friends. *American Sociological Review, 34,* 465-481.

Matteson, M., & Ivancevich, J. (1982). *Managing job stress and health. New York: Collier Macmillan.*

McClelland, A.C. (1976). Sources of stress in the drive for power. In B. Serban (Ed.), *Psychopathology of human adaptation.* New York: Plenum.

Norbeck, J. (1985). Types and sources of social support for managing job stress in critical care nursing. *Nursing Research, 34,* 225-230.

Pines, M. (1980). Psychological hardiness: the role of challenge in health. *Psychology Today, 14*(7), 34-44, 98.

Selye, H. (1978). Interviewed by Laurence Cherry, on the real benefits of eustress. *Psychology Today, 11,* 60-70.

Index

A

Achievement-motivation theory, 238-244
  case study for, 238
    analysis of, 240-241
  characteristics of, 239-240
  research on, 241-244
Adams, J. Stacy, 256-263
Adjourning stage, 64
Aesthetic needs, 213
Affinito, M., 199
Aldag, R.J., 121, 141, 142
Alderfer, Clayton P., 137, 216, 217, 222-227
Alderfer's ERG theory, 218; *see also* Existence, re-
    latedness, and growth (ERG) theory
Alexander, E.L., 242, 253
Alexander, J.E., 181
Alexander, J.W., 100, 120
Alidina, S., 111
Allison, S.E., 182
Allocative efficiency, 85
Allport, F.H., 185
Anderson, A.S., 178
Anderson B., 306
Anderson, D., 276
Anderson, R., 318
Andrews, I.R., 260-261
Andrica, D.C., 315
Antonovsky, A., 348
Appraisal Interviewing Model, 322, 325-328
  case study on, 325
    analysis of, 327-328
  interviewing techniques and, 326
  research on, 328
Arad, R., 167
Argote, L., 120
Argyris, Chris, 148, 152, 189, 288-292
Ari, O.N., 189
Aristotle, 37, 39, 40, 50
Armandi, B.R., 218
Armstrong, G.D., 181
Arndt, M.J., 200
Arnold, H.J., 251
As, D., 126
Atkinson, John W., 166, 232, 238-244

Attribution theory, 58-61
  case study on, 58
    analysis of, 59-61
  nursing process and, 60
  research on, 61
Authority
  charismatic, 96, 99
  hierarchy of, 97, 98
  personal, 104
  professional, 96
  rational-legal, 95, 96, 98, 99
  statutory, 104
  traditional, 95, 98, 99
Autocratic style, 102
Autocratic system, 186, 189
Automation, 97, 100
Autonomy, 137, 138, 140
  principle, of, 33, 37, 38

B

Bailey, M.M., 242
Bakke, E. Wright, 288
Baldes, J.J., 274
Bandura, Albert, 303-307
Bar Tal, D., 59, 61
Bardwell, R., 58
Bargaining model, 50
Barhyte, D.Y., 127
Baron, R.M., 261
Barriers, 193
Bartolke, K., 190
Bases of social power, 192-202
  case study on, 192
    analysis of, 196-197
  coercive, 192, 195
  expert, 192, 195
  legitimate, 192, 195
  referent, 192, 195
  research on, 197-202
  reward, 192, 194
Basic human needs, 223
Bass, B., 197-199
Bass, R.I., 275
Batchelor, G.J., 135

Batchley, M.E., 286
Batey, M.V., 276
Batten, D.B., 276
Bauerschmidt, 100
Baumler, J.V., 276
Bavelos, A., 27
Beauchamp, T.L., 31, 33, 34, 35
Beck, M.L., 323
Bedeian, A.G., 110
Behavior modification, 141, 293-301
  case study on, 293
    analysis of, 298
  ethics and, 297
  intervention strategies for, 294-295
  principles of, 293, 295
  research on, 299-301
  rules of, 295
Behavioral contingency management, 295-297
Bell, C.H., 141, 271, 276, 277
Beneficence, principle of, 33, 37-38
Benevolent authoritative management, 124
Benne, K.D., 20, 27, 28
Benner, Patricia, 252, 335
Bennis, W.G., 20, 27, 28, 151, 189, 199
Benson, J.K., 50
Benson, J.T., 68
Bentham, Jeremy, 33
Berger, M.S., 323
Berkowitz, N., 199
Berscheid, E., 260
Bertalanffy, Ludwig von, 129-135
Best fit, 115, 116, 120, 150
Bevis, E.O., 23
Beyers, M., 286
Biddle, B.J., 331
Birkenbach, X.C., 252
Birkofer, J.R., 314
Bishop, R.C., 142
Bishoprick, D.W., 94, 96
Bizman, A., 217, 226
Blake, R.R., 338, 339, 340, 341
Blanchard, Kenneth, 174-182
Blau, Peter, 96, 97
Blumer, Herbert, 43, 44, 45, 54-57
Bonjean, C.M., 188, 291
Boje, D.M., 43, 51
Boseman, F.G., 118
Boulding's hierarchy of system complexity, 51
Boundary, 193
Bowers, D.G., 126-127
Bowman, B., 323
Braaten, L.J., 64
Brandt, R.B., 32, 34
Brass, D.J., 271
Breeze, J.D., 103
Brennan, E., 22
Breu, C., 28
Bridwell, L.G., 216-217, 218, 226
Brief, A.P., 141, 142
Brink, P.T., 16

Brodie, M.B., 103, 104, 105, 106
Broedling, L.A., 251
Bronstein, J., 310
Brooten, D.A., 21, 23
Brown, B., 276
Brown-Stewart, P., 277
Brownell, P., 311, 316, 317
Bryan, J.F., 271, 274, 275
Buccheri, R.C., 262
Budgen, C.M., 307
Budget, 309-318
  case study on, 309-310
    analysis of, 312-316
  research on, 316-318
  theory of, 310-312
Budgets
  imposed, 314
  participative, 314, 316
Buhlman, R., 61
Buller, P.F., 271
Bureaucracy, theory of, 93-101, 184
  case study on, 93-94
    analysis of, 98-100
  characteristics of, 95
  dysfunctional nature of, 96
  limitations of, 99-100
  professionals and, 96
  research on, 100-101
Bureaucratic model, 50
Bureaucratization, 94
Burke, M., 120
Burke, R., 127
Burke, R.J., 292, 328
Burkhardt, C.S., 28
Burkman, K.A., 20, 28
Burns, H., 318
Burns, T., 116
Butterfield, D.A., 127
Buttrick, R., 261
Byrnes, K.A., 323

C

Calkin, J.D., 328
Campbell, D.B., 218
Campbell, D.J., 251, 274
Campbell, D.T., 232
Campbell, J.D., 230
Campbell, J.P., 223, 225, 274
Campbell, K.M., 251
Caplan, E., 152
Carey, A., 152
Carlston, D.E., 59
Carroll, J., 59, 61
Carroll, S.J., 273, 284, 285, 286
Carroll, T.L., 315, 316
Cartledge, N., 167, 271
Caruth, D., 109
Cashman, J. 250
Casio, W.F., 269
Castellano, J.J., 141

Centralization, 105, 117, 121
Ceteris paribus, 71, 75, 77, 80
Chain of command, 104; *see also* Authority, hierarchy of; Scalar chain
Chandler, A., 116
Chandler, G., 208
Chandra, G., 311, 314
Change, planned; *see* Planned change
Change agent, 22, 23
Change process, 22, 23
Change theory, classical, 20
Chemers, M., 155, 163, 164
Chenhall, R.H., 311, 316, 317
Chesney, A.A., 276
Childress, J.F., 31, 33, 35, 38
Chin, R., 20, 27, 28
Christman, L.P., 127, 277
Clark, C., 64
Clark, N., 208
Clarke, B.A., 307
Classical management theory, 102-111
  case study on, 102-103
    analysis of, 108-110
  elements of, 107-108
  research on, 110-111
Client information, 139
Coch, L., 126
Code of ethics, 98
Cognitive dissonance, 257
Cognitive evaluation theory, 266
Cognitive needs, 213
Cognitive role theory, 331
Commanding, 107
Communication, 193
Competition, 31
Complement goods, 72, 74
Comstock, D.E., 119-120
Conflict
  management of, 124
  negative, 338
  positive, 338
Conflict mode model, 337-343
  case study on, 337-338
    analysis of, 340
  research on, 341-343
Conflict styles, 339, 342
Conflict theory, 338-340
  criteria for, 338
Conformity, 331
Congruence, 121
  contingency vs., 121
Consensus, 331
Consultative management, 124
Consumer expectations, 75
Consumer income, 75
Consumer tastes, 75
Consumers, 70
Contingency theory, 113-121, 150
  case study on, 113
    analysis of, 115

Contingency theory—cont'd
  criticism of, 121
  hypotheses for, 114-115
  research on, 115-121
  terminology in, 113-114
Contingency theory of leadership, 154-164
  case study on, 154-155
    analysis of, 159-161
  criticism of, 164
  research on, 162-164
Continuous reinforcement schedule, 294
Control graph, 188
Control theory, 183-190
  case study on, 183-184
    analysis of, 187-188
  definition of, 184
  research on, 188-190
Controlling, 108
Conway, M.E., 330, 332, 333, 334, 335
Cook, K.S., 261
Cooke, A.A., 186, 188, 189
Coordinating, 107-108
Coordination, 134
Corder, J., 188
Cornell, D., 242-243
Corwin, R.G., 100
Cost analysis, 86
Couillard, N.A., 22
Counte, M.A., 127
Courtemanche, J., 243
Covaleski, M., 315, 316, 317
Craigie, D., 235
Cronbach's alpha, 199
Cronenwett, L.R., 318
Crowley, J., 178
Cuff, R.D., 100
Cummings, L.L., 118-119, 142, 166, 231, 233, 249, 275
Curry, 97
Curtain, Leah L., 52
Cycle of events, 133

D

Dachler, H.P., 250
Dalton, D.R., 110
Dandridge, T., 50
Dansereau, F., 250
Darling, C.W., 335
Darr, K., 32
Davidhizar, E., 235
Davidhizar, R., 60
Davis, A.J., 41
Davis, T.R.V., 297, 298
Davis-Sharts, J., 219
De Cosmo, J.L., 95
Decentralization, 117
Deci, Edward L., 264-269
Decision-making model, 1-18
  case study on, 1
    analysis of, 3, 9, 16

Decision-making model — cont'd
  outcomes of, 10-15
  problem attributes in, 2, 4-8, 10-12, 14, 15
  research on, 16
  strengths of, 3
  utility of, 3
  weaknesses of, 16-17
Decker, P.J., 253, 301, 306, 307
Deets, C., 200
Deficiency needs, 213
Degree of formalized structure, 114
Delegation, 104-105
Demand
  derived, 81
  law of, 71-76
Demand curve, 70, 72, 75
Dennis, K.E., 100
Deontology, 33
Dependence-independence, 194
Desire for award theory, 277
Dessler, G., 108
DeVitt, H., 231, 233
Dewer, R., 292
Dickerson, G.L., 181
Diers, Donna, 52
Dieterly, D., 199, 200, 201
Dietrich, B., 23
Differentiation, 115, 117, 118, 134
  definition of, 114
Dill, W.R., 117
Direct costs, 88
Dirsmith, M., 315, 316, 317
Discipline, 105
Distributive justice, 257
Division of work, 104
Domination, 94, 95
Donnelly, J.H., 285
Dossett, D.L., 275
Douglass, L.M., 23, 251
Dowd, R.P., 317
Downey, H.K., 121
Dracup, Kathleen, 28
Drazin, R., 121
Dressler, G., 97
Drew, D.J., 181
Drucker, Peter F., 273, 282, 284
Ducette, J., 61
Duchon, D.J., 276
Duldt, B.W., 55, 56, 57
Duncan, R.B., 118, 121
Dunham, R.B., 141, 227
Dunne, R.S., 336
Dunnette, M.D., 215, 230, 261
Duxbury, M.L., 181

E

Earley, P.C., 167, 275
Eason, F.R., 234, 235
Economic efficiency, 85

Economic theories, 68-90, 310
  case study on, 68-69
    analysis of, 87-89
  limitations of, 86, 87
  research on, 90
Edminister, R.O., 276
Edwards, M., 298
Edwardson, S.R., 318
Effective supply, 76
Effort, 249-250
Egalitarianism, 34, 35-36, 38, 39
Ehrlich, S.A., 336
Eiven, R.B., 232
Ellis, D.J., 28
Empowerment, 209
Engelhardt, H.T., 34, 35, 36, 37, 38, 39
Entropy, 130
  negative, 133
Equifinality, 134
Equilibrium, market, 79-81, 83, 84
Equity, 106
Equity theory, 256-263, 300
  case study on, 256-257
    analysis of, 259-260
  propositions of, 260
  research on, 260-263
Erez, M., 167, 169
Erickson, H.C., 307
Eriksen, C.W., 232
Eschweiler, W., 190
Esprit de corps, 106
Esteem needs, 212
Ethical statement, 32
Ethics, 31-34
  biomedical, 33
  definition of, 32
  law and, 32
  normative, 33
Evans, M., 167, 171
Exchange, 257
Exchange theory, 300
Existence needs, 223
Existence, relatedness, and growth (ERG) measures,
  217
Existence, relatedness, and growth (ERG) theory,
  137, 222-227
  case study on, 222
    analysis of, 225-226
  major propositions of, 223
  Maslow's hierarchy of needs theory and, 223-224
  research on, 226-227
Expectancy theory, 137, 245-253, 272, 300
  case study on, 245-246
    analysis of, 247-249
  goal setting and, 272
  motivation and, 246
  research on, 249-253
Expectancy theory of motivation, 166
Experienced meaningfulness, 138

Experienced responsibility, 138
Exploitative authoritative management, 124
External locus of control, 141
Extinction, 294
Extraorganizational factors, 345

F

Factors of production, 76
Falasco, P.R., 276
Farley, M.J., 208
Farmer, R., 348
Farr, J.L., 251
Farris, G.F., 127
Faulconer, D.R., 349
Fayol, Henri, 102-111
Fear of penalty theory, 277
Feathers, N.T., 232
Feedback, 137, 138, 139, 140, 144, 208
Feeney, E.J., 299
Fein, M., 143
Feistritzter, K., 199
Feldman, D.C., 208
Feldman, H., 59
Ferguson, M.J., 276
Fernandez, T.M., 328
Festinger, Leon, 257
Fiedler, Fred, 154-164
Field, 20-21, 24, 27
Field theory, 20
Field value system, 22
Fielding, G.J., 110
Finch, F.E., 251, 328
Fine, R.B., 276
Finn, R.H., 261
Fixed costs, 86, 88
Fixed-interval schedule, 295
Fixed-ratio schedule, 294
Flechenberger, D., 190
Fleishman, E.A., 126
Focal position, 332
Folkman, S., 347
Force field, 193, 194
Force-field analysis, 20, 65
Forces, driving and restraining, 20-21, 24-25
Ford, Robert N., 231, 234
Fouraker, L.E., 116
Fraker, S., 208
Frank, L.L., 143
Frankena, W.K., 32
Franklin, R.L., 275
Frederick, E.A., 274
Freedman, S., 260, 261
Frelin, A.J., 318
French, John R.A., 126, 192-202, 284, 328, 348
Frieze, I., 59, 61
Froberg, D., 335
Frost, P., 50
Frost, P.J., 274
Fry, S.T., 41

Fryer, F.W., 274
Functional role theory, 331
Funke-Furber, J., 111
Fuszard, B., 140, 220

G

Galbraith, J., 166, 249
Gallant, B.W., 181-182
Gamboa, V.U., 299, 300
Gannon, M.J., 110
Ganong, J., 286
Ganong, W., 286
Gardner, D.L., 318
Gardner, G., 126
Garner, W.K., 232
Gentleman, C., 349
George, S., 200
Georgopoulos, B.S., 166, 185, 249
Ghiselli, E.E., 152
Gibbard, G., 64
Gier, J.A., 275
Giffin, K., 55, 56, 57
Giges, J.N., 235
Gillies, D.A., 20
Gillon, R., 36, 37, 39, 40
Ginsberg, A., 121
Giovanneti, P.E., 318
Gipson, D.L., 110
Gjerdingen, D., 335
Glass ceiling, 208
Glassman, R., 95
Glusko, G., 310
Goal congruence theory, 288-292
    case study on, 288
        analysis of, 291
    propositions of, 289
    research on, 291-292
Goal orientation, 114
Goal-setting theory, 144, 270-277
    case study on, 270
        analysis of, 273-274
    participation in, 275
    research on, 274-277
Gochnauer, A., 56
Goddard, N.L., 315
Goertzen, I., 41, 315
Goldberg, M., 217, 226
Goldman, V.B., 349
Goldstein, A.P., 305, 306
Golembiewski, R.T., 127
Goode, W.J., 332, 334
Goodin, M.F., 181
Goodwin, L.D., 28
Gordon, M.E., 231, 232
Gorman, S.J., 208
Gouldner, A.W., 97
Graen, G., 166, 250
Graham, J.V., 200
Gray, E.R., 152

Green, J.P., 151
Greenfield, J., 310
Grenier, M., 208
Grey, J.F., 318
Grier, M., 99
Grigaliunas, B.S., 231, 233
Grillot, A., 41
Grimes, R.M., 120
Group process, 63-66
  case study on, 63-64
    analysis of, 65-66
  research on, 66
Group standard, 21
Grove, S.K., 318
Growth needs, 213, 223
Growth satisfaction, 224
Gudykunst, W., 208
Guest, R.H., 181

H

Hackman, J. Richard, 136-144, 208
Haire, M., 152
Hake, H.W., 232
Hakel, M.D., 230
Hall, D.T., 217-218
Hall, J., 340, 341
Hall, J.W., 127
Halloran, E.J., 318
Hambleton, R., 175
Hamner, E.P., 299, 300
Hamner, W.C., 271, 276, 294, 295, 299
Hardy, M.E., 330, 332, 333, 334, 335
Harnett, D.L., 271, 276
Harp, R., 163, 164
Harris, B.V., 231, 232
Harris, C.W., 28
Harrison, J.K., 315, 316
Hartman, J., 64
Harvey, J., 58, 59, 60
Harwood studies, 126, 127
Haussman, R.K., 120
Hawthorne effect, 143
Haymna, L., 23
Hayne, A.N., 41, 140
Hazlett, C.B., 100, 119, 120
Hedlund, R.D., 171
Hedonism, 246
Hegyvary, S.T., 120
Heider, Fritz, 58-61
Hekeler, R., 348
Henemen, H.G., 231, 233
Henley, S.J., 181
Henry, B., 52, 277, 317
Hersey, Paul, 174-182
Hexum, J., 318
Hierarchy of needs, 137, 211-220, 223-224, 226, 227
  case study on, 211-212
    analysis of, 214-215
  research on, 215-220

High-growth-needs individual, 138, 140, 141, 142
High-growth-needs profession, 144
Hilker, R.R.J., 348
Hill, J.W., 142
Hinshaw, A.S., 307, 317
Hirst, M.K., 271-272, 311
Hoffman, F.M., 310
Hollee, M.L., 286
Hollenbeck, J.R., 168
Homans, George, 257
Homeostasis, 134
Hospers, J., 32, 34, 35, 36
House, J.W., 348
House, Robert J., 166-172, 230, 251
Howard, R.H., 275
Hsi, B.P., 120
Huber, G.P., 120
Huckabay, L.M.D., 40, 317-318, 348, 349
Hulin, C.L., 142
Human relations theory, 17
Human resources theory of participation, 17
Humanistic nursing communication, 56
Hunter, J.E., 217, 227
Huntsman, A.J., 323
Huston, C.J., 286
Hygiene factors, 230, 232, 236

I

"I," 56
Ickes, W., 58
Ilgen, D.R., 274
Incentives, 23, 216
Indirect costs, 88
Inequity, 257, 258, 260, 261, 262
Inferior good, 75
Information, 208
Initiative, 106
Inputs, 76, 85, 130, 132, 133, 257-258, 260
  prices of, 76-77
Instrumentality, 246-247, 250, 251, 253
Integration, 116, 118, 134
  definition of, 114
Integrative stress theory, 344-349
  case study on, 344
    analysis of, 346-348
  goals of, 345
  research on, 348-349
Interaction-influence bond, 189
Intermittent reinforcement schedule, 294
Internal locus of control, 141
Interpretive-interactionist perspective, 43, 49
Intraorganizational factors, 345
Intraorganizational strain, 185
Israel, J., 126
Ivancevich, J.M., 275, 276, 284, 285, 344-349

J

Jacobsen, B., 59, 61
Jacobsen, P.R., 260
Jacox, A.K., 318

Jagla, B., 349
Jago, Arthur G., 1-18, 164
Janis, I., 348
Jargon, 44, 49, 51, 53
Jensen, Mary Ann, 64, 66
Job characteristic theory, 136-144
  case study on, 136
    analysis of, 139-140
  dimensions of, 137-138
  model of, 137
  psychological states of, 138
  research on, 140-144
Job Description Index (JDI), 217, 226
Job design, 227
Job Diagnostic Survey (JDS), 138, 141, 144
Job dissatisfiers, 230, 231, 232
Job enlargement theory, 140, 226
Job enrichment, 136, 138, 139, 227, 231, 234
Job redesign, 138-139, 143, 250
  benefits of, 138
  purposes of, 139
Job satisfaction, 252
Job Satisfaction Scale, 262
Job satisfiers, 229-230, 231, 232
Johnson, M.R., 318
Johnson, S., 179
Jones, K.R., 317
Jones, N., 166
Jones, N.W., 249
Jorgenson, D.O., 261
Jungian functions, 341
Justice, B., 120
Justice
  comparative, 31-32
  distributive, 31-32, 34
  noncomparative, 32
  principle of, 34
  theories of, 30-41
    case study on, 30-31
      analysis of, 39-40
    ethics and, 31-34
    research on, 40-41
    types of, 34-39

K

Kabanoff, Boris, 341-342
Kagawa, M., 251
Kahn, Robert L., 97, 125, 129-130, 132, 134, 188,
    189, 230, 231
Kaluzny, M.A., 41
Kanfer, F.H., 305
Kanfer, R., 275
Kant, Immanuel, 33
Kanter, Roasabeth Moss, 204-209
Kaplan, R.F., 227
Karren, R.J., 271, 272, 273
Katz, Daniel, 97, 125, 129-130, 132, 134
Katz, N.H., 338
Katz, R., 142
Katzell, R.A., 126

Kavanagh, M., 261
Kavcic, B., 190
Kay, A., 151
Kay, E., 284, 328
Keane, A., 61
Kelley, H., 59
Kelly, E.A., 318
Kemp, V.H., 28
Kendall, L.M., 271, 275
Khandwalla, P.N., 117
Kidd, R., 58
Kilmann, R.H., 337
Kim, H.S., 57
Kim, J.S., 300
King, B.W., 219
King, E., 22
King, I.M., 130-132
King, N., 231, 232
King, P.J., 323
King's framework for nursing administration, 132, 135
    major concepts in, 132
King's theory of goal attainment, 130-132, 135
Kinley, J., 318
Kinne, S.B., 274
Kirby, S., 126
Kirchhoff, B.A., 285
Kirk, R., 283, 286
Klein, H.J., 168
Klein, S.M., 251
Knerr, C.S., 167, 271
Knowledge of results, 138
Kobasa, S.C., 348
Komaki, J., 299
Koontz, H., 108
Kopelman, R.E., 250
Korman, A., 243
Kotter, John P., 22, 208, 336
Koys, D.J., 276
Kraft, W.P., 136
Kramer, C.C., 314
Kramer, M., 100, 335
Kreitner, R., 294, 295, 298
Krizek, M.B., 252
Kronman, G., 120
Krusell, J., 269

L

L organization, 116
La Monica, E., 252, 325
La Rocco, J.M., 348
Lacoursiere, R., 64
Laissez-faire system, 186, 189
Lammert, M., 66
Lancaster, J., 234, 236
Langton, J., 94, 95
Language, 42-53
  case study on, 42
    analysis of, 47-49
  leadership and, 48
  organization and, 49

Language — cont'd
  people and, 48-49
  research on, 49-53
Lant, T.K., 274
Larwood, L., 261
Latham, G.P., 168, 169, 271, 274, 275, 276, 304, 306
Law, 32
Lawler, Edward E., III, 136-144, 166, 215, 218, 249, 250, 251, 261
Lawrence, M., 64
Lawrence, Paul R., 22, 113-121, 135, 189, 340, 341
  hypotheses of, 114-115
Lawrence-Lorsch uncertainty scale, 121
Lawyer, J.W., 338
Lazarus, R., 347
Le Clair, H., 52
LEAD-Other, 180
LEAD-Self, 180
Leader-member relations, 156, 158, 164
Leadership, 48
Leadership behavior, 155
Leadership style, 2, 17, 155, 156, 161, 163-164, 175, 176, 179, 180, 251, 291, 306
  group situation and, 163-164
Least Preferred Co-worker (LPC) scale, 156, 157
Leatt, P., 119, 120
Leavitt, H.J., 117
Lee, B.T., 234, 235
Lee, I.M., 261
Lee, R.M., 100
Lee-Villsenor, 181
Leifer, R., 120
Lenz, C.L., 234, 235
Leventhal, G.S., 261
Levine, E.L., 185, 189
Levine, R., 261
Levinger, G., 194
Lewin, Kurt, 19-28, 65, 193, 194, 200, 270
  classical change theory and, 20
  field theory and, 20
  force-field analysis and, 20, 27, 28
Libertarianism, 34, 36-37, 38, 39
Lied, T.R., 251
Life cycle model, 64
Life cycle theory, 175
Life space, 20, 21, 193, 194, 201
Liert, Rensis, 123-127, 148, 184, 188, 189, 262
Likert scale, 2, 158, 201
Lincoln, J., 208
Lindeman, C., 317
Linking pin function, 124, 126
Litwack, E., 349
Lobb, M., 66
Locke, Edwin, 142, 167, 168, 169, 270-277, 300
Locomotion, 193, 194
Locus of cause, 59
Long, G., 261
Longest, B.B., 32
Lorber, R., 179

Lorsch, Jay W., 113-121, 135, 150, 185, 340, 341
  hypotheses of, 114
Lottery
  natural, 38
  social, 38
Love needs, 212
Low-growth-needs individual, 141
Lowery, B., 59, 61
Luthans, Fred, 293-294, 295, 297, 298, 299
Lyon, H.L., 285

M

MacAfree, R.B., 323
Maciag, W.S., 294
Mackenzie, R.A., 311
Mager, Robert F., 320-323
Mahar, L., 155
Mahmoudi, H., 97
Mahoney, G., 166
Mahoney, G.A., 249
Mahoney, T.A., 274
Maier, Norman R.F., 2, 322, 325-328
Mainiero, L., 208
Mali, P., 282, 283
Malone, E., 151, 152
Malone, M., 199
Malone, M.F., 98, 99
Management by objectives (MBO), 180, 273, 281-286
  basic elements of, 282-283
  case study on, 281
    analysis of, 283-284
  phases of, 283
  research on, 284-286
Managerial Style Questionnaire (MSQ), 285
Manager's rating form, 180
Mann, F.C., 123
Mann, R.D., 64
Mansfield, E., 310
Mark, B., 120, 121, 134
Market, 70
Market clearing price, 80, 82
Markham, W.T., 188
Markov chain, 217
Marquis, B.L., 286
Marriner, A., 233, 261, 262, 338, 343
Marriner-Tomey, A., 16, 23, 220, 230, 247, 259, 267, 269
Marrow, A.J., 126, 127
Marxism, 34, 36, 39
Maslow, A.H., 137, 147, 151, 211-220, 225, 241
Mathapo, J., 233
Matsui, T., 251
Matteson, Michael T., 344-349
Maturity level, 175-176, 180
  components of, 175-176
Mausner, B., 230, 231
Mawhinney, T.C., 300
Mayberry, M.A., 40

Mayers, M., 323
Mayo, Elton, 152
McBride, A., 60
McCauley, K., 59
McClelland, A.C., 348
McClelland, David C., 238-243
McCloskey, J.C., 318
McClure, M.L., 127
McDonald, B.R., 318
McDonald, M.J., 298
McGivern, D.O., 310
McGrath, L.G., 335
McGregor, Douglas, 147-153, 282
McIntire, S.A., 276
McIntyre, R.M., 251
McLane, A.M., 181-182
McMahon, J.T., 190, 275
"Me," 56
Mead, George Herbert, 56, 331
Meaning, 45, 49
Mechanistic system, 116
Meisenholder, J., 335
Mensch, L., 252
Mento, A.J., 271, 272, 273
Merit pay, 235
Metaethics, 33
Meyer, H.H., 284, 328
Meyer, M.W., 97
Meyers-Briggs Type Personality Indicator, 341
Mia, L., 311, 316
Michaels, J.W., 261
Michlitsch, J.F., 110
Microallocation, 37
Middi, S.R., 348
Miles, R.E., 217, 226
Mill, John Stuart, 33
Miller, C.L., 200
Miller, G., 216
Miller, G.A., 97
Miller, J., 208
Miller, K., 56
Mills, T.M., 64
Miner, J.B., 95, 96, 97, 100, 108, 125, 127, 136, 140, 162, 184, 186, 188, 213, 225, 226-227, 229, 242, 249, 250, 251, 257, 258, 260, 266, 270, 271, 272, 275, 281, 297
Minimalist theory of justice, 37
Misener, T.R., 318
Mitchell, B.S., 336
Mitchell, T.R., 141, 171, 260, 275, 276, 277, 300
Mitchell, V.F., 217, 226
Mitroff, I.I., 51
Mobley, W.H., 250
Modeling, 297, 298, 301, 304, 306
Monahan, L., 348
Moore, L.M., 261
Moran, S., 22
Morgan, G., 50
Morrison, H.W., 194

Morse, D.D., 110
Morse, J.J., 115, 150, 184
Morse, J.L., 300, 306
Morse, N.C., 126
Motivating Potential Score (MPS), 138
Motivation, 239
    extrinsic, 264-269
        case study on, 264-265
            analysis of, 267-268
        research on, 268-269
    intrinsic, 264-269
        case study on, 264-265
            analysis of, 267-268
        categories of, 265
        effects of external rewards on, 266
        research on, 268-269
Motivation-hygiene theory, 136, 137, 229-236
    case study on, 229
        analysis of, 230
    mental illness and, 231, 233
    research on, 230-236
    Theories 1, 2, 3, 4, and 5 and, 232
Moudgill, P., 217, 226
Mouton, J.S., 338, 339, 340, 341
Mowday, R.T., 142
Mulkowsky, G.P., 261
Munson, R., 33, 36, 37
Munzenrider, R., 127

N

Nadler, D.A., 139
Nagamatsu, J., 251
Natemeyer, W.E., 176, 180
Natural units of work, 139
Naylor, M., 23
Need
    for achievement (n-Ach), 238
    for affiliation (n-Aff), 239
    for power (n-Pow), 238
Neely, A.E., 178
Negandhi, A.R., 117
Negative feedback, 134
Negative reinforcement, 294
Nelson, J.R., 126
Nelson, R., 335
Nemeroff, W.F., 300
Network, 208
New, J.R., 22
Nightingale, Florence, 277
Non-Linear Systems, Inc., 151-152
Nonmaleficence, principle of, 33
Norbeck, J., 348-349
Nord, W.R., 297-298
Nordland, R., 44
Normal good, 75
Norrgren, F., 185, 190
Norton, B., 315, 316
Nougaim, K.E., 217-218
Novak, J.L., 276

Nozick, Robert, 36
Numerof, R., 20, 21
Nursing by objectives (NBO), 286
Nursing process, 60
Nystrom, P.C., 144

O

Observation, 304
Odiorne, G.S., 282, 284
O'Donnell, C., 108
O'Donnell, D., 323
O'Gara, P.W., 261
Ohtsuka, Y., 251
Oldfield, S., 64
Oldham, Greg R., 136-144, 208, 274, 275, 276
Operant conditioning; *see* Behavior modification
Order, 106
Orem, Dorothea, 177-182
Orem's self-care deficit theory, 177-182
  levels of care, 177
Organ, D.W., 295
Organization, 49
  definition of, 113
Organizational assessment inventory, 120
Organizational climate, 125, 251
Organizational design, 250, 251
Organizational flexibility, 185
Organizational performance, 114
Organizational productivity, 185
Organizational role theory, 331
Organizing, 107
Orientation of members toward others, 114
Orife, J.N., 141
Orthodox Job Enrichment Program, 231
Osborn, R.N., 118
Other, 258
Otteman, R., 299
Outputs, 85, 130, 132, 133
Overreward hypothesis, 262
Overton, P., 100, 119, 120

P

Paine, F.T., 110
Paris, B.J., 213
Park, A.K., 274
Parse, R.R., 51, 52
Parse's Man-Living-Health model, 51, 52
Participative goal setting, 167
Participative management, 2, 102, 123-127, 149-150,
  151, 152
Path-goal perception, 249
Path-goal theory of leadership, 166-172
  case study on, 166
    analysis of, 169-171
  definition of, 166
  origins of, 166
  research on, 171-172
Paths, 193
Pavett, C.M., 252

Pay, 105, 144, 251, 253, 262, 297
Pearce, J.L., 138, 142
Pearce, M.G., 299
Pearlin, L.I., 199
Pedalino, E., 299, 300
Peer leadership, 125
Peltz, D.C., 126
Pennings, J.M., 118, 291
People, 48-49
Performance evaluation, 284
Performance problems, 320-323
  case study on, 320
    analysis of, 321-323
  research on, 323
Perritt, G.W., 190
Perrow, J.L., 188
Person, 258-259
Peters, T., 316
Peterson, L., 59
Pfeffer, J., 141, 208, 218, 226
Phillips, C., 286
Physiological needs, 212
Pierce, J.L., 227
Pierce, L.L., 276
Pincus, J.D., 52
Pinder, C.C., 250
Pines, M., 348
Pipe, Peter, 320-323
Planned change, 19-28
  applications of, 23
  case study on, 19-20
    analysis of, 23-27
  definition of, 20
  process of, 23
  research on, 27-28
Planning, 107
Podsakoff, P.M., 197-199, 201-202
Pollard, H.R., 105, 108
Polyarchic organizations, 185, 186, 187, 189
Pondy, Louis R., 42-53
  conceptual models of, 50
Porac, J.F., 275
Porras, J.I., 306
Porter, L.W., 110, 142, 152, 166, 216, 217, 218, 249,
  250, 275
Position power, 159
Position power scale, 158, 159, 162
Positive reinforcement, 294, 299, 300
Poteet, G.W., 315
Power, 194, 240, 243
  elements associated with, 240
  women and, 241
Powers, R., 298
Pratto, D., 335
Prescott, P.A., 28
Pressley, T.A., 109
Prest, W., 167
Preston, J.G., 309
Preston, M., 335

Preston, S.J., 285
Price, J., 72-74
Price, V.J., 276
Pridham, K., 52
Pritchard, R.D., 223, 251, 261, 274
Problem-solving method, 326-327
Producers, 70, 76, 85
Productive resources theory of value, 36
Production theory, 84-86
Productivity, 77, 141
Profit motive, 86, 87
  health industry and, 87
Prospero, G.D., 275
Protestant ethic, 142
Proxy measure, 87
Pryor, N.M., 231, 232
Psychodrama, 331
Psychological change, 194
Punishment, 294

Q

Quantity demanded, change in, 76
Queen Bee Syndrome, 206

R

Ragan, J., 164
Raia, A.P., 281, 286
Rakish, J.S., 32
Randolph, W.A., 120
Range, 194
Ratio-of-cost-to-charge (RCC) accounting
    method, 87
Rational scientific world view, 95
Rationalization, 94-95
Rauschenberger, J., 217, 227
Raven, Bertram, 192-202
Rawls, J., 35-36, 39
  "original position" and, 35
  theory of justice and, 35-36
  "veil of ignorance" and, 35
Reality shock, 335
Reasoning, deductive and inductive, 46
Reference group, 257-258
Regions, 193
Reimann, B.C., 117
Reimer, E., 126, 184
Reinforcement
  negative, 294, 301
  positive, 294, 299, 300, 301
Reinforcement schedules, 294-295
Reinharth, L., 250-251
Relatedness needs, 223, 224
Relationship behavior, 175, 180
Resistance to change, 22
Resources, 208
Restructuring, 193
Resultant force, 194
Rewards, 294
Rhodewalt, F., 163, 164

Rice, G.H., 94, 96
Rice, J.M., 335
Richards, M., 318
Rider, M., 64
Riehl, J., 51-52, 56, 57
Riehl interaction model, 51-52, 56, 57
Rinker, G., 178
Ritchie, R.J., 300, 306
Roach, K.L., 298
Roberts, K.H., 217, 226
Robey, D., 142
Robinson, M.E., 323
Rodman, H., 335
Roe, A., 216
Roedel, R.R., 144
Roethlisberger, Fritz, 152
Rogers' theory of unitary man, 57
Role ambiguity, 333
Role bargaining, 334
Role competence, 332
Role conflict, 331, 333
Role expectations, 332
Role identity, 332
Role incongruity, 333
Role making, 334
Role occupant, 332
Role overload, 333
Role overqualification, 333
Role partner, 332
Role performance, 332
Role set, 332
Role strain, 332, 333
Role stress, 332, 333, 336
Role taking, 332, 334
Role theories, 330-336
  case study on, 330
    analysis of, 334-335
  concepts of, 331-332
  perspectives on, 331
  research on, 335-336
Role transition, 332, 336
Role underload, 333
Role underqualification, 333
Rompre, R.M., 335
Ronen, S., 276
Rose, A.M., 56
Rosen, M., 275
Rosenbaum, H.L., 318
Rosenbaum, W.B., 260
Rosenberg, M., 199
Rosengren, W.R., 134
Rosenkrantz, S.A., 294
Ross, I.C., 126
Ross, P., 164
Rossel, R.D., 292
Roth, P.A., 315, 316
Rousseau, D.M., 138, 143
Rowland, B.L., 187, 286, 310
Rowland, H.S., 187, 286, 310

Rubenowitz, S., 185, 190
Ruble, T.L., 339-340
Rudd, J.R., 275
Rudy, E.B., 61
Runkel, P.J., 64
Rush-Medicus Nursing Process Monitoring Method-
    ology, 120
Rutkowski, B., 286
Ryan, Thomas, 270-271

S

Saari, L.M., 168, 304, 306
Sadock, B., 64
Safety needs, 212
Salancik, G.R., 141, 168, 218, 226
Sanford, C., 261
Sauers, D.A., 275
Saywell, R.M., 68
Scalar chain, 104, 105-106
Scalzi, C., 336
Schempp, C.M., 335
Schlesinger, L., 22
Schmidt, S.M., 118-119
Schmidt, W.H., 2, 314
Schmitt, N., 217, 227
Schneck, R., 100, 119, 120
Schneider, B., 217, 226
Schneider, J.M., 276
Schneider, K., 323
Schneider, M.J., 276
Schneier, C.E., 297
Schnitzler, C.P., 99
Schoolar, J.C., 120
Schoonhoven, C.B., 121
Schriesheim, C.A., 172, 197-199, 201-202
Schriesheim, J.F., 172
Schutz, M., 52
Schwab, D.P., 142, 231, 233, 275
Schwartz, R.D., 232
Schwirian, P.M., 277
Scott, W.R., 119-120
Searight, M., 164
Seashore, S.E., 126-127
Sechrest, L., 232
Self-actualization, 212-214, 216-217, 218
Self-rating form, 180
Selye, Hans, 348
Sexton, W.P., 95, 142
Seybolt, J.W., 252, 253
Shalley, 274, 275
Shaping, 297
Shaver, A.V., 298
Shaw, N.K., 168
Shenkar, O., 276
Sheridan, D., 310
Shiplett, S., 164
Shipley, T.E., 242
Shortage, 79-80
Sietsema, M.R., 40
Silva, M.C., 41

Simms, L., 315
Simonds, R.H., 141
Simonetti, J.L., 118
Sims, H.P., 141, 143-144, 171, 227, 251
Singleton, E.K., 315, 316
Sirota, D., 142
Situational attributes, 2
Situational control, 156-159
Situational leadership, 174-182
    case study on, 174-175
        analysis of, 178-180
    model of, 177
    research on, 180-182
Skill variety, 137, 138
Skinner, B.F., 293-301
Slocum, J.W., 121
Smelzer, C., 317
Smith, C.G., 189
Smith, E., 208
Smith, P.C., 261
Smith, R.K., 226
Smyth, P., 126
Snyderman, B.S., 230, 231
Social learning theory, 303-307
    case study on, 303-304
        analysis of, 305-306
    process of, 304-305
    research on, 306-307
Socialization deficit, 333
Sonberg, V., 316
Sondak, A., 219
Sorcher, M., 300, 306
Specialization, 104
Spencer, D.G., 141
Spendolini, M.J., 110
Spitz, H., 64
Spradley, B.W., 40
Stability of tenure of personnel, 106
Stalker, G.M., 116
Stark, P.L., 310, 315, 316
Status set, 332
Staw, B., 50
Steel, R.P., 271, 272, 273
Steers, R., 141, 275
Stein, G.A., 242
Stevens, B.J., 251, 310
Stewart, L., 208
Stewart, R., 110
Stolz, S.B., 297-298
Stone, E.F., 142
Storey, R., 121
Storrs, Constance, 104
Straser, L., 127, 310, 312
Stressors, 345
Stroking, 235
Structural role theory, 331
Structural theory, 204-209
    case study on, 204-205
        analysis of, 206-207
    research on, 207-209

Structured normative ethical theory, 33
Stull, M.K., 276-277
Subenvironment, 114
Substitute good, 72, 74, 89
Subsystem, 114
Sullivan, E.J., 253, 301, 306, 307
Supervisor scale, 262
Supervisor Support subscale of the Work Environment Scale, 262
Supervisory relationship training, 306
Supplier expectations, 79
Suppliers, number of, 79
Supply and demand, 70-79
   changes in, 81-84
Supply curve, 70, 76, 78
Supportive relationships, principle of, 123-124
Surplus, 80
Suttle, J.L., 218
Symbolic interactionism, 43-46, 51, 54-57, 331, 334
   case study on, 54-55
      analysis of, 56
   research on, 56-57
System, open, 129
   characteristics, of, 132
   definition of, 129
System 4, theory of, 123-127
   case study on, 123
      analysis of, 125
   research on, 125-127
   systems 1, 2, and 3 and, 124
Systems model, 50
Systems theory, 129-135
   case study on, 129
      analysis of, 132-134
   characteristics of, 132
   definition of, 129
   research on, 134-135
Swain, M.A.P., 307
Szelenyi, I., 349
Szilagyi, A.D., 141, 143-144, 171, 227, 251

T

T organization, 116
Tannenbaum, Arnold S., 183-190
Tannenbaum, R., 2, 314
Tappen, R.M., 20, 22, 26
Task behavior, 175, 180
Task combination, 139
Task-goal attributes, 275
Task identity, 137, 138, 140, 144
Task significance, 137, 138, 140
Task structure, 158-159, 164, 172
Task structure scale, 158, 159, 160-161
Taves, M.J., 100
Taylor theory of management, 2
Technical efficiency, 85
Technology, 77
Tell and listen, 326
Tell and sell, 326
Terborg, J.R., 275

Thematic Apperception Test (TAT), 241
Theory X and Y, 147-153
   beliefs of, 148
   case study on, 147
      analysis of, 150
   propositions of, 148
   research on, 150
Thomas, K.W., 253, 338-343
Thomas and Kilmann Conflict MODE Instrument, 339, 341
   criticisms of, 341-342
Thompson, M., 208
Thompson, P.H., 250
Thompson, Victor, 96
Throughputs, 130, 132, 133
Time orientation, 114
Todor, W.D., 110
Tomlin, E.M., 307
Tosi, H., 121, 273, 284, 285, 286
Tuckman, Bruce W., 63-66
Tuckman's inductive model, 64-65
Tung, R.L., 118
Tuttle, W.C., 317
Tuzzolino F., 218
Twist, P.A., 318
Two-factor theory, 232, 236
Two-tiered system of health care, 38, 39, 40
Tyndall, A., 180
Type A behavior, 168

U

Udell, J., 111
Udy, S., 117
Ulrich, R.A., 234
Umstot, D.D., 141, 276, 277
Uncertainty, 114
Unity
   of command, 105
   of direction, 105
Utilitarianism, 32, 33, 34, 37, 39

V

Valence, 246-247, 250, 251, 253
Valle, V., 59
Van de Van, A.H., 121
Van Fleet, D.D., 110
Vance, G.G., 291
Vance, R.J., 251
Vander Merwe, R., 252
Vanderzee, H., 310
Variable costs, 86, 88
Variable-interval schedule, 295
Variable-ratio schedule, 295
Variables
   causal, 124
   end-result, 124
   intervening, 124
Venkatraman, N., 121
Vermeersch, P.E.H., 318
Veroff, Joseph, 238-244

Vertical loading, 139
Vestal, K.W., 316
Vogel, G., 66
Vraciu, R.A., 311
Vroom, Victor H., 1-18, 166, 167, 189, 231, 245-253
Vroom and Yetton decision-making model, 2, 3, 26, 251

W

Waddell, W.M., 298
Wagner, F.R., 110
Wahba, M.A., 216, 217, 218, 226, 250-251
Wakefield-Fisher, M., 181
Walker, C.R., 253
Walker, D., 310
Walker, D.D., 252
Walker, W.B., 328
Walster, E., 260
Walster, G., 260
Walter, G.A., 217, 226
Walters, L., 34
Walton, R.E., 143
Wanous, J.P., 142, 218, 227
Ward, C.R., 335
Ward, M., 22
Warren, J.B., 234, 235-236
Wasch, R.S., 314
Watson, S., 323
Weary, G., 59
Weaver, D.J., 199
Webb, E.J., 232
Weber, Max, 93-101
Weick, A., 22
Weiner, Bernard, 61
Weinman, M.L., 120
Weir, T., 127, 292
Weiss, H.M., 300, 306
Weiss, R.M., 94, 96
Weiss, T., 261
Weitzel, A.R., 323
Welch, L., 21
Weldon studies, 127
Werbel, J., 292
Wesley, W., 323
Wexley, K.N., 300
Whall, A.L., 219

White, J.K., 141, 142
White, S.E., 276
Wickens, J.D., 285
Wiener, Y., 233
Wiesen, L., 233
Wigdon, L.A., 230
Wilcox, D.S., 328
Wilets, J.M., 123
Willert, T.M., 318
Williams, K.L., 136
Wilson, J.S., 277
Winter, D., 241
Winter, L.L., 97
Wofferd, J., 164
Wojnaroski, P., 167
Wolf, G., 318
Wolf, M.G., 231, 232
Wolfson, A.D., 142
Wolkenheim, B., 323
Women in management, 204-209
Wong, J., 252
Wong, S., 252
Wood, Marilyn J., 16, 57
Woods, J.R., 68
Woodtli, A.O., 340, 342, 343
Woodward, J., 116
Work personality, 250
Work role, 250
Wortman, C., 61
Wren, D.A., 186
Wyer, R., 59
Wysocki, J., 163, 164

Y

Yalom, I., 64
Yankelovich, D., 120, 252
Yinon, Y., 217, 226
Young, L.C., 41, 140
Yukl, G.A., 271, 275, 276
Yura, H., 219, 226, 227

Z

Zantra, A., 231, 234
Zedeck, S., 261
Zimmerman, D.K., 126
Zwang, A., 218, 227

/

M

f